Handbook of Clinical Pediatric Endocrinology

EDITED BY

Charles G.D. Brook MA MD FRCP FRCPCH

Emeritus Professor of Paediatric Endocrinology
University College London
London, UK

Rosalind S. Brown MD CM

Associate Professor of Pediatrics
Harvard Medical School
Director, Clinical Trials Research, Endocrine Division
Children's Hospital Boston
Boston, MA, USA

FIRST EDITION

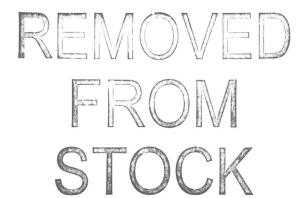

Blackwell
Publishing

© 2008 Charles Brook, Rosalind Brown
Blackwell Publishing, Inc., 350 Main Street, Malden, Massachusetts 02148-5020, USA
Blackwell Publishing Ltd, 9600 Garsington Road, Oxford OX4 2DQ, UK
Blackwell Publishing Asia Pty Ltd, 550 Swanston Street, Carlton, Victoria 3053, Australia

First published 2008

Library of Congress Cataloging-in-Publication Data
Brook, C. G. D. (Charles Groves Darville)
   Handbook of clinical pediatric endocrinology / Charles G.D. Brook, Rosalind S. Brown. –
1st ed.
      p. ; cm.
   ISBN 978-1-4051-6109-1
   1. Pediatric endocrinology–Handbooks, manuals, etc. I. Brown, Rosalind S. II. Title.
   [DNLM: 1. Endocrine System Diseases–Handbooks. 2. Adolescent. 3. Child. 4. Infant.
WK 39 B871h 2008]
   RJ418.B727 2008
   618.92′4–dc22

                                                                        2007025837

ISBN-13: 978-1-4051-6109-1

A catalogue record for this title is available from the British Library

Set in 8.75/12pt Meridien by Charon Tec Ltd (A Macmillan Company), Chennai, India
Printed and bound in Singapore by Markono Print Media Pte Ltd

Commissioning Editor: Alison Brown
Editorial Assistant: Jennifer Seward
Development Editor: Rob Blundell
Production Controller: Debbie Wyer

For further information on Blackwell Publishing, visit our website:
http://www.blackwellpublishing.com

Contents

Preface

This book is a distillation of the most relevant and practical clinical advice from the 5th edition of Brook's Clinical Pediatric Endocrinology (Blackwell 2005). That book is intended for specialists in pediatric endocrine practice but this one is aimed to assist pediatricians who may encounter endocrine problems and endocrinologists who may encounter children.

Each chapter is headed by a series of what we have called learning points. These are intended to draw attention to the commonest clinical issues and to indicate that further guidance on them will be found later in the chapter.

We have tried to make sure that all concentrations are shown in both SI and traditional units and have highlighted differences in the availability of drugs and tests in Europe and USA. In the Appendices we have provided a compendium of growth charts for common syndromes and a table of normal values with conversion coefficients from SI to traditional units. Since this is a first edition, we should be very glad to have our attention drawn to any errors.

From Wiley-Blackwell, we thank Alison Brown, whose idea this book was, and Rob Blundell for assisting in its production. We hope that you will find it useful and easy to use.

Charles Brook
Rosalind Brown
September 2007

1 The Application of Science to Clinical Practice

Learning Points

- There are endocrine, paracrine and autocrine hormones
- They comprise three groups, those derived from tyrosine, protein and peptide hormones and steroids
- Two different types of cell synthesize either peptide and protein hormones or steroid hormones

- Hormones elicit effects on target cells by interacting with receptors either at the cell surface or within the cytoplasm and nucleus
- Both traditional and non-traditional inheritance play a major part in human health and disease

---

Hormones belong to a class of regulatory molecules synthesized in special cells. These cells may be collected into distinct glands or may be found as single cells within some other organ, such as the gastrointestinal tract. Endocrine hormones are released from the cells that make them into the adjacent extracellular space, whence they enter a local blood vessel and circulate to their target cells. Some cells secrete hormones that act on themselves (autocrine hormones); some (paracrine hormones) affect nearby cells without entering the bloodstream. Molecules secreted by neurones that excite or inhibit other neurones or muscle by means of synapses are called neurotransmitters. Sometimes, however, both neurotransmitters and hormones are secreted by neurones, thus forming the neuroendocrine system.

From the chemical standpoint, there are three groups of hormones: the first are derived from the amino acid tyrosine, the second are peptide and protein hormones and the third are steroid hormones.

Handbook of Clinical Pediatric Endocrinology, 1st edition. By Charles G. D. Brook and Rosalind S. Brown. Published 2008 by Blackwell Publishing, ISBN: 978-1-4501-6109-1.

Hormones derived from tyrosine include epinephrine, which is secreted by the adrenal medulla, and norepinephrine, which can be produced in the adrenal medulla but is also produced at sympathetic nerve endings, where it acts as a neurotransmitter. Dopamine, another derivative of tyrosine, is a neurotransmitter that can also act as a hormone when released from the median eminence to suppress the secretion of prolactin (PRL) from the anterior pituitary. The thyroid hormones (thyroxine and triiodothyronine) each have two fused molecules of tyrosine; thyroxine has four iodine atoms attached to the amino acid rings, while triiodothyronine has three iodine atoms substituted in the two aromatic rings (Fig. 1.1).

Protein and peptide hormones vary considerably in size. Thyrotrophin-releasing hormone (TRH) has only three amino acid residues while many of the hormones from the gastrointestinal tract, such as secretin from the duodenum and gastrin from the stomach, are larger, with up to 34 amino acids, while parathyroid hormone (PTH) is larger still, with 84. Ring structures linked by disulphide bridges are present in some hormones (Fig. 1.2). An intrachain disulphide bond to form a

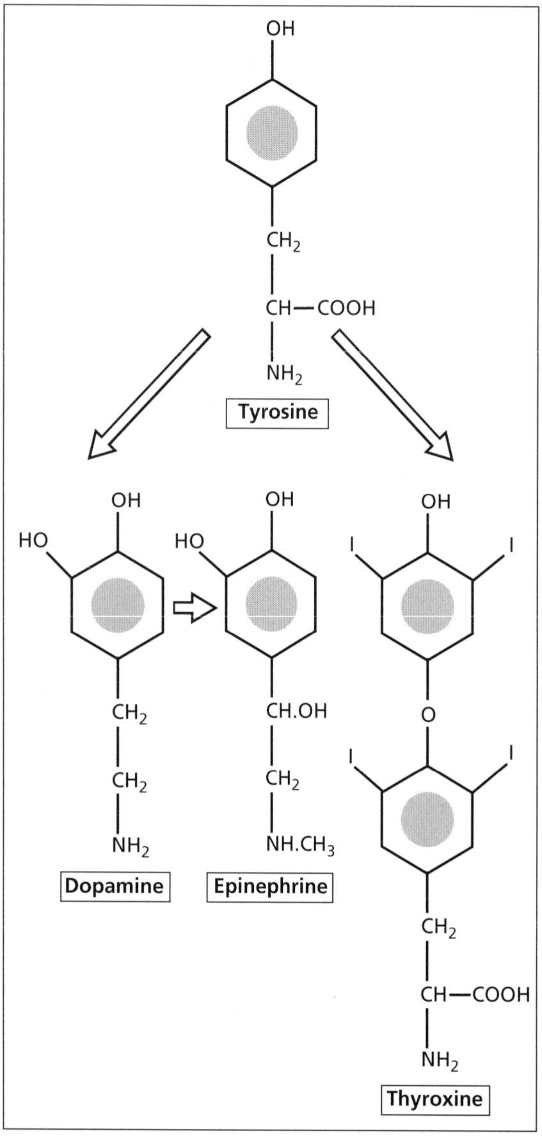

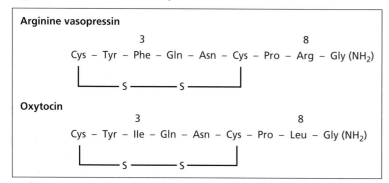

Figure 1.1 Hormones derived from tyrosine.

ring of seven amino acids at the amino-terminus is also found in calcitonin. Insulin may be regarded as a small protein or a large peptide; it consists of A-chains and B-chains linked by interchain disulphide bonds. Insulin is synthesized as a large precursor molecule (proinsulin) in a single chain of which a section, the connecting- (or C-) peptide, is subsequently removed by enzymatic hydrolysis after the disulphide bonds have been formed: the remaining two linked chains make up the insulin molecule. A number of other peptide hormones are also synthesized in larger precursor forms that are modified prior to secretion.

Some hormones are quite large proteins, such as the glycoprotein hormones from the anterior pituitary, each of which has two peptide chains. Follicle-stimulating hormone (FSH), luteinizing hormone (LH) and thyrotrophin-stimulating hormone (TSH) each have two chains, referred to as the α- and β-subunits. The two subunits are synthesized quite separately; the α-subunit in each is very similar but the β-subunits are different and confer the biological specificities on the hormones. Within a given species, there may be considerable microheterogeneity of the structures of these hormones, so that a number of naturally occurring variants coexist. The variability of the glycoprotein hormones is largely due to differences in their carbohydrate composition, and the variants are referred to as isohormones or isoforms.

Steroids are a class of lipids derived from cholesterol and include cortisol, aldosterone, testosterone, progesterone and oestradiol. Small changes in the basic chemical structure (Fig. 1.3) cause dramatic changes in the physiological action of this group of hormones.

Arginine vasopressin

$$\text{Cys} - \text{Tyr} - \overset{3}{\text{Phe}} - \text{Gln} - \text{Asn} - \text{Cys} - \text{Pro} - \overset{8}{\text{Arg}} - \text{Gly (NH}_2)$$

Oxytocin

$$\text{Cys} - \text{Tyr} - \overset{3}{\text{Ile}} - \text{Gln} - \text{Asn} - \text{Cys} - \text{Pro} - \overset{8}{\text{Leu}} - \text{Gly (NH}_2)$$

Figure 1.2 Structures of arginine vasopressin and oxytocin. Note the minor differences in chemical structure which confer major differences in action.

Biosynthesis of peptide hormones

Protein or peptide hormone synthesis starts with the transcription of a gene, proceeds through translation of a messenger ribonucleic acid (mRNA) and culminates in post-translational modification of the peptide or protein hormone (Fig. 1.4). The gene consists of double-stranded (ds) deoxyribonucleic acid (DNA).

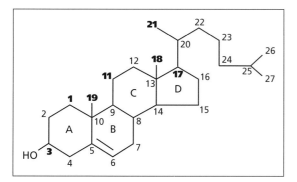

Figure 1.3 Structure of cholesterol, which is the base of the steroid nucleus. Cholesterol itself has a side chain on C17 (making it a C27 compound) which is removed in the biosynthesis of classic steroid hormones but retained in vitamin D.

At its 5′ end (the 'upstream' side) is the regulatory region known as the promoter, which includes the TATA box (a sequence of seven thymidine–adenosine bases). This is followed by a variable number of exons (expressed sequence regions) and introns (intervening sequences), which make up the structural gene.

RNA polymerase produces an RNA transcript of the exons and introns in the form of pre-mRNA. Removal of the RNA sequences derived from the introns is followed by splicing together of the exon-derived sequences. Further post-transcriptional changes include the addition of a 7-methyl guanosine (7-meg) cap at the 5′ end and a poly a (a series of adenosine residues) tail on the 3′ end. When the mature mRNA is bound to a ribosome, translation occurs to give a peptide precursor that includes the signal peptide of the prehormone (or preprohormone). Post-translational processing is needed before the hormone is ready for secretion.

Storage

Protein- or peptide-hormone-secreting cells store the newly synthesized hormone in small vesicles or secretory granules scattered around the periphery of

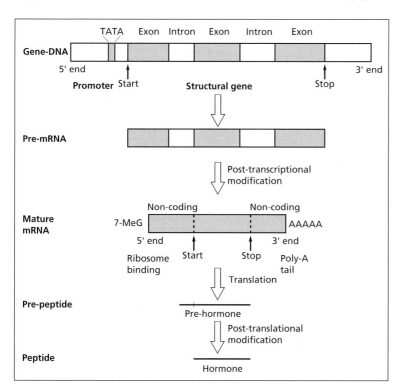

Figure 1.4 Schematic representation of a gene and of the events leading to the synthesis of a peptide hormone.

3

the cells just inside the cell membrane. Movement of the vesicles from the Golgi apparatus to a position near the cell membrane is influenced by two types of filamentous structure, called microtubules and microfilaments, which are found in all cells.

Secretion

The cell requires a stimulus before the stored prohormone is activated and released. The stimulation may be hormonal and usually involves a change in permeability of the cell to calcium ions which are required for interaction between the vesicle and plasma membranes and for the activation of enzymes, microfilaments and microtubules. Specific endopeptidases in the storage vesicle are activated during the secretory process and produce the active form of the hormone for release from the cell.

The mode of secretion in the cell is by exocytosis. The membrane of an intracellular storage granule fuses with the plasma membrane of the cell which parts near the point of fusion so that the content of the vesicle is secreted into the extracellular space surrounding the blood vessels. The membrane that originally surrounded the vesicle is recycled within the cell.

Steroid hormones

Cholesterol is the precursor of all steroid hormones. All the steroid-hormone-synthesizing cells of the body, the adrenal cortex, placenta, testis and ovary, contain intracellular fat droplets in the cytoplasm composed principally of cholesterol esters, the storage form of the hormone precursor. Cholesterol moves to the mitochondria to be converted to pregnenolone. This is transported to the surrounding smooth endoplasmic reticulum where it is transformed into the appropriate steroid hormone by a series of reactions (see Chapter 6, page 99). It is not known how the hormones get out of the cell but steroid-secreting cells, unlike protein- and peptide-producing cells, do not store hormone in a state ready for secretion but synthesize it for secretion as required.

Transport of hormones in the blood

Most peptide and protein hormones circulate in the bloodstream with little or no association with serum proteins. There are specific transport proteins (thyroxine-, cortisol- and sex-hormone-binding globulins) in the circulation that bind thyroxine and many of the steroid hormones. The high specificity of these transport proteins is such that minor changes in the structure of hormones affect binding. For example, aldosterone is only weakly bound to cortisol-binding globulin. Many hormones may also loosely associate with other circulating proteins, especially albumin.

Protein-bound hormone is in equilibrium with 'free' (or unbound) hormone. The free hormone can diffuse to tissues more readily and so the physiological state usually corresponds more closely with the concentration of the free hormone. As a result of changes in the concentration of binding protein, the total and bound concentrations of hormone may alter quite markedly, even though this is accompanied by only a small change in the free hormone concentration with the result that the physiological status remains unaltered.

Hormone action

Hormones elicit their effects on target cell function by interacting with receptors either at the cell surface or within the cytoplasm and nucleus (Fig. 1.5). Receptors for the pituitary-derived proteins, insulin and the catecholamines are present at the plasma membrane; steroid and thyroid hormones access intracellular-binding sites.

The concentration of each receptor can vary and a cell may become more or less sensitive to a given extracellular concentration of ligand. Sensitization can occur by increasing the number of binding sites available through a combination of increased receptor synthesis and decreased degradation. Cells can become refractory (desensitized) by altering receptor localization (e.g. by internalizing cell-surface receptors), reducing receptor levels or recruiting molecules that deactivate intracellular signaling pathways.

Cell-surface receptors

Of the two major groups of cell-surface receptors, the first relies upon tyrosine kinase for the initiation of signaling and the second group tends to activate serine or threonine kinases by coupling to G-proteins.

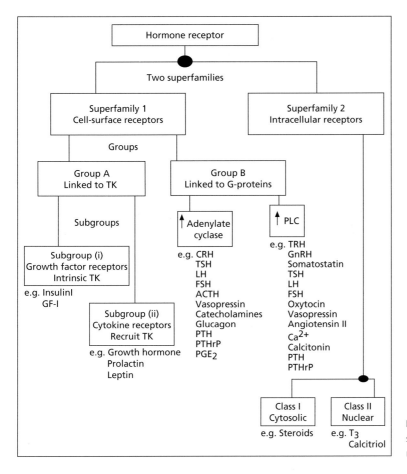

Figure 1.5 A composite diagram showing the different classes of hormone receptors.

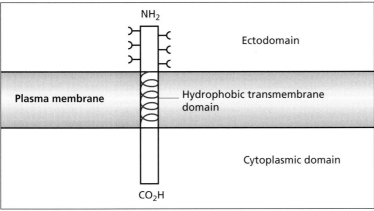

Figure 1.6 Schematic representation of a membrane-spanning cell-surface receptor with three clearly identifiable domains.

However, there is an underlying structural unity in all cell-surface receptors because each is made up of three segments, an extracellular domain, a transmembrane region and a cytoplasmic domain (Fig. 1.6).

The N-terminus of the protein forms the extracellular component of the receptor, which is responsible for hormone recognition and binding. The transmembrane region varies in structure from a simple linear stretch

Table 1.1 Examples of G-protein-coupled receptors (GPCRs).

Family	Examples	G-protein
A	TRH receptor	
	GnRH receptor	Gqα
	Oxytocin	
	Biogenic amine receptors	
	FSH receptor	
	LH receptor	Gsα/Gqα
	TSH receptor	
	Vasopressin	
	Somatostatin	Giα/Gqα
	Melanocortin receptor	Gsα
B	Calcitonin receptor	Gsα/Giα/Gqα
	CRH receptor	
	Glucagon receptor	Gsα
	PTH receptor	
	PTHrP receptor	Gsα/Gqα
C	Calcium receptors	Gqα/Giα
	Glutamate receptors	Gsα/Gqα

CRH, corticotrophin-releasing hormone; GnRh, gonadotropin-releasing hormone; PTHrP, parathyroid hormone-related protein

of amino acids to a more complex arrangement that threads the plasma membrane. This segment is often regarded as a passive anchor but it can influence receptor function as, for example, mutations in the transmembrane region of the fibroblast growth factor (FGF) receptor are associated with achondroplasia. The cytoplasmic C-terminus of the receptor forms the effector region of the molecule because it initiates an intracellular signaling cascade that eventually results in the cellular response.

G-protein-coupled receptors (GPCRs) form a superfamily of more than 1000 membrane proteins. These receptors transduce hormonal signals and also mediate the cellular response to neurotransmitters, lipids, nucleotides, ions and sensory stimuli, such as light, smell and taste.

As their name suggests, activation of GPCRs generally leads to the recruitment of intracellular G (guanine)-proteins and then the generation of second messengers, for example cyclic adenosine monophosphate (cAMP) and inositol 1,4,5-triphosphate (IP_3). Some of these receptors can signal through G-protein-independent pathways.

Although GPCRs have the same basic design as the tyrosine kinase-linked receptors, in that they possess extracellular, transmembrane and intracellular domains. They can be grouped into three families, A, B and C (Table 1.1) on the basis of sequence similarity within the transmembrane region. There is little similarity between the groups, apart from the characteristic tertiary structure facilitated by the seven transmembrane helices.

Defects

Given their numerous and varied ligands, it is not surprising that mutations in GPCRs or their interacting G-proteins are associated with endocrine disease. Mutations that alter the extracellular (ligand-binding) domains of the receptor lead to hormone resistance (e.g. the TSH receptor), whereas aberrations in the transmembrane region of the receptor can result in altered receptor function.

Germline mutations in Xq28, which codes for the vasopressin V2 receptor, cause receptor misfolding and loss of receptor function so that circulating vasopressin, despite being present at very high levels, cannot

Table 1.2 Examples of defects in intracellular receptors that are associated with endocrine disease.

Receptor	Clinical effects	Which are due to decreased
ARs	Partial or complete AR insensitivity syndromes	Receptor number
		AR binding
		AR dimerization
	Kennedy syndrome	Expanded CAG repeat in N-terminus
	Breast cancer	AR dimerization
	Prostate cancer	AR response to progesterone
Glucocorticoid	Generalized inherited glucocorticoid resistance	Hormone binding
		GR number
		DNA binding
ER	Usually lethal	Hormone binding
	ER resistance	DNA binding
T_3 (TR)	Resistance to thyroid hormone	TRβ gene defects
		T_3 binding
Calcitriol (VDR)	Calcitriol-resistant rickets	VDR dimerization

Calcitriol (VDR) Calcitriol-resistant rickets VDR dimerization AR, androgen; ER, estrogen; GR, glucocorticoid receptor, VDR, vitamin D receptor.

increase urine concentration and nephrogenic diabetes insipidus results. Some cases of early onset severe obesity may be explained by functional defects in the melanocortin-4 receptor.

Activating mutations are also detrimental, presumably by altering crucial helix–helix interactions so that the receptor is active even in the absence of ligand. Familial male precocious puberty (testotoxicosis) is the result of such a mutation in the gene coding for the LH receptor (LHR), and activating mutations in the transmembrane domain of the TSH receptor have been reported in association with neonatal hyperthyroidism and toxic thyroid adenomas in adults.

Mutations resulting in the loss of Gsα function are linked to pseudohypoparathyroidism (Albright's hereditary osteodystrophy). If the mutation is maternally transmitted, resistance to the multiple hormones that activate Gsα in their target tissues occurs. Mutations resulting in the constitutive activation of Gsα cause McCune–Albright syndrome and some cases of acromegaly.

Intracellular receptors

Receptors for hormones such as the sex steroids, glucocorticoids, thyroxine and aldosterone are part of a large family of receptors (>150 members) that are located inside the cell (Fig. 1.5). These receptors function as hormone-regulated transcription factors and control the expression of specific target genes by interacting with regions close to the gene promoters. Consequently, the cellular response to these hormones takes longer than the quickfire cell-surface receptor/second-messenger systems described above.

Defects

Mutations in the genes coding for intracellular receptors are responsible for numerous endocrinopathies as they can result in hormone resistance (Table 1.2). Studies of the glucocorticoid receptor suggest that defects resulting in abnormal interactions with co-activator molecules, and indeed problems with the co-activators themselves, may also be the cause of hormone resistance syndromes.

Target tissue metabolism

Some of the hormones that work through intracellular receptors are converted by enzymes expressed in their target cells to metabolites that are more potent because of their higher affinity for the receptor. For example, tissue-specific deiodinases convert T_4 to T_3, 5α-reductase metabolizes testosterone to dihydrotestosterone and 1α-hydroxylase in the mitochondria

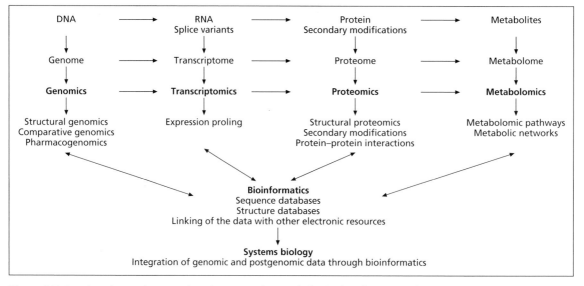

Figure 1.7 Overview of genomics, transcriptomics, proteomics, metabolomics, bioinformatics and systems biology.

of cells in the renal tubule converts 25-OH vitamin D to calcitriol. These 'activation' steps offer a way of achieving a range of effects, and various disorders can result from defects in target tissue metabolism. The best-known example is androgen insensitivity.

11β-hydroxysteroid dehydrogenase (11βHSD), which is expressed by aldosterone responsive cells in the kidney, converts cortisol to cortisone to prevent the overstimulation of the mineralocorticoid receptor that would otherwise occur as a result of the high concentration of cortisol in relation to the circulating level of aldosterone. Deficiency or impaired function of this enzyme leads to the hypertension and hypokalemia characteristic of the apparent mineralocorticoid excess (AME) syndrome.

Measurement of the concentrations of hormones in blood

Hormones are generally measured by immunoassays, although other techniques, particularly bioassays, play significant roles. All assays rely on a comparison between responses produced in the assay system by the sample and those produced by different known concentrations of a reference preparation. For immunoassays and bioassays, a calibration curve is generated with the reference preparation, and the unknown concentration of the hormone in the sample can then be interpolated from this.

Bioassays, which measure the potency of a hormone by quantifying its biological effect, suffer many practical problems so their use is limited to research. Immunoassays, which rely on the recognition of a hormone by an antibody, are capable of high sample throughputs, which has resulted in their widespread use. The four main attributes that account for their successful application in diagnostic services are their sensitivity, specificity, precision and convenience.

Genetics (Fig. 1.7)

With the exception of simple trauma, almost every disease has a genetic component. In *monogenic disorders*, such as congenital adrenal hyperplasia (CAH), the genetic component is the major etiological factor. In *complex disorders*, multiple genes, in conjunction with environmental and lifestyle factors, contribute to the pathogenesis; hence their designation as *polygenic* or *multifactorial* disorders. In other instances, genetic factors influence the manifestation of disease indirectly by defining the host's susceptibility and resistance as, for example, in infectious disease.

The term *genome*, introduced before the recognition that DNA is the genetic material, designates the totality of all genes on all chromosomes in the nucleus of a cell. *Genomics* refers to the discipline of mapping, sequencing and analyzing genomes. Because of the rapidly growing list of mapped and sequenced genomes of numerous organisms, genomics is currently undergoing a transition with increasing emphasis on functional aspects.

Genome analysis can be divided into *structural genomics* and *functional genomics*. The analysis of differences among genomes of individuals of a given species is the focus of *comparative genomics*. The complement of mRNAs transcribed by the cellular genome is called the *transcriptome* and the generation of mRNA expression profiles is referred to as *transcriptomics*.

The term *proteome* has been coined to describe all the proteins expressed and modified following expression of the entire genome in the lifetime of a cell. *Proteomics* refers to the study of the proteome using techniques of protein separation and identification. The emerging field of *metabolomics* aims at determining the composition and alterations of the *metabolome*, the complement of low-molecular-weight molecules. The relevance of these analyses lies in the fact that proteins and metabolites function in *modular networks* rather than linear pathways. Hence, any physiological or pathological alteration may have many effects on the proteome and metabolome.

The growth of biological information has required computerized databases to store, organize, annotate and index the data. This has led to the development of *bioinformatics*, the application of informatics to (molecular) biology. Computational and mathematical tools are essential for the management of nucleotide and protein sequences, the prediction and modeling of secondary and tertiary structures, the analysis of gene and protein expression and the modeling of molecular pathways, interactions and networks. Numerous continuously evolving databases provide easy access to the expanding information about the genome of man and other species. The integration of data generated by transcriptomic, proteomic and metabolomic analyses through informatics, *systems biology*, is aimed at understanding phenotypic variations and creating comprehensive models of cellular organization and function. These efforts are based on the expectation that an understanding of the complex and dynamic changes in a biological system may provide insights into pathogenic processes and

the development of novel therapeutic strategies and compounds.

Mutations and human disease

Mutations are an important cause of genetic diversity as well as disease. A *mutation* is any change in the nucleotide sequence of DNA, regardless of its functional consequences. Mutations can affect one or a few nucleotides or consist of gross numerical or structural alterations in individual genes or chromosomes. Large deletions may affect a portion of a gene or an entire gene or, if several genes are involved, they may lead to a *contiguous gene syndrome*. Occasionally, mispairing of homologous sequences leads to *unequal cross-over*. This results in gene duplication on one of the chromosomes and gene deletion on the other chromosome. For example, a significant fraction of growth hormone (*GH*) gene deletions involves unequal crossing-over.

Mutations involving single nucleotides are referred to as *point mutations*. Substitutions are called *transitions* if a purine is replaced by another purine base (A to G) or if a pyrimidine is replaced by another pyrimidine (C to T). Changes from a purine to a pyrimidine or vice versa are referred to as *transversions*. Certain DNA sequences, such as successive pyrimidines or CG dinucleotides, are particularly susceptible to mutagenesis. Therefore, certain types of mutations (C to T or G to A) are relatively common. Moreover, the nature of the genetic code results in over-representation of certain amino acid substitutions. If the DNA sequence change occurs in a coding region and alters an amino acid, it is called a *missense mutation*. Depending on the functional consequences of such a missense mutation, amino acid substitutions in different regions of the protein can lead to distinct phenotypes. Small deletions and insertions alter the reading frame if they do not represent a multiple of three bases. Such *frameshift* mutations lead to an altered carboxy-terminus. Mutations may also be found in the regulatory sequences of genes and result in reduced gene transcription. Mutations in intronic sequences or in exon junctions may destroy or create splice donor or splice acceptor sites.

Some mutations are lethal, some have less deleterious yet recognizable consequences and some confer evolutionary advantage. Mutations in germ cells (*germline mutations*) can be transmitted to the progeny. Mutations also occur during embryogenesis (*somatic mutations*). Mutations that occur during development lead to *mosaicism*, a situation in which tissues are composed of cells with different genetic constitutions, as illustrated by Turner or McCune–Albright syndromes. If the germline is mosaic, a mutation can be transmitted to some progeny but not others, which some-times leads to confusion in assessing the pattern of inheritance. Some somatic mutations are associated with neoplasia because they confer a growth advantage to cells by activating (proto)oncogenes or inactivating tumor suppressor genes.

Polymorphisms are sequence variations that have a frequency of at least 1% and do not usually result in an overt phenotype. Often they consist of single base pair substitutions that do not alter the protein coding sequence but some alter mRNA stability, translation or the amino acid sequence. Silent base substitutions and single-nucleotide polymorphisms (SNPs) are encountered frequently during genetic testing and must be distinguished from mutations that alter protein expression or function. Some SNPs or combinations of SNPs may play a pathogenic role in complex disorders by conferring susceptibility for the development of the disease.

Functional consequences of mutations

Mutations can broadly be classified as gain- and loss-of-function mutations. The consequences of an altered protein sequence often need experimental evaluation *in vitro* to determine that the mutation alters protein function.

Gain-of-function mutations are typically dominant and result in phenotypic alterations when a single allele is affected. *Loss-of-function* (inactivating) mutations are usually recessive, and an affected individual is homozygous or compound heterozygous (i.e. carrying two different mutant alleles) for the disease-causing mutations. Mutation in a single allele can result in *haploinsufficiency*, a situation in which one normal allele is not sufficient to maintain a normal phenotype. Haploinsufficiency is a commonly observed mechanism in diseases associated with mutations in transcription factors. For example, monoallelic mutations in the transcription factor TTF1 are associated with transient congenital hypothyroidism, respiratory distress and ataxia.

The clinical features among patients with an identical mutation in a transcription factor often vary significantly. One mechanism underlying this variability consists of the influence of modifying genes. Haploinsufficiency can affect the expression of rate-limiting enzymes. For example, in MODY 2 (maturity onset diabetes of the young 2), heterozygous glucokinase mutations result in haploinsufficiency with a higher threshold for glucose-dependent insulin release and mild hyperglycemia.

Mutation of a single allele can result in loss-of-function due to a dominant-negative effect. In this case, the mutated allele interferes with the function of the normal gene product by several different mechanisms. The mutant protein may interfere with the function of a multimeric protein complex, as illustrated by Liddle syndrome, which is caused by mutations in the β- or γ-subunit of the renal sodium channel. In thyroid hormone resistance, mutations in the thyroid hormone receptor β lead to impaired T_3 binding; the receptors cannot release co-repressors and they silence transcription of target genes. The mutant protein can be cytotoxic, as in autosomal-dominant neurohypophyseal diabetes insipidus, in which abnormal folding leads to retention in the endoplasmic reticulum and degeneration of the arginine vasopressin (AVP)-secreting neurons.

An increase in dosage of a gene product may also result in disease. For example, duplication of the *DAX1* gene results in dosage-sensitive sex reversal.

Genotype and phenotype

An observed trait is referred to as a *phenotype*. The genetic information defining the phenotype is called the *genotype*. Alternative forms of a gene or a genetic marker are referred to as alleles, which may be polymorphic variants of nucleic acids that have no apparent effect on gene expression or function. In other instances, these variants may have subtle effects on gene expression, thereby conferring adaptive advantages or increased susceptibility. Commonly occurring allelic variants may reflect mutations in a gene that clearly alter its function, as illustrated, for example, by the DF508 deletion in the cystic fibrosis conductance regulator.

Because each individual has two copies of each chromosome, an individual can have only two alleles at a given locus. However, there can be many different alleles in the population. The normal or common allele is usually referred to as *wild type*. When alleles at a given locus are identical, the individual is *homozygous*. Inheriting such identical copies of a mutant allele occurs in many autosomal-recessive disorders, particularly in circumstances of consanguinity. If the alleles are different, the individual is *heterozygous* at this locus. If two different mutant alleles are inherited at a given locus, the individual is referred to as a *compound heterozygote*. *Hemizygous* is used to describe males with a mutation in an X-chromosomal gene or a female with a loss of one X-chromosomal locus.

A *haplotype* refers to a group of alleles that are closely linked together at a genetic locus. Haplotypes are useful for tracking the transmission of genomic segments within families and for detecting evidence of genetic recombination, if the cross-over event occurs between the alleles.

Allelic and phenotypic heterogeneity

Allelic heterogeneity refers to the fact that different mutations in the same genetic locus can cause an identical or similar phenotype. *Phenotypic heterogeneity* occurs when more than one phenotype is caused by allelic mutations. For example, different mutations in the androgen receptor can result in a wide phenotypic spectrum. In some cases, the receptor is deleted or mutated in a manner that inactivates it completely which leads to complete androgen insensitivity syndrome in a karyotypic male. By contrast, the phenotype may be milder if the androgen receptor is only partially inactivated. In these patients, the phenotype may include infertility, gynecomastia or epispadias. Allelic heterogeneity is explained by the fact that many different mutations are capable of altering protein structure and function. Allelic heterogeneity creates a significant problem for genetic testing because the entire genetic locus must be examined for mutations, as these can differ in each patient.

Locus or non-allelic heterogeneity and phenocopies

Non-allelic or *locus heterogeneity* refers to the situation in which a similar disease phenotype results from mutations at different genetic loci. This occurs when more than one gene product produces different subunits of an interacting complex or when different genes are involved in the same genetic cascade or physiological pathway. For example, congenital hypothyroidism associated with dyshormonogenesis can arise from mutations in several genes located on different chromosomes. The effects of inactivating mutations in these genes are similar because the protein products are all required for normal hormone synthesis. Similarly, the genetic forms of diabetes insipidus can be caused by mutations in several genes. Mutations in the AVP-NPII gene cause autosomal-dominant or -recessive forms of neurohypophyseal diabetes insipidus. The nephrogenic forms can be caused by mutations in the X-chromosomal AVPR2 receptor gene, whereas mutations in the aquaporin-2 (AQP-2) gene cause either autosomal-recessive or -dominant nephrogenic diabetes insipidus.

Recognition of non-allelic heterogeneity is important because the ability to identify disease loci in linkage studies is reduced by including patients with similar phenotypes but different genetic disorders. Genetic testing is more complex because several different genes need to be considered along with the possibility of different mutations in each of the candidate genes.

Phenocopies designate a phenotype that is identical or similar but results from non-genetic or other genetic causes. For example, obesity may be due to several Mendelian defects or have a primarily behavioral origin. As in non-allelic heterogeneity, the presence of phenocopies has the potential to confound linkage studies and genetic testing. Patient history, subtle differences in clinical presentation, and rigorous testing are key in assigning the correct phenotype.

Variable expressivity and incomplete penetrance

Penetrance and *expressivity* are two different yet related concepts that are often confused. Penetrance is a qualitative notion designating whether a phenotype is expressed for a particular genotype. Expressivity is a quantitative concept describing the degree to which a phenotype is expressed. It is used to describe the phenotypic spectrum in individuals with a particular disorder. Thus, expressivity is dependent on penetrance.

Penetrance is *complete* if all carriers of a mutant express the phenotype; it is *incomplete* if some individuals do not have any features of the phenotype. Dominant conditions with incomplete penetrance are characterized by skipping generations with unaffected carriers transmitting the mutant gene. For example, hypertrophic obstructive cardiomyopathy (HOCM) caused by mutations in the *myosin-binding protein C* gene is a dominant disorder with clinical features in only a subset of patients who carry the mutation. Incomplete penetrance in some individuals can confound pedigree analysis. In many conditions with postnatal onset, the proportion of gene carriers affected varies with age so it is important to specify age when describing penetrance. Variable expressivity is used to describe the phenotypic spectrum in individuals with a particular disorder.

Some of the mechanisms underlying expressivity and penetrance include modifier genes, gender and environmental factors. Thus, variable expressivity and penetrance illustrate that genetic and/or environmental factors do not influence only complex disorders, but also 'simple' Mendelian traits. This has to be considered in genetic counseling, because one cannot always predict the course of disease, even when the mutation is known.

Sex-influenced phenotypes

Certain mutations affect males and females quite differently. In some instances, this is because the gene resides on the X or Y sex chromosomes. As a result, the phenotype of mutated X-linked genes will usually be expressed fully in males but variably in heterozygous females, depending on the degree of X inactivation and the function of the gene. Because only males have a Y chromosome, mutations in genes such as *SRY* (which causes male-to-female sex reversal) or *DAZ* (*deleted in azoospermia*, which causes abnormalities of spermatogenesis) are unique to males.

Other diseases are expressed in a sex-limited manner because of the differential function of the gene product in males and females. Activating mutations in the LHR cause dominant male-limited precocious puberty in boys. The phenotype is unique to males because activation of the receptor induces testosterone production in the testis, whereas it is functionally silent in the ovary. Homozygous inactivating mutations of the FSH receptor cause primary ovarian failure in females because the follicles do not develop in the absence of FSH action but, because testosterone production is preserved, sexual maturation occurs in affected males in whom spermatogenesis is impaired.

Chromosomal disorders

Chromosomal (cytogenetic) disorders are caused by numerical or structural aberrations in chromosomes.

Molecular cytogenetics has led to the identification of more subtle chromosome abnormalities referred to as *microdeletion* and *imprinting* syndromes.

Errors in meiosis and early cleavage divisions occur frequently. Some 10–25% of all conceptions harbor chromosomal abnormalities, which often lead to spontaneous abortion. Numerical abnormalities are much more common than structural defects, especially trisomy, which is found in about 25% of spontaneous abortions and 0.3% of newborns.

Numerical abnormalities in sex chromosomes are relatively common. Males with a 47XXY karyotype have Klinefelter syndrome and females with trisomy 47XXX may be subfertile. Autosomal monosomies are usually incompatible with life; 45XO is present in 1–2% of all conceptuses but leads to spontaneous abortion in 99% of all cases. Mosaicism (e.g. 45XO/45XX, 45XO/45XXX), partial deletions, isochromosomes and ring chromosomes all cause Turner syndrome. Sex chromosome monosomy usually results from loss of the paternal sex chromosome. The 47XXY can result from paternal or maternal nondisjunction, while the autosomal trisomies are most commonly caused by maternal non-disjunction during meiosis, a defect that increases with maternal age. Trisomies are typically associated with alterations in genetic recombination.

Structural rearrangements involve breakage and reunion of chromosomes. Rearrangements between different chromosomes (*translocations*) can be *reciprocal* or *Robertsonian*. Reciprocal translocations involve exchanges between any of the chromosomes; Robertsonian rearrangements designate the fusion of the long arms of two acrocentric chromosomes. Other structural defects include deletions, duplications, inversions and the formation of rings and isochromosomes. Deletions affecting several tightly clustered genes result in *contiguous gene syndromes*, disorders that mimic a combination of single gene defects. They have been useful for identifying the location of new disease-causing genes. Structural chromosome defects can be present in a 'balanced' form without an abnormal phenotype. They can, however, be transmitted in an 'unbalanced' form to offspring and thus cause a hereditary form of chromosome abnormality.

Paternal deletions of chromosome 15q11-13 cause Prader–Willi syndrome (PWS), while maternal deletions are associated with the Angelman syndrome.

The difference in phenotype results from the fact that this chromosomal region is imprinted, that is, differentially expressed on the maternal and paternal chromosomes.

Acquired somatic abnormalities in chromosome structure are often associated with malignancies and are important for diagnosis, classification and prognosis. Deletions can lead to loss of tumor suppressor genes or DNA repair genes. Duplications, amplifications and rearrangements, in which a gene is put under the control of another promoter, can result in gain-of-function of genes controlling cell proliferation. For example, rearrangement of the 5′ regulatory region of the *PTH* gene located on chromosome 11q15 with the *cyclin D1* gene from 11q13 creates the *PRAD1* oncogene, resulting in overexpression of *cyclin D1* and the development of parathyroid adenomas.

2 The Endocrine Problems of Infancy

Learning Points

- Non-specific symptoms in infancy can be caused by any endocrine disorder
- Hypoglycemia with high glucose consumption (>10 mg/kg/min) is probably due to hyperinsulinism
- Hypoglycemia with low glucose consumption is associated with hypothalamo-pituitary problems
- Fits, jitteriness and hyperactivity may all be caused by hypoglycemia or hypocalcemia
- Conjugated hyperbilirubinemia may be due to cortisol deficiency; unconjugated hyperbilirubinemia may be due to hypothyroidism
- Congenital hypothyroidism due to iodine deficiency is the commonest preventable cause of mental retardation worldwide. Screening can eliminate this cause
- Vomiting may be due to cortisol deficiency, especially in males with congenital adrenal hyperplasia, whose genitalia are normal, and to hypercalcemia
- Congenital adrenal hyperplasia is the commonest cause of ambiguous genitalia

Hypothalamo-pituitary problems

Clinical features of hypopituitarism may appear in the neonatal period, often with a stormy perinatal course, or later with growth failure; they vary in severity according to the number of hormone deficiencies. Hormonal deficits can be one part of a syndrome, with patients manifesting abnormalities in extra-pituitary structures, usually in structures sharing a common embryological origin, such as the eye and forebrain. Mutations involved in human hypothalamo-pituitary disease are listed in Table 2.1.

The presentation of hypopituitarism in the neonatal period may be non-specific with poor feeding, lethargy,

Handbook of Clinical Pediatric Endocrinology, 1st edition. By Charles G. D. Brook and Rosalind S. Brown. Published 2008 by Blackwell Publishing, ISBN: 978-1- 4501-6109-1.

apnea, jitteriness and poor weight gain. Hypoglycemia is present in the majority of patients with multiple pituitary hormone deficiency (MPHD), probably due to adrenocorticotrophic hormone (ACTH) deficiency, although it has also been reported in patients with isolated growth hormone (GH) deficiency. Measurement of capillary blood glucose is routine in sick neonates and measurement of true blood glucose should be undertaken if the capillary glucose is <2.6 mmol/L (47 mg/dL). At the same time, blood should also be taken for measurement of random GH, cortisol, insulin, non-esterified fatty acids and ketone bodies.

Low serum insulin in the presence of hypoglycemia will rule out hyperinsulinemia but low serum GH and/or cortisol concentrations should point to a possible diagnosis of hypopituitarism. Infants with thyroid-stimulating hormone (TSH) deficiency may present with temperature instability and prolonged unconjugated hyperbilirubinemia. Conjugated hyperbilirubinemia

Table 2.1 Human mutations causing abnormal hypothalamo-pituitary development and function.

Gene	Phenotype	Inheritance
Isolated hormone abnormalities		
GH1	Isolated growth hormone deficiency	R, D
GHRHR	Isolated growth hormone deficiency	R
TSH-β	Isolated TSH deficiency and secondary hypothyroidism	R
TRHR	Isolated TSH deficiency and secondary hypothyroidism	R
T-PIT	ACTH deficiency	R
PC 1	ACTH deficiency, hypoglycemia, impaired glucose tolerance, HH, obesity	R
POMC	ACTH deficiency, obesity, red hair	R
DAX1	Adrenal hypoplasia congenital and HH	XL
GnRHR	Isolated gonadotropin deficiency and HH	R
KAL-1	Kallman syndrome	XL
FSH-β	Primary amenorrhea; defective spermatogenesis	R
LH-β	Delayed puberty	R
AVP	Diabetes insipidus	R, D
Combined pituitary hormone deficiency (CPHD)		
PIT1	GH, TSH, prolactin deficiencies	R, D
PROP1	GH, TSH, LH, FSH, prolactin, evolving ACTH deficiency	R
Specific syndrome		
HESX1	Septo-optic dysplasia	R, D
LHX3	CPHD (GH, TSH, LH, FSH, prolactin), short neck, limited rotation	R
LHX4	CPHD (GH, TSH, ACTH) with cerebellar abnormalities	D
SOX3	IGHD and mental retardation	XL
GLI2	Holoprosencephaly and multiple midline defects	D
GLI3	Pallister-Hall syndrome	D
Pitx2	Rieger syndrome	D

D, dominant; HH, hypogonadotrophic hypogonadism; R, recessive; XL, X-linked.

is a marker of cortisol deficiency and, together with recurrent sepsis, apnea and seizures, should prompt investigation for hypopituitarism.

Occasionally, neonates present with diabetes insipidus (DI), although this is much more common in patients with associated midline defects. The symptoms are polyuria and polydipsia with weight loss but cortisol is essential for the excretion of a water load and the diagnosis of DI may be masked in patients with ACTH deficiency. Treatment with hydrocortisone will unmask DI and caution should be exercised in patients with multiple pituitary hormone abnormalities when they are commenced on glucocorticoid replacement treatment, with careful monitoring for DI.

DI in neonates is best managed with fluid therapy alone. However, if an infant with DI cannot concentrate urine to reach an osmolality greater than the renal solute concentration of the feed, excessive urine output and hypernatremia will result. Large volumes of added free water required to reduce the renal solute concentration of standard infant formulas may result in inadequate calorie intake and poor growth. Decreasing the solute load with low-solute formula or breast milk can reduce the obligate urine output, allowing fluid balance to be achieved with modest free water supplementation in infants who can concentrate their urine to between 70 and 100 mOsm/L. If DI is severe and urine cannot be spontaneously concentrated to 70 mOsm/L, addition of a thiazide diuretic is helpful in increasing urine osmolality and reducing urine output.

A history of breech delivery or other instrumental delivery is commoner in patients with hypopituitarism.

Patients with gonadotropin deficiency, particularly luteinizing hormone (LH), may present with undescended testes and a micropenis, since growth of the penis is dependent upon normal secretion of LH and testosterone in the second and third trimesters.

Patients with hypopituitarism and visual abnormalities should be reviewed by an ophthalmologist to rule out optic nerve hypoplasia.

Management of MPHD

The mainstay is replacement therapy with the appropriate hormones as soon as deficiencies are confirmed.

If a mutation within *PROP1* is documented and cortisol secretion is normal, it should be reassessed at regular intervals since cortisol deficiency may develop. If a pituitary mass is present, serial magnetic resonance imaging (MRI) scans are indicated in order to monitor the size of the mass. In patients with septo-optic dysplasia (SOD), ophthalmological, neurological, educational and social support should be offered to the patients and their families, given the visual disability that is part of the condition.

Thyroid

Marked changes occur in thyroid physiology at birth. One is an abrupt rise in serum TSH within 30 min of delivery due to the relative hypothermia of the extrauterine environment. Concentrations of 60–70 mU/L are reached resulting in a 50% increase in serum T_4 and a three- to fourfold increase in serum T_3 within 24 h.

The premature infant

Thyroid function in the premature infant reflects the immaturity of the hypothalamic–pituitary–thyroid axis found in comparable gestational age infants *in utero*. In samples obtained by umbilical cord sampling, there is a progressive increase in the TSH, thyroxine-binding globulin (TBG), T_4 and T_3 concentrations in fetuses with increasing maturity. Following delivery, there is a surge in T_4 and TSH like that observed in term infants but the magnitude is less in premature neonates and there is a more dramatic fall in T_4 concentration over the next 1–2 weeks. This decrease is particularly marked in very low-birthweight infants (<1.5 kg, approximately equivalent to

<30 weeks' gestation), in whom the serum T_4 may occasionally be undetectable. In most cases, total T_4 is more affected than free T_4 because of abnormal protein binding and/or the decreased TBG in babies with immature liver function. Serum T_3 is reduced for a longer period in the premature newborn.

The causes of the postnatal decrease in T_4 in premature infants are complex. In addition to the clearance of maternal T_4 from the neonatal circulation, preterm babies have decreased iodide stores and are less able to regulate iodide balance.

Iodide uptake by the thyroid can be demonstrated at 10–11 weeks' gestation but the capacity of the fetal thyroid to reduce iodide trapping in response to excess iodide does not appear until near term. Thus, premature infants are much more likely than full-term babies to develop hypothyroidism when exposed to the excess iodine found in some skin antiseptics and drugs to which these babies are frequently exposed.

Despite the reduced total T_4 observed in some preterm babies, TSH concentrations are not significantly elevated in most. Transient elevations are seen in some, a TSH concentration >40 mU/L being more frequent the greater the degree of prematurity. Although an elevated TSH concentration may reflect true primary hypothyroidism, the increase in TSH seen in preterm infants may also reflect the elevated TSH of adults recovering from severe illness.

Congenital hypothyroidism

Congenital hypothyroidism (CH) is the commonest treatable cause of mental retardation. Worldwide, the most common cause is iodine deficiency, which affects almost 1 billion people. In areas where iodine deficiency is severe, CH is endemic ('endemic cretinism') and is characterized clinically by mental retardation, short stature, deaf mutism and specific neurological abnormalities.

Screening for CH

In iodine-sufficient areas and in areas of borderline iodine deficiency, CH occurs in 1 in 3000–4000 infants. In order to achieve optimal neurological outcome, treatment must be initiated soon after birth before affected infants are recognizable clinically. Neonatal screening programs have therefore been introduced in most industrialized areas of the world and detect about 6000 cases annually.

Screening strategies for CH

Measurement of T_4 and/or TSH is performed on an eluate of dried whole blood collected on filter paper by skin puncture on days 1–4 of life. Because of the neonatal TSH surge and the dynamic changes in T_4 and T_3 concentrations that occur within the first few days of life, early discharge increases the number of false-positive results.

Two screening strategies for the detection of CH have evolved. In both, a two-tiered approach is used. In much of North America, primary screening of T_4 is performed with TSH reserved for those specimens with a low T_4 (usually the lowest 10th–20th percentile). In most of Europe and Japan, a primary TSH/backup T_4 is employed. Recently, with the development of more sensitive, non-radioisotopic TSH assays, Canada and some states in the United States have switched to a primary TSH program.

Babies whose initial TSH is >50 mU/L are most likely to have permanent CH, whereas a TSH between 20 and 49 mU/L may be a false-positive result or represent transient hypothyroidism. Transient CH is particularly common in premature infants in borderline iodine-deficient areas.

A primary T_4/backup TSH program detects primary, secondary or tertiary hypothyroidism (1 in 50 000 to 1 in 100 000 live births), babies with a low T_4 but delayed rise in the TSH, TBG deficiency and hyperthyroxinemia but may miss compensated hypothyroidism. A primary TSH strategy detects overt and compensated hypothyroidism but misses secondary or tertiary hypothyroidism, a delayed TSH rise, TBG deficiency and hyperthyroxinemia. There are fewer false positives with a primary TSH strategy.

Both strategies miss the rare infant whose T_4 and TSH levels are normal on initial screening but who later develops low T_4 and elevated TSH concentrations (<0.5% of infants).

Thyroid dysgenesis

The causes of non-endemic CH and their relative frequencies are listed in Table 2.2. The most common cause (~90%) is sporadic thyroid dysgenesis. Thyroid dysgenesis may result in the complete absence of thyroid tissue (agenesis) or it may be partial (hypoplasia), often accompanied by a failure to descend into the neck (ectopy). Females are affected twice as often as males.

Inborn errors of thyroid hormonogenesis

Decreased T_4 synthesis due to an inborn error of thyroid hormonogenesis is responsible for most of the remaining cases (10–15%) of CH. Different defects have been characterized and include: (1) failure to concentrate iodide; (2) defective organification of iodide due to an abnormality in the thyroid peroxidase (TPO) enzyme or in the H_2O_2 generating system; (3) defective thyroglobulin (Tg) synthesis or transport and (4) abnormal iodotyrosine deiodinase activity. The association of a partial organification defect with sensorineural deafness is known as Pendred syndrome. All inborn errors of thyroid hormonogenesis are associated with a normally placed thyroid gland of normal or increased size and this feature distinguishes this cause from thyroid dysgenesis.

Inborn errors of thyroid hormonogenesis tend to have an autosomal-recessive form of inheritance consistent with a single gene mutation and many of these abnormalities have been identified.

TSH resistance

Babies with TSH resistance have a normal or hypoplastic gland or, in rare cases, no thyroid gland at all. Because the TSH gene is expressed only after the thyroid gland has migrated into the neck, loss-of-function mutations could explain hypoplasia or apparent aplasia but not ectopy. The clinical findings in TSH resistance vary from compensated to overt hypothyroidism, depending on the severity of the functional defect.

Decreased TSH synthesis or secretion

TSH deficiency may be isolated or it may be associated with other pituitary hormone deficiencies. Familial cases of both TSH and TRH (thyrotrophin-releasing hormone) deficiencies have been described. TSH deficiency as part of MPHD may be associated with abnormal midline facial and brain structures (particularly cleft lip and palate and absent septum pellucidum and/or corpus callosum).

Thyroid hormone resistance

Resistance to the action of thyroid hormone, although usually diagnosed later in life, may be identified in the newborn period by neonatal screening programs that determine TSH. Affected babies are not usually symptomatic. Most cases result from a mutation in the TRβ gene and follow an autosomal-dominant pattern of inheritance.

Table 2.2 Differential diagnosis of permanent congenital hypothyroidism (CH).

Thyroid dysgenesis (1 in 4500)
Isolated thyroid aplasia, hemiagenesis or hypoplasia ± ectopy
  Transcription factor defect (PAX-8)
  Unknown*
Associated with other developmental abnormalities
  Transcription factor defect (TTF-2, SHH, Tbx1)

Inborn errors of thyroid hormonogenesis (1 in 35 000)
Failure to concentrate iodide
Abnormal organification of iodine
  Abnormal TPO enzyme
  Abnormal H_2O_2 generation (THOX)
  Pendred syndrome
Defective Tg synthesis or transport
Abnormal iodotyrosine deiodinase

Secondary and/or tertiary hypothyroidism (1 in 50 000 to 100 000)
Hypothalamic abnormality
  Isolated TSH deficiency
    TRH deficiency
  Multiple hypothalamic hormone deficiencies
    Isolated hypothalamic defect
    Associated with other midline facial/brain dysmorphic features (e.g. SOD, cleft lip/palate)
Pituitary abnormality
  Isolated TSH deficiency
    TRH resistance
    Abnormal TSHβ molecule
  Multiple pituitary hormone deficiencies
    Posterior pituitary eutopic (transcription factor defect, e.g. POU1F-1, PROP1, LHX)
    Posterior pituitary ectopic

TSH resistance
TSH receptor gene mutation
Post-receptor defect?
Gsα gene mutation

Thyroid hormone resistance (1 in 100 000)

*Most common.

Abnormal thyroid hormone action can also result from failure of T_4 to enter cells. This occurs when there is an abnormality on one of the thyroid hormone transporters.

Transient congenital hypothyroidism

Estimates of the frequency of transient CH vary greatly depending on how this condition is defined. Causes are listed in Table 2.3. Iodine deficiency, iodine excess and drugs are common causes of transient hypothyroidism but the cause may be unknown.

Maternal antithyroid medication

Transient neonatal hypothyroidism may develop in babies whose mothers are being treated with antithyroid medication (propylthiouracil (PTU), methimazole (MMI) or carbimazole) for Graves' disease. Babies with antithyroid drug-induced hypothyroidism usually develop a goiter which may cause respiratory embarrassment, especially with higher doses. Both the hypothyroidism and the goiter resolve spontaneously with clearance of the drug from the baby's circulation and replacement therapy is not usually required.

Maternal thyrotrophin receptor antibodies

Maternal TSH receptor-blocking antibodies, a population of antibodies closely related to the TSH receptor-stimulating antibodies in Graves' disease, may be transmitted to the fetus in sufficient titer to cause transient CH.

Table 2.3 Differential diagnosis of transient CH.

Primary hypothyroidism
Prenatal or postnatal iodine deficiency or excess
Maternal antithyroid medication
Maternal TSH receptor-blocking antibodies

Secondary or tertiary hypothyroidism
Prenatal exposure to maternal hyperthyroidism
Prematurity (particularly <27 weeks' gestation)
Drugs
  Steroids
  Dopamine

Miscellaneous
Isolated TSH elevation
Low T$_4$ with normal TSH
  Prematurity
  Illness
  Undernutrition
Low T$_3$ syndrome

Transient secondary and/or tertiary hypothyroidism

Occasionally, babies born to mothers who were hyperthyroid during pregnancy develop transient hypothalamo-pituitary suppression. This hypothyroxinemia is usually self-limited but it may last for years and require replacement therapy.

Clinical manifestations of CH

Clinical evidence of hypothyroidism is difficult to appreciate in the newborn. Many of the classic features (large tongue, hoarse cry, facial puffiness, umbilical hernia, hypotonia, mottling, cold hands and feet and lethargy) are subtle and develop only with the passage of time. Figure 2.1 shows a baby with untreated CH diagnosed clinically compared with an infant in whom the diagnosis was made at 3 weeks of age in the early days of newborn screening.

Non-specific signs that suggest CH include prolonged, unconjugated hyperbilirubinemia, gestation longer than 42 weeks, feeding difficulties, delayed passage of stools, hypothermia or respiratory distress in an infant weighing over 2.5 kg. A large anterior fontanelle and/or a posterior fontanelle >0.5 cm is frequently present.

The extent of the clinical findings depends on the cause, severity and duration of the hypothyroidism. Babies in whom severe hypothyroidism was present

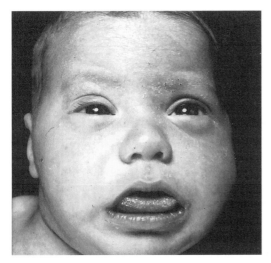 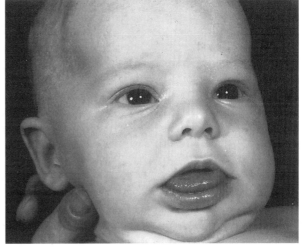

Figure 2.1 Infant with severe, untreated CH diagnosed clinically prior to the advent of newborn screening (a), compared with an infant with CH identified through newborn screening (b). Note the striking difference in the severity of the clinical features.

in utero tend to be the most symptomatic at birth. Babies with athyreosis or a complete block in thyroid hormonogenesis have more signs and symptoms at birth than infants with an ectopic thyroid, the most common cause of CH.

Babies with CH are of normal size at birth but, if diagnosis is delayed, linear growth becomes impaired. The presence of a goiter suggests an abnormality in thyroid hormonogenesis or in thyroid hormone action or suggests that it will be transient.

Laboratory evaluation

The diagnosis of primary CH is confirmed by decreased free T_4 and elevated TSH concentrations. Thyroid imaging provides information about the location and size of the thyroid gland. A radionuclide scan (either ^{123}I or [99m]pertechnetate) has long been the standard approach but color Doppler ultrasonography is almost as sensitive as ^{123}I in identifying ectopic thyroid tissue which may be located anywhere along the pathway of thyroid descent from the foramen cecum to the anterior mediastinum. Thyroid imaging is helpful in verifying whether a permanent abnormality is present and helps genetic counseling since thyroid dysgenesis is almost always sporadic, whereas abnormalities in thyroid hormonogenesis are autosomal recessive.

Treatment

Thyroxine replacement should begin as soon as the diagnosis of CH has been confirmed. Parents should be counseled regarding the causes of CH, the importance of compliance and the excellent prognosis in most babies if therapy is initiated early. Treatment need not be delayed in anticipation of performing a thyroid scan as long as this is done within 5–7 days of initiating treatment.

An initial dose of 10–15 µg/kg is commonly recommended to normalize the T_4 as soon as possible but there is a current trend to use higher doses (12–17 µg/kg). Babies with compensated hypothyroidism may be started on the lower dose, while those with severe CH (e.g. $T_4 < 5$ mg/dL (64 nmol/L)), such as those with thyroid agenesis, should be started on a higher dose. Thyroid hormone may be crushed and administered with water, juice or formula but care should be taken that all the medicine has been swallowed. It should not be given with substances that interfere with its absorption, such as iron, soy or fiber. Many babies will swallow the pills whole or chew the tablets with their gums even before they have teeth. Liquid preparations are less stable than tablets and therefore less reliable.

The aims of therapy are to normalize the serum T_4 concentration as soon as possible, to avoid hyperthyroidism and to promote normal growth and development. On the conventional doses, serum T_4 concentrations normalize in most infants within 1 week and the TSH within 1 month but more rapid normalization may improve outcome in the most severely affected infants. Subsequent adjustments in dose are made according to the results of thyroid function tests and the clinical picture.

Normalization of the TSH concentration may be delayed because of relative pituitary resistance. In such cases, characterized by a normal or increased serum T_4 and an inappropriately high TSH level, the T_4 value is used to titrate the dose of medication but non-compliance is the most common cause and should be excluded.

Current recommendations are to repeat T_4 and TSH at 2 and 4 weeks after the initiation of L-thyroxine treatment, every 1–2 months during the first year of life, every 2–3 months between 1 and 3 years of age and every 3–12 months thereafter until growth is complete. In hypothyroid babies in whom an organic basis was not established at birth and in whom transient disease is suspected, a trial of stopping replacement therapy can be initiated after the age of 3 years when most thyroid hormone-dependent brain maturation has occurred.

Whether or not premature infants with hypothyroxinemia should be treated remains controversial.

Prognosis

The cognitive outcome of babies with CH detected on newborn screening has been extensively studied. In the initial reports, despite the eradication of severe mental retardation, the intellectual quotient (IQ) of affected infants was 6–19 points lower than that of control babies. Although this IQ deficit was small, it was nonetheless significant as judged by a fourfold increase in the need for special education in affected children. In addition, sensorineural hearing loss, attention problems and various neuropsychological variables were noted, although the frequency and severity of these abnormalities were much less than in the prescreening era. Babies most likely to have permanent intellectual sequelae were infants with the most severe *in utero* hypothyroidism as determined by initial T_4 level (<5 mg/dL (64 nmol/L)) and skeletal maturation at birth. These findings led to the widely held conclusion at the time that some cognitive deficits in the most severely affected babies might not be reversible by postnatal therapy.

In the initial programs, a T_4 dose of 5–8 µg/kg was used and treatment was not initiated until 4–5 weeks of age. By contrast, accumulating data from a number of different studies have demonstrated that, when a higher initial treatment dose is used and treatment is initiated earlier (before 2 weeks), this developmental gap can be closed, irrespective of the severity of the CH at birth. Whether a higher starting dose is associated with increased temperamental difficulties and attention problems, particularly in less severely affected infants, remains controversial. Combined therapy with T_4 and T_3 offers no advantage over T_4 alone.

Neonatal hyperthyroidism

Transient neonatal hyperthyroidism (neonatal Graves' disease)

Unlike CH, which is usually permanent, neonatal hyperthyroidism is almost always transient. It results from the transplacental passage of maternal TSH receptor-stimulating antibodies. Hyperthyroidism develops only in babies born to mothers with the most potent stimulatory activity in serum, which can, of course, persist after maternal thyroidectomy. This amounts to 2–3% of mothers with Graves' disease. Most babies born to mothers with Graves' disease have normal thyroid function.

Clinical manifestations
Fetal hyperthyroidism is suspected because of tachycardia (pulse >160/min), especially if there is failure to thrive. Signs and symptoms in the infant include tachycardia, irritability, poor weight gain and prominent eyes. Goiter may be related to maternal antithyroid drug treatment as well as to the neonatal Graves' disease itself. Rarely, infants with neonatal Graves' disease present with thrombocytopenia, hepatosplenomegaly, jaundice and hypoprothrombinemia,

a picture that may be confused with congenital infections. Dysrhythmias and cardiac failure may develop and may cause death, particularly if treatment is delayed or inadequate. The half-life of TSH receptor antibodies is 1–2 weeks. The duration of neonatal hyperthyroidism, a function of antibody potency and metabolic clearance rate, is usually 2–3 months but may be longer.

Laboratory evaluation
The diagnosis of hyperthyroidism is confirmed by the demonstration of an increased concentration of T_4, free T_4, T_3 and free T_3 accompanied by a suppressed TSH. Fetal ultrasonography may be used to detect a goiter and monitor fetal growth.

Therapy
Maternal administration of antithyroid medication is used to treat the mother and the fetus. The lowest dose of PTU or MMI necessary to normalize the fetal heart rate and render the mother euthyroid or slightly hyperthyroid is usually chosen. After birth, treatment is expectant. PTU (5–10 mg/kg/day) or MMI (0.5–1.0 mg/kg/day) can be used, initially in three divided doses. If the hyperthyroidism is severe, a strong iodine solution (Lugol's solution or SSKI, one drop every 8 h) is added to block the release of thyroid hormone immediately because the effect of PTU and MMI may be delayed for several days. Therapy with both PTU and iodine is adjusted subsequently, depending on the response. Propranolol (2 mg/kg/day in two or three divided doses) is added if sympathetic overstimulation is severe, particularly in the presence of pronounced tachycardia. If cardiac failure develops, treatment with digoxin should be initiated and propranolol discontinued.

Rarely, prednisone (2 mg/kg/day) is added for immediate inhibition of thyroid hormone secretion and decreased generation of T_3 from T_4 in peripheral tissues.

Lactating mothers can continue nursing as long as the dose of PTU or MMI does not exceed 400 or 40 mg, respectively. As the milk–serum ratio of PTU is one-tenth that of MMI, a consequence of pH differences and increased protein binding, PTU is preferable to MMI although relatively low doses of MMI can be given to nursing mothers with no adverse effects on the baby. At higher doses of antithyroid medication, close supervision of the infant is advisable.

Permanent neonatal hyperthyroidism

Rarely, neonatal hyperthyroidism is permanent due to a germline mutation in the TSH receptor resulting in its constitutive activation. A gain-of-function mutation of the TSH receptor should be suspected if persistent neonatal hyperthyroidism occurs in the absence of detectable TSH receptor antibodies in the maternal circulation. Early recognition is important because the thyroid function of affected infants is frequently difficult to manage medically. When diagnosis and therapy are delayed, irreversible sequelae, such as cranial synostosis and developmental delay, may result. For this reason, early aggressive therapy with either thyroidectomy or radioablation has been recommended.

Fetal and neonatal calcium metabolism

The parathyroid glands are active in the human fetus from about 12 weeks of gestation. Thereafter, a positive gradient of calcium of 0.25–0.5 mmol/L is maintained across the placenta. Studies of parathyroid hormone (PTH) have demonstrated that very little is detectable in fetal plasma.

The normal full-term infant contains approximately 27 g of calcium, most of it acquired during the last trimester, and the net transfer of calcium across the placenta is 300–400 mg/day at term. Turnover of calcium amounts to more than 1% per day of total body calcium, compared with about 1/50th of this rate in adults. Fetal bone is very active.

The supply of calcium from the mother is terminated at birth which results in a rapid fall in plasma calcium to a nadir of 1.8–2.0 mmol/L (7.2–8.0 mg/dL) by 48 h. The normal concentration (2.2–2.6 mmol/L, 8.8–10.4 mg/dL) is achieved toward the end of the first week as the supply of calcium is resumed in milk and the normal physiological mechanisms are established.

Post-neonatal calcium, phosphate and magnesium metabolism

Following the establishment of normal physiological concentrations of calcium in plasma, there is little variation throughout life despite a 50-fold increase in bone mineral. By contrast, concentrations of phosphate vary considerably, being highest during periods of greatest demand for bone mineral, particularly during the neonatal period and adolescence. Concentrations of magnesium are also maintained within a narrow range (0.6–1.2 mmol/L, 1.2–2.4 mEq/L) with little variation.

Four factors maintain normal calcium physiology: PTH, vitamin D and its metabolites, parathyroid receptor peptide (PTHrP) and calcitonin. The first two are the most important outside fetal life. Magnesium has an important part to play since deficiency interferes with PTH secretion.

Neonatal hypocalcemia

Hypocalcemia may occur within the first 2–3 days of life because the physiological fall in plasma calcium is exaggerated, especially in preterm infants, following birth asphyxia, in sick infants and in those born to diabetic mothers. The mechanisms are unclear but may represent a delayed response to the rise of PTH following hypocalcemia. Magnesium deficiency may be a factor and magnesium concentration should be measured and corrected if necessary. Early onset hypocalcemia usually corrects itself spontaneously within the first week but additional calcium supplements may be required if symptoms persist. Hypophosphatemia is frequently present in preterm infants and may contribute to the development of bone disease of prematurity.

Hypocalcemia occurring toward the end of the first week is usually symptomatic. It can be the first manifestation of hypoparathyroidism but vitamin D deficiency or primary hyperparathyroidism in the mother must be considered. In the former, hypocalcemia can present at any time after birth depending on the severity of the deficiency and is not necessarily associated with radiological evidence of rickets, particularly if the presentation is soon after birth. It is almost entirely confined to infants of mothers from ethnic minority groups and routine vitamin D supplementation of 400 IU/day may not be sufficient to prevent neonatal hypocalcemia in these infants.

Hyperparathyroid mothers may be asymptomatic and the presence of hypocalcemia in the infant may be a clue to maternal disease. Measurement of bone profile in the mother and of vitamin D in mother and infant should form part of the investigation.

Neonatal hypocalcemia that is symptomatic requires treatment with intravenous 10% calcium gluconate (0.225 mmol/mL) given as a slow infusion of 1–3 mL/kg. This can be continued as an infusion of 1–2 mmol/kg/day or as oral supplements. It is important to ensure that the infusion is given into a secure intravenous site since extravasation causes unsightly burns. In the event of vitamin D deficiency, additional vitamin D supplements of 1000–1500 IU/day are required.

Hypercalcemia

Symptoms of hypercalcemia are age dependent. Mild hypercalcemia may be asymptomatic but, as the calcium concentration rises above 3.0 mmol/L (12 mg/dL), symptoms become more common. Infants present with poor feeding, failure to thrive, vomiting, constipation and irritability. Treatment consists of giving a low-calcium diet. A low-calcium milk (e.g. Locasol where available) is useful but, where patients live in hard water areas, there may be sufficient calcium in the water to negate its effect. If symptoms are severe, a short course of prednisolone, 1 mg/kg/day, is useful and can usually be stopped after a few weeks.

Idiopathic infantile hypercalcemia was originally described in infants born to mothers who had been ingesting large quantities of vitamin D and the incidence declined with a general reduction in vitamin D supplementation but some cases continue to occur with no evidence of excess vitamin D intake. Familial cases have been described.

Some of the features of this condition show similarities to Williams syndrome and can include hypertension, strabismus and radioulnar synostosis with failure to thrive, poor feeding, etc. Dysmorphic features are usually absent and correction of the hypercalcemia allows normal development, although the tendency to hypercalcemia may last beyond the first year. Lack of mutations in the elastin gene allows this condition to be distinguished from Williams syndrome.

Treatment consists of lowering the plasma calcium with a calcium- and vitamin D-restricted diet, steroids and bisphosphonates if necessary. Cellulose phosphate has been used to limit calcium absorption.

Neonatal primary hyperparathyroidism is usually caused by a homozygous inactivating mutation in the calcium-sensing receptor (CaSR) gene and occurs mostly in consanguineous families. Newborns feed poorly, fail to thrive and suffer constipation and atonia shortly after birth. Gross hypercalcemia, often in excess of 5.0 mmol/L (20 mg/dL), and hypophosphatemia are present. PTH is markedly elevated and hyperparathyroid bone disease develops such that respiratory

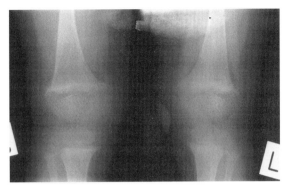

Figure 2.2 Radiographic image of lower end of femur and upper tibia in an infant suffering from severe neonatal primary hyperparathyroidism. Note the "moth-eaten" appearance and the similarity to that of rickets. This infant's chest radiograph showed the presence of multiple rib fractures and cystic areas, and he was ventilator dependent for several weeks prior to parathyroid gland removal. He then developed a severe "hungry bone" syndrome requiring infusion of large quantities of calcium to prevent symptomatic hypocalcemia.

distress necessitating assisted ventilation may result from poor rib compliance. The bones become thin and develop a moth-eaten appearance because of the severe hyperparathyroidism (Fig. 2.2). Multiple fractures may occur and the condition may be mistaken for rickets. A 'hungry bone' condition usually develops requiring infusion of large quantities of intravenous calcium to prevent hypocalcemia until the bones recover.

Once the diagnosis has been established, total parathyroidectomy is required to eliminate the hypercalcemia. Bisphosphonates may be useful temporarily to restore normocalcemia before surgery.

Disorders of sex development

In the vast majority of infants at birth, sex assignment is instantaneous. Parents faced with a situation in which that may not be the case find this unbelievable but there is a spectrum between male and female genitalia (Fig. 2.3). The neonatologist and, in turn, the pediatric endocrinologist must institute a series of investigations to try to establish a cause, although it should be recognized from the outset that a cause may not be found, especially in the XY infant with

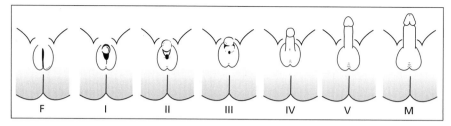

Figure 2.3 A recognized scoring system for the degree of virilization of the external genitalia in a female infant with congenital adrenal hyperplasia (Prader score I–V). F, normal female; M, normal male. The Quigley score for androgen insensitivity to quantify the degree of undermasculinization has a similar basis.

ambiguous genitalia. There should not be undue delay in sex assignment but a decision on sex of rearing may need to be delayed in some circumstances.

Newborn infants with the following features should be investigated:
- Infants with ambiguous genitalia.
- Severe hypospadias with or without undescended testes, micropenis or bifid scrotum or shawl scrotum.
- An apparent male infant with non-palpable testes.
- Female infant with inguinal herniae.
- Isolated clitoromegaly and/or labial fusion (examine for maternal virilization).
- Genital anomalies associated with syndromes.

Clinical assessment requires a history and physical examination. Family history and exposure to potential reproductive tract teratogens are particularly relevant.

Examination of the external genitalia should record:
- *Phallus* – size and presence of chordee, is it a micropenis or clitoromegaly?
- *Site of urethral opening* – has a urine stream been observed?
- *One or two external orifices on the perineum?*
- *Development of labioscrotal folds* – whether there is a bifid scrotum, fused labia, rugosity and pigmentation of skin.
- *Whether gonads are palpable and their position.*

Labial adhesion

Although this condition has nothing to do with ambiguous genitalia, it causes confusion and anxiety since it occurs in 3% of prepubertal girls with peak incidence in the first year of life. It is never present at birth.

The appearance is typical, with fusion of the labial skin extending from the posterior fourchette toward the urethral opening. A thin membranous line in the midline where the tissues fuse is clearly visible. The urethra may be a pinhole opening in extensive fusion. The etiology is unknown, but lack of estrogen is probably contributory.

Most infants are asymptomatic. If symptoms do occur, they are usually urinary: urine may pool behind the vaginal adhesions and cause post-micturition dribble, soreness and vulval irritation. Parents may be anxious about the possibility of an absent vagina (see Chapter 4) but the diagnosis can be made on examination alone and no investigations are indicated, although the ultrasound demonstration of a uterus may be reassuring.

Spontaneous resolution is common, and treatment is not necessary in the absence of symptoms. Estrogen cream applied topically to the midline fusion for no longer than 6 weeks will cause the labia to buttonhole and then separate but recurrence after discontinuing estrogen is common. Estrogen absorbed through the vagina can cause breast swelling and tenderness. Surgical separation is rarely needed unless urinary symptoms are persistent and estrogen therapy has failed but recurrence is common even after surgery and can lead to children having multiple surgical procedures.

Terminology

True hermaphroditism, defined as the presence of both ovarian and testicular tissue in the one individual, may be in the form of separate gonads or combined as an ovotestis. The diagnosis can be confirmed only by histology.

The terms pseudohermaphroditism prefaced by female and male to describe causes of masculinization in females and undermasculinization in males, respectively, have long been used but are confusing and should be replaced by plain English, masculinized female or undermasculinized male.

Causes of ambiguous genitalia are shown in Table 2.4.

The masculinized female

The placenta contains an aromatase enzyme system that is generally extremely efficient in protecting a female fetus from the effects of androgens in the maternal circulation: placental aromatase deficiency is a recognized cause of ambiguous genitalia in a female infant whose mother is also virilized during pregnancy.

In the context of ambiguous genitalia, congenital adrenal hyperplasia (CAH) is the commonest cause and the most straightforward diagnosis to establish. This must be undertaken promptly (if not made by newborn screening) in view of the potential life-threatening consequences to the infant of glucocorticoid and mineralocorticoid deficiency. Giving dexamethasone to the mother from early in pregnancy can successfully prevent or diminish masculinization of the external genitalia in an affected female infant but long-term effects on the brain are not known. This is a unique example of preventing a major congenital malformation by medical intervention.

Table 2.4 Causes of ambiguous genitalia.

Type/cause
Masculinized female
Fetal androgens (e.g. CAH, placental aromatase deficiency)
Maternal androgens (e.g. ovarian and adrenal tumors)
Undermasculinized male
Abnormal testis determination (e.g. Partial (XY) and mixed (XO/XY) gonadal dysgenesis)
Androgen biosynthetic defects (e.g. LH receptor-inactivating mutations, 17βOH-dehydrogenase deficiency, 5α-reductase deficiency)
Androgen insensitivity syndrome variants
True hermaphroditism
Presence of testicular and ovarian tissue
Syndromal (e.g. Denys–Drash, Frasier and Smith–Lemli–Opitz syndromes)

The undermasculinized male: defects in gonadal development

Complete gonadal dysgenesis occurs when normal development and function of Sertoli cells and Leydig cells, which are essential for hormone-mediated sex differentiation of the internal and external genitalia in the male, fail. A dysgenetic gonad results in the clinical disorder, gonadal dysgenesis. When both gonads are streaks, the phenotype is female, whatever the karyotype. Consequently, XY complete gonadal dysgenesis (Swyer syndrome) leads to complete sex reversal and no ambiguity in sex development. Approximately 15–20% of patients have a mutation of the *SRY* gene. There are familial cases of XY complete gonadal dysgenesis in which the genetic cause is unknown and the pattern of inheritance can be X-linked or autosomal recessive. There is a high risk of gonadal tumors such as gonadoblastoma and germinoma.

Partial gonadal dysgenesis gives rise to ambiguity of the genitalia because of the preservation of some Leydig cell function with an XY karyotype. There are generally Müllerian duct remnants, reflecting inadequate Sertoli cell production of anti-Müllerian hormone (AMH). These appearances are not dissimilar from those of an early developing testis so dysgenetic gonads in partial gonadal dysgenesis syndromes represent a failure in gonad maturation.

Mixed gonadal dysgenesis is the term used when there is 45,XO/46,XY chromosomal mosaicism. Gonadal morphology is typically a testis on one side and a streak gonad on the contralateral side. A wide spectrum of phenotypes can result from XO/XY sex chromosome mosaicism with varying degrees of sex reversal. Abnormalities of the external genitalia may be in the form of a severe hypospadias with cryptorchidism but the penis may be normal in size. Alternatively, the degree of undermasculinization can be manifest solely as a hypertrophied clitoris. There is no correlation between the phenotype and the proportion of XO vs. XY cell lines, whether this is determined in blood or fibroblasts. In later childhood, stigmata of Turner syndrome may appear.

Examples of eponymous syndromes associated with gonadal dysgenesis include the *Denys–Drash and Frasier syndromes*, both caused by mutations in *WT1*, a gene essential for gonadogenesis and nephrogenesis. In the Denys–Drash syndrome, there are usually genital anomalies at birth in XY cases, a characteristic nephropathy resulting from diffuse mesangial sclerosis and a predisposition to Wilms' tumor with a median age of onset by 12 months. Frasier syndrome differs with respect to a more severe gonadal dysgenesis generally resulting in complete XY sex reversal, a nephropathy characterized by focal segmental glomerulosclerosis and a predisposition to gonadoblastoma rather than Wilms' tumor.

SOX9, an SRY-related protein, is a transcription factor involved in both chondrogenesis and early testis determination. Heterozygous mutations in the SOX9 gene can cause campomelic dysplasia, a multiskeletal disorder, with sex reversal in the majority of affected males. Not all affected patients have both gonadal dysgenesis and genital anomalies.

Another key gene in development of the gonads is *SF1* (steroidogenic factor 1). The gene is also required for development of the adrenals and the hypothalamus. Disruption of the gene causes combined XY sex reversal and adrenal insufficiency.

ATRX syndrome is another multisystem disorder associated with XY gonadal dysgenesis. The syndrome comprises β-thalassemia, mental retardation and multiple congenital anomalies.

Defects in androgen biosynthesis

Fetal Leydig cell androgen synthesis is initially placental human chorionic gonadotropin (hCG) dependent but depends later on LH stimulation from the fetal pituitary. Fetal serum concentrations of testosterone rise into the normal adult male range toward the end of the first trimester when Wolffian duct stabilization occurs, followed later by growth of the external genitalia. The timing and magnitude of the rise in androgen and AMH concentrations are critical for normal male sex differentiation. Abnormalities in a number of biosynthetic steps can result in inadequate androgen production and an undermasculinized male infant. Some of these abnormalities also affect adrenal steroidogenesis.

Enzymes relevant to testis-specific defects are 17β-hydroxysteroid dehydrogenase and 5α-reductase enzyme deficiencies. Both these defects present at birth with severe undermasculinization, often to the extent of complete sex reversal, but a remarkable degree of virilization of the external genitalia may occur with the onset of puberty.

Defects in androgen action

Failure of development of the external genitalia in a male with a 46,XY karyotype and testes that produce age-appropriate circulating concentrations of androgens defines tissue-specific resistance to the action of androgens. This is the commonest cause of male undermasculinization.

Total resistance leads to complete XY sex reversal and no ambiguity of the external genitalia. This is the complete androgen insensitivity syndrome (CAIS), also known as testicular feminization. Some response to androgens results in partial androgen insensitivity syndrome (PAIS). The degree of response may be manifest as mild clitoromegaly, true ambiguity of the genitalia, hypospadias alone or impaired fertility in an otherwise normal male.

Testosterone is elevated and LH levels are unsuppressed in CAIS and PAIS. Androgens aromatized to estrogens result in breast development in XY males unopposed by androgen action. Thus, the patient with CAIS has a normal female phenotype at puberty, except for absent or scanty pubic and axillary hair. Clinical presentation is usually in adolescence with primary amenorrhea but the condition may present in infancy with inguinal herniae, which are found to contain testes at the time of surgical repair. The patient with PAIS and a more male phenotype frequently develops gynecomastia at puberty and breast cancer has been reported.

The pathophysiology of CAIS and PAIS is related to a defect in the intracellular action of androgens. A mutation in the androgen receptor gene is identified in about 80% of XY sex-reversed females who have clinical, biochemical and histological evidence of CAIS but in only about 15–20% of patients with PAIS.

There is a risk of gonadoblastomas, seminomas and germ cell tumors developing in the gonads of patients with CAIS or PAIS. For this reason gonadectomy has often been performed. Delaying gonadectomy until later in life will allow spontaneous puberty without the need for exogenous estrogen administration. Delaying until after puberty may lead to improved adult bone density. If the testes are retained, assiduous follow-up is necessary although monitoring is difficult. Clinical palpation is possible only if the gonads are in the groin or inguinal canal. Ultrasound is not accurate enough reliably to detect early malignant changes.

The gynecological management of CAIS focuses on psychological support and treatments for vaginal hypoplasia. The psychological aspects of living with CAIS are paramount to successful management. There are few long-term data but the initial strong reactions of shock, anger, grief and shame can persist for many years in affected individuals and their families.

Vaginal development in CAIS is variable but vaginal hypoplasia is common. The vagina is composed of a lower urogenital portion and an upper portion derived from Müllerian structures. Owing to the effects of AMH, the Müllerian portion of the vagina will not develop. Normal vaginal length in the general population is about 11 cm, whereas vaginal lengths within a CAIS population range from 2 cm upwards leading to a high prevalence of sexual dysfunction exacerbated by psychological factors.

Treatments concentrate mainly on vaginal self-dilation to increase vaginal length. Small retrospective studies have shown this to be a beneficial approach but there are no prospective studies on this treatment and its impact on sexual function. The advantages of this method are that risks and side-effects of treatment are low and the patient is in charge of her own treatment. However, the time taken to create a vagina can be several months and some women find dilators difficult and unpleasant to use. There are several surgical options available but outcome studies are scarce and there is little information about the comparative risks and benefits of the various techniques available.

True hermaphroditism and other sex chromosome anomalies

The term hermaphroditism should be applied only to individuals possessing both well-differentiated testicular tissue and ovaries that contain follicles. The most frequent karyotype is 46,XX followed by a third of cases with 46,XX/XY mosaicism and <10% having a 46,XY karyotype. Most patients have ambiguous genitalia with perineal hypospadias, bifid scrotum and usually a normal-sized phallus. Ovotestis is the most common gonad.

The XX male generally has normal differentiation of the external genitalia, although hypospadias may occur. The testes are small and firm, height is below the average for normal males (unlike Klinefelter syndrome) and gynecomastia is usual. There is an increased risk of carcinoma of the breast. Affected males are infertile.

Klinefelter syndrome (47,XXY) affects around 1 in 600 males and is not usually associated with ambiguous genitalia. However, there are single case reports of genital anomalies comprising hypospadias, penoscrotal transposition and even a few cases with complete sex reversal consistent with androgen insensitivity.

Investigations

A karyotype with a sufficient number of mitoses analyzed to exclude mosaicism is required.

The commonest cause of newborn ambiguous genitalia is CAH due to 21-hydroxylase deficiency. Measurement of serum 17OH-progesterone is a reliable test for 21-hydroxylase deficiency. In a 46,XX infant with ambiguous genitalia, elevated 17OH-progesterone (generally >300 nmol/L, 100 μg/dL) and a uterus visualized on pelvic ultrasound, the diagnosis is CAH. Ancillary biochemical tests should establish whether the infant is also a salt loser. It may be necessary to perform a synacthen/cortrosyn stimulation test, especially if CAH is suspected in a preterm infant or there is a possibility of one of the rarer enzyme defects. Male infants with non-palpable testes must have a karyotype; it is unacceptable to miss this opportunity to establish a diagnosis of CAH in a female masculinized to a Prader score V degree.

In the XY or XO/XY infant with ambiguous genitalia, investigations are aimed at establishing the location and function of testes if present. The hCG stimulation test is pivotal in this situation, coupled with imaging and laparoscopy to identify gonad site and histology. hCG is given as 1500 units daily for 3 days, with a post-hCG blood sample collected 24 h after the last injection. Occasionally, a longer test is needed using a twice weekly injection regimen for 2 weeks. Pre- and post-hCG blood samples should be analyzed for androstenedione, testosterone and dihydrotestosterone (DHT).

Sertoli cell function can be assessed by measurement of AMH and inhibin B. Both proteins are elevated in serum during infancy. Circulating levels of AMH remain high until puberty when they fall in response to the effect of testosterone. Hence, AMH levels are elevated in intersex states associated with androgen insensitivity but low in disorders of gonadal dysgenesis. An undetectable value suggests anorchia, so this is a useful test in the investigation of an XY infant with ambiguous genitalia with no palpable gonads. Inhibin B is also undetectable in anorchia and the levels correlate with the increment in testosterone following an hCG stimulation test in boys with gonadal dysgenesis and androgen insensitivity. Basal measurements of AMH and inhibin B alone may be sufficient for confirming anorchia but baseline LH and follicle-stimulating hormone (FSH) measurements together with a suitably performed hCG stimulation test should not be omitted from the protocol.

Imaging with ultrasound and MRI is used to delineate the internal genital anatomy, including localizing the site and, possibly, the morphological nature of the gonads. Only histology will provide precise details of the gonads and many infants with ambiguous genitalia require a laparoscopy to reach a diagnosis.

Management

Early management is focused on establishing a diagnosis, particularly for the infant who may have a life-threatening disorder with adrenal insufficiency. If this is the case, treatment with appropriate replacement of glucocorticoids, mineralocorticoids, glucose and fluid is required.

The XY infant with ambiguous genitalia poses more difficulties in management. It is possible that a definitive diagnosis may not be reached, even after extensive investigation. Sometimes, a trial of testosterone treatment can give an indication about androgen responsiveness and future treatment options. A decision about sex assignment may be delayed until such a trial is complete. Infants with disorders of inadequate fetal androgen production are likely to respond to androgens with an increase in phallic growth. This can also happen in PAIS due to some missense mutations, so a positive response to androgens should not assume that androgen insensitivity is excluded.

Despite the anxiety about how to manage intersex disorders, there is consensus that the newborn infant with ambiguous genitalia should be sex assigned as soon as is practicable after birth. When surgery should be undertaken the nature of the procedure are issues that remain to be resolved. The results of some adult outcome studies of intersex patients are beginning to alter early surgical practice. Thus, surgery is not performed so readily for the enlarged clitoris, creating a vagina is not necessary before puberty and an XY infant with a micropenis should not necessarily be sex assigned female. The early management of ambiguous genitalia is undertaken by engaging the family fully in a climate of openness. This must include explaining the current limitations in knowledge about diagnosis and longer-term outcome studies. Above all, professional staff have a responsibility to support the family in reaching a decision on sex assignment and to continue that support as appropriate through childhood and adolescence.

Genetic lesions in steroidogenesis

Autosomal-recessive disorders disrupt each of the steps in the pathway of steroidogenesis (see Chapter 6). Most result in diminished synthesis of cortisol. In response to adrenal insufficiency, the pituitary synthesizes increased amounts of ACTH, which promotes increased steroidogenesis and stimulates adrenal hypertrophy and hyperplasia. Thus, the term CAH refers to a group of diseases traditionally grouped together on the basis of the most prominent finding at autopsy.

In theory, CAH is easy to understand. A genetic lesion in one of the steroidogenic enzymes interferes with normal steroidogenesis. The signs and symptoms of the disease derive from deficiency of the steroidal endproduct and the effects of accumulated steroidal precursors proximal to the blocked step.

In practice, CAH can be confusing both clinically and scientifically. Because each steroidogenic enzyme has multiple activities and many extra-adrenal tissues contain enzymes that have similar activities, the complete elimination of a specific adrenal enzyme may not result in the complete elimination of its steroidal products from the circulation.

Thus, for example, in the case of a baby with an abnormality of cholesterol transport due to a defective steroid acute-regulatory (StAR) protein, there is no delivery of cholesterol to the side-chain cleavage enzyme and no steroids can be produced. Such a baby will not have been able to differentiate as a male, even if there are testes present but such testes will produce AMH; the baby will be born with a short vagina and absent uterus and fallopian tubes. At birth, he will be apparently female but will rapidly lapse into a salt-losing crisis, become profoundly ill

Table 2.5 Varieties of CAH and their effects.

Defect	Ambiguous genitalia in genotypic		Salt loss	Hypertension	Puberty
	Males	Females			
StAR protein	+	−	+	−	Absent
3β-hydroxysteroid dehydrogenase	+	+	+	−	Absent
17α-hydroxylase	+	−	−	+	Absent
21-hydroxylase	−	+	+	−	Precocious
11β-hydroxylase	−	+	−	+	Precocious

and die unless steroids are administered. This condition, known as congenital lipoid adrenal hyperplasia, is characterized by an accumulation of lipid droplets in the cells of the adrenal cortex.

Contrast this with the effects of 11β-hydroxylase (CYP11B1) deficiency. Such a patient will be unable to make cortisol but corticotrophin-releasing factor (CRH)–ACTH drive will force the overproduction of deoxycorticosterone, a mineralocorticoid that can lead to malignant hypertension. There will also be excessive production of sex steroids, leading to masculinization of a female fetus *in utero* or to precocious puberty in a boy exposed to excessive androgen stimulation.

All varieties of enzymatic block have been recognized and Table 2.5 shows the clinical effects of the loss of the various enzyme systems. The most common is due to a deficiency of 21-hydroxylase, accounting for some 90% of the cases. Identification of the enzyme deficiency depends on measuring circulating steroids and identifying those that are deficient and those that are produced in excess.

For all of these conditions, treatment is available with either mineralocorticoid or glucocorticoid replacement or both and some of them will, of course, require sex-steroid treatment at puberty. The consequences of making the wrong diagnosis are very considerable for the individual patient.

Clinical forms of 21-OHD

Salt-wasting 21-OHD is due to a complete deficiency of P450c21 activity, effectively eliminating both glucocorticoid and mineralocorticoid synthesis. Females are frequently diagnosed at birth because of masculinization of the external genitalia. Males are not generally

diagnosed at birth and come to medical attention as a result of neonatal screening for 17-OHP, during the salt-losing crisis that follows 5–15 days later or they die, not having been diagnosed.

Virilized females with elevated concentrations of 17-OHP who do not suffer a salt-losing crisis have the simple virilizing form of CAH. Males often escape diagnosis until age 3–7 years, when they develop pubic, axillary and facial hair and phallic growth.

Prenatal diagnosis and treatment of 21-OHD

The prenatal diagnosis and therapy of 21-OHD are being actively pursued but prenatal therapy remains experimental and controversial. The fetal adrenal is active in steroidogenesis from early in gestation, so a diagnosis can be made by cordocentesis or amniocentesis and measurement of 17-OHP in fetal plasma or amniotic fluid.

Prenatal treatment requires early and accurate prenatal diagnosis. Female fetuses affected with 21-OHD begin to become virilized at about 6–8 weeks' gestation at the same time that a normal male fetal testis produces large amounts of testosterone. This causes fusion of the labioscrotal folds, enlargement of the genital tubercle into a phallus and the formation of the phallic urethra. If fetal adrenal steroidogenesis is suppressed in an affected fetus, the virilization can be reduced or eliminated.

Several studies have reported the successful application of this approach by administering dexamethasone to the mother in doses of 20 mg/kg maternal body weight as soon as pregnancy is diagnosed. This dose is 3–6 times the physiological replacement dose. This can be done only when the parents are known to be heterozygotes by having already had an affected child.

Even in such pregnancies, only one in four fetuses will have CAH. Furthermore, as no prenatal treatment is needed for male fetuses affected with CAH, only one in eight pregnancies of heterozygous parents would harbor an affected female fetus that might potentially benefit from prenatal treatment and seven would have been treated unnecessarily. The efficacy, safety and desirability of such prenatal treatment remain highly controversial.

Treatment of pregnant rats with 20 mg/kg dexamethasone predisposes the fetuses to hypertension in adulthood and some studies indicate that even moderately elevated concentrations of glucocorticoids can be neurotoxic. Thus, prenatal treatment of CAH remains an experimental and controversial therapy that should be done only in research centers. Follow-up studies of very long duration are needed to evaluate its effects fully, especially on the seven fetuses treated unnecessarily.

Treatment

The management of this disorder remains difficult. Overtreatment with glucocorticoids causes delayed growth, even when the degree of overtreatment is insufficient to produce signs and symptoms of Cushing syndrome. Undertreatment results in continued overproduction of adrenal androgens, which hastens epiphyseal maturation and closure, again resulting in compromised growth and other manifestations of androgen excess.

Doses of glucocorticoids should be based on the expected normal cortisol secretory rate. Widely cited classic studies have reported that the secretory rate of cortisol is 12.5 ± 3 mg/m^2/day and have led most authorities to recommend doses of 10–20 mg/m^2/day hydrocortisone. However, the cortisol secretory rate is actually substantially lower, at $6–7 \pm 2$ mg/m^2/day. Newly diagnosed patients, especially newborns, do require substantially higher initial doses to suppress their hyperactive CRH/ACTH/adrenal axis: simple physiological replacement is usually insufficient to suppress adrenal androgens.

Most authorities favor the use of oral hydrocortisone or cortisone acetate in three divided daily doses in growing children. Only one oral mineralocorticoid preparation, fludrocortisone (9α-fluorocortisol),

is generally available. It must be given as crushed tablets, not as a suspension, which delivers the medication unreliably.

Additional salt supplementation, usually 1–2 g of NaCl per day in the newborn, is also needed.

Blood glucose homeostasis

The fetus receives a constant intravenous supply of glucose across the placenta, fetal glucose uptake being directly related to both the maternal blood glucose concentration and the transplacental gradient. The transition from a transplacental supply of nutrients to intermittent feeding and fasting with the introduction of milk feeds into the gut is accomplished by the normal infant at term with little external evidence of the magnitude of the changes taking place. The process of adaptation is, however, incomplete and is compromised when the infant is born prematurely or following intrauterine growth retardation.

A normal infant at term has an immediate postnatal fall in blood glucose concentration during the first 2–4 h from values close to maternal levels to around 2.5 mmol/l (45 mg/dL), which implies that one or more of the mechanisms required for fasting adaptation are not fully developed at birth but this fall is necessary to induce the hormonal surges involved in stimulating enzymic activation.

In all mammalian species there is a major and abrupt increase in plasma glucagon concentrations within minutes to hours of birth accompanied by a surge in catecholamine secretion. Plasma GH concentration are considerably elevated at birth. This changing hormonal milieu mobilizes glucose from glycogen and substrate delivery through lipolysis and proteolysis. The release of free fatty acids into the circulation is followed by an abrupt increase in the production of ketone bodies from the liver. The role of cortisol remains enigmatic.

Severe hypoglycemia occurs if the normal relationship of these hormones is disturbed but the net effect of the changes is to stabilize the blood glucose concentration at a lower level during the first few hours while milk feeding is initiated. The availability of ketone bodies allows a sparing effect of glucose for brain utilization.

Hypoglycemia

The recognition and diagnosis of hypoglycemia in the neonatal period depend on routine monitoring of blood glucose levels at frequent intervals after birth in asymptomatic infants at risk and in any infant who demonstrates a symptom that might suggest hypoglycemia. Groups at particular risk are shown in Table 2.6. It is important to monitor blood glucose in relation to the time of feeds. A blood glucose concentration that increases after a feed is less worrying than one that is persistently low. If low concentrations are obtained during routine monitoring in asymptomatic high-risk infants or at the time of symptoms in symptomatic infants, the result should be confirmed in the laboratory but intervention does not need to wait for the result. Resolution of symptoms after glucose confirms that they were due to hypoglycemia.

In investigating hypoglycaemia in the neonatal period, the clinical history should include details of pregnancy and delivery, birthweight, gestational age of the infant, noting in particular any evidence of fetal distress, birth asphyxia and smallness for dates. The relationship of a hypoglycemic episode to the most recent meal can be important. Hypoglycemia occurring after a short fast (2–3 h) may suggest a glycogen storage disease but hypoglycemia occurring after a long fast (12–14 h) may suggest a disorder of gluconeogenesis. Post-prandial hypoglycemia may indicate galactosemia or hereditary fructose intolerance. A family history of

sudden infant deaths may be a clue to an unrecognized, inherited metabolic disorder. Provocation factors such as an upper respiratory tract infection or an episode of gastroenteritis leading to hypoglycemia should be documented. From the history and physical examination, certain groups of infants at risk of transient hypoglycemia who need monitoring can be identified.

The presence or absence of maternal diabetes or rhesus incompatibility is important. Increased birthweight and macrosomia should raise the possibility of neonatal hyperinsulinism. Distinctive physical signs such as transverse ear lobe creases, exomphalos and macroglossia should raise the possibility of the Beckwith–Wiedemann syndrome, whereas the presence of micropenis and undescended testes might indicate the presence of hypopituitarism. Midline defects, including cleft palate, could indicate congenital hypopituitarism, while ambiguous genitalia could indicate CAH.

Hepatomegaly should always be sought but may be absent at birth. Hepatomegaly is associated with abnormal glycogen metabolism, defects in gluconeogenesis and galactosemia. Moderate hepatomegaly due to glycogen accumulation may, however, develop in infants with hyperinsulinism who are receiving high infusion rates of glucose to maintain normo-glycemia. Particular attention should be paid to the rate of growth, micropenis, undescended testes, skin pigmentation, blood pressure and weight loss in childhood.

Congenital hyperinsulinism of infancy (HI) is by far the most difficult to manage. It is associated with a high incidence (up to 25%) of neurological handicap, which has not changed over the course of the last 20 years. Hyperinsulinism causes hypoglycemia primarily as a result of increased utilization of glucose with a decreased rate of endogenous glucose production. These effects are due to inappropriate secretion of insulin, which has been called a variety of names, including idiopathic hypoglycemia of infancy, leucine-sensitive hypoglycemia, neonatal insulinoma, microadenomatosis, focal hyperplasia, nesidioblastosis and persistent hyperinsulinemic hypoglycemia of infancy (PHHI).

Sporadic and familial variants of congenital HI are recognized, with sporadic forms being relatively uncommon (incidence 1 per 40 000 live births) and familial forms being common (as high as 1 in 2500 live births) in communities with high rates of consanguinity. The genetic basis of many of these cases has been

Table 2.6 Groups at risk from hypoglycemia.

Premature infants
Intrauterine growth-retarded infants
Infants born to diabetic (insulin-dependent and gestational) mothers
Infants subjected to perinatal asphyxia
Infants born with erythroblastosis fetalis
Infants with Beckwith–Wiedemann syndrome
Maternal administration of some drugs such as sulfonylureas/β-blockers
Macrosomic infants
Any 'sick' infant
Polycythemic infants
Hypothermic infants
Infants with congenital heart disease
Infants with 'metabolic' conditions
Older children with infections such as malaria

identified and includes mutations in the components of the K_{ATP} channel and of other intracellular enzymes important in insulin secretion.

The condition presents in the newborn period or during the first 2–6 months after birth in term and preterm neonates. Many neonates have a characteristic appearance strikingly resembling that of an infant of a diabetic mother. This suggests that the hyperinsulinism has been present for some time before birth. Very rarely, HI may present in an older child when it is likely to be due to an insulinoma.

The characteristic metabolic and endocrine profile of a blood sample drawn at the time of hypoglycemia is hyperinsulinemia, hypoketotic, hypofatty acidemic hypoglycemia with inappropriately raised insulin accompanied by high concentrations of connecting- (or C-) peptide levels. High intravenous infusion rates of glucose may be required to maintain a blood glucose concentration above 3 mmol/L (55 mg/dL). Because of the anabolic effects of insulin, the hypoglycemia occurs despite a liver engorged with glycogen that can be mobilized by administration of glucagon. The glycemia can usually be improved by an infusion of somatostatin that will switch off insulin secretion. Neonates with hyperinsulinemic hypoglycemia fail to generate an adequate serum cortisol counter-regulatory hormonal response, which appears to be related to inappropriately low plasma ACTH concentrations at the time of hypoglycemia.

The level of insulin in the blood may not be particularly high but what is an appropriate insulin concentration for normoglycemia becomes inappropriate in the presence of hypoglycemia. The demonstration of measurable insulin in a hypoglycemic sample is strong evidence for a failure of basal insulin control.

The immediate imperative of management is to give glucose sufficient to maintain blood glucose concentrations above 3 mmol/L (55 mg/dL). Infusion rates in excess of 4–6 mg/kg/min, even >20 mg/kg/min, may be necessary. Having stabilized the blood glucose concentration, it is imperative to determine whether the patient will respond to conventional medical therapy with diazoxide and a thiazide diuretic. Both drugs should be given concurrently to overcome the tendency of diazoxide to cause fluid retention and to capitalize on the fact that the drugs have synergistic effects in increasing blood glucose concentration. A convenient starting dose of diazoxide is 5–10 mg/kg/day in three 8-hourly aliquots, increasing to a maximum of 20 mg/kg/day.

In the light of understanding the defect in the molecular physiology of congenital hyperinsulinism, the use of a calcium channel-blocking agent, such as nifedipine, has been promoted, with some patients showing good response. However, as some patients also have impairments in voltage-gated calcium entry, nifedipine may not always be beneficial. Glucagon given by continuous infusion (starting dose 1.0 mg/kg/h) concurrently with the somatostatin analog octreotide (initial dose 10 mg/kg/day) may confer substantial benefit.

The pediatrician is faced with an important challenge when managing a child who proves to be unresponsive to conventional therapy with diazoxide. The options are either to contemplate the long-term combined continuous subcutaneous infusion of glucagon and somatostatin or to consider surgical resection of the pancreas. Few centers have experience of the first of these treatments and the practical aspects of the management may be considerable.

Partial pancreatectomy is not without risk and not a procedure to be undertaken lightly. The operation most commonly performed is a 95% pancreatectomy in the first instance but some children still remain hypoglycemic and a further attempt can then be made to control the procedure with diazoxide. In a minority of cases, total pancreatectomy may be necessary to control the severe hyperinsulinism, which may be exacerbated by regeneration of the pancreatic remnant.

HI has been classified into diffuse and focal disease. The recognition of 'focal' disease has led to performing preoperative percutaneous transhepatic pancreatic vein catheterization with the withdrawal of multiple blood samples to identify 'hotspots' of insulin secretion. Rapid-frozen sections are used to identify areas of focal hyperplasia at surgery, which are then resected.

Congenital hypopituitarism may present with life-threatening hypoglycemia, abnormal serum sodium concentrations, shock, microphallus and later growth failure. Causes include SOD, other midline syndromes and mutations of transcription factors involved in pituitary gland development. Children with acquired hypopituitarism typically present with growth failure and may have other complaints depending on the etiology and the extent of missing pituitary hormones. Appropriate replacement therapy with hydrocortisone and GH can alleviate hypoglycemia.

3 Problems of Growth in Childhood

Learning Points

- After the completion of fetal growth, postnatal growth is divided into three components: infantile, childhood and pubertal

- Nutrition is the predominant influence on infantile growth, growth hormone on childhood growth and sex steroids on pubertal growth

- Normal growth is defined by a normal growth rate, regardless of height achieved, so accurate measurement is essential for growth assessment

- Estimation of bone age does not provide diagnostic information, only an estimate of height prognosis

- An abnormal growth velocity is the most important indication for investigation of short or tall children but the extent of the deviation of height from normal is an additional consideration

- Short stature can occur as part of a dysmorphic syndrome and Turner syndrome should be considered in any female with unexplained short stature

Growth occurs by accretion of tissue through cell hyperplasia (an increase in cell number), cell hypertrophy (an increase in cell size) and apoptosis (programmed cell death). Hyperplasia and apoptosis are genetically regulated to limit the size of an organ or the body. The speed and success of growth depend on the relative rates of these three cellular events.

Prenatal growth

During the first trimester, the fetus establishes tissue patterns and organ systems. From weeks 1 to 3, the ectoderm, mesoderm and endoderm are formed within the embryonic disk. From weeks 4 to 8, there is rapid growth and differentiation to form all the major organ systems in the body. In the second trimester, the fetus undergoes major cellular hyperplasia and, in the third, organ systems mature in preparation for extra-uterine life.

From weeks 4 to 12, crown-rump growth velocity is 33 cm/year, from 12 to 24 weeks 62 cm/year and from 24 weeks to term 48 cm/year. Weight gain over the same intervals shows a different pattern with modest gains initially (0.1 kg/year from weeks 4 to 12) followed by 2.7 kg/year in weeks 12 to 24, escalating in the last 16 weeks to 8.7 kg/year. Length velocity is maximal in the second trimester but maximal weight gain is achieved in the third trimester, although there is a declining weight velocity in the last weeks of pregnancy.

The orchestration of these processes is dependent in part on a class of developmental genes belonging to the homeobox family. The homeobox (a 180-base pair DNA sequence, encoding a 60-amino-acid homeodomain) was originally discovered in the genome of the fruit fly *Drosophila* but is present in all multicellular organisms. Homeobox-containing genes encode for proteins that include a homeodomain and bind DNA,

Handbook of Clinical Pediatric Endocrinology, 1st edition. By Charles G. D. Brook and Rosalind S. Brown. Published 2008 by Blackwell Publishing, ISBN: 978-1-4501-6109-1.

Table 3.1 Examples of homeobox gene mutations causing human growth/developmental disorders.

PAX 6	Aniridia; Peter's anomaly (defect of anterior chamber of the eye); anophthalmia
MSX-1	Craniosynostosis
SHOX	Short stature in Turner syndrome; rare cause of idiopathic short stature; Leri–Weill dyschondrosteosis
HESX-1	Familial septo-optic dysplasia
PIT-1	Combined GH, TSH and prolactin deficiencies
PROP-1	Congenital hypopituitarism

thereby controlling gene expression and hence cell differentiation and organ development.

Class I *Hox* (homeobox) genes are involved in patterning embryonic structures such as the axial skeleton, the limbs, digestive and genital tracts and in craniofacial and nervous system development. Abnormalities in human homeobox genes usually give rise to specific organ malformation but there are also genes that have a wider impact on whole body growth (Table 3.1).

Fetal growth is constrained by maternal factors and placental function but is co-ordinated by growth factors acting locally in a paracrine manner (e.g. insulin-like growth factor (IGF)-I and IGF-II, fibroblast growth factor (FGF), epidermal growth factor, transforming growth factors α and β) or as endocrine hormones (e.g. insulin). Curiously, hormones important in postnatal growth (e.g. growth hormone (GH) and thyroxine) do not play a role in prenatal growth.

Nutrition plays a rate-limiting role. Placental transport of nutrients and metabolites can occur by simple diffusion, where transfer is limited by blood flow through the placenta and placental surface area (e.g. oxygen, carbon dioxide, urea), by carrier-mediated facilitated diffusion down a concentration gradient not requiring energy (e.g. glucose and lactate) and by active transport using carrier proteins and energy (e.g. amino acids).

Understanding factors that can control fetal growth has assumed increasing importance since epidemiological studies have established links between intrauterine and early extrauterine growth retardation (IUGR/EUGR) and the risk of developing a host of health problems in later life, which include hypertension, cardio- and cerebrovascular disease, insulin resistance and non-insulin-dependent diabetes mellitus. The link between early growth and later disease is postulated to occur through programming, where an insult

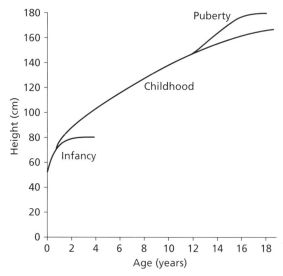

Figure 3.1 The ICP model of growth for boys. Data shown are the mean height values (cm) for age.

(e.g. maternal undernutrition) at a critical period in fetal development leads to a permanent deleterious metabolic alteration rendering the individual prone to specific disease later in life. Hormones and growth factors are potential targets for programming. Evidence is accumulating that insulin and the GH–IGF axis are modified in those born with IUGR and leptin may also be important but how these changes translate into disease is not known.

Postnatal growth

The growth trajectory of each stage of growth (fetal, infant (I), childhood (C) and pubertal (P)) can be represented mathematically by the 'ICP growth model' (Fig. 3.1). Growth during the first 3 years

Table 3.2 Requirements for normal human growth.

Absence of chronic disease
Emotional stability, secure family environment
Adequate nutrition
Normal hormone actions
Absence of defects impairing cellular/bone growth

results from a combination of a rapidly decelerating infancy component and a slowly decelerating childhood component. The latter dominates the mid-childhood years but is altered by the pubertal contribution, which is modeled on a sigmoid curve.

Throughout the growing years, a stable environment is required for normal growth (Table 3.2).

The infant

During the first year, infants grow rapidly but at a sharply decelerating rate (Fig. 3.2b). A similar pattern is observed for weight gain. Although hormones and receptors within the GH–IGF axis play their part, nutritional input is the principal regulator of growth in infancy and alterations in dietary intake have the greatest impact on growth during this period. Early onset of obesity in an otherwise normal infant leads to tall stature in childhood whereas obesity developing later in childhood has much less effect.

The correlation between length and weight at birth and mean parental size is poor, reflecting the dominant influence of the intrauterine environment over the genotype. Once this effect is removed, a period of 'catch-up' or 'catch-down' growth commonly occurs during the first 2 years, while the infant establishes its own growth channel. Catch-up growth starts soon after birth and is completed over 6–18 months, while catch-down growth commences between 3 and 6 months and is completed by 9–20 months. By 2 years of age, this process has increased the correlation between length and mid-parental height to an r-value of 0.7–0.8. Likewise, the correlation between an individual's birth length and their adult height has an r-value of only 0.3 but the correlation between height and final height has increased to an r-value of 0.8 by 3 years of age.

Although growth charts give the impression that growth is linear, most studies of short-term growth (day to day, week to week) find it to be saltatory, occurring in short bursts separated by periods of growth stasis.

The child

By 4 years of age, average growth velocity has declined to 7 cm/year and the prepubertal nadir in average velocity is 5–5.5 cm/year (Fig. 3.2b). On an individual basis, there is a well-recognized mid-childhood growth spurt. Additionally, if an individual is measured throughout childhood, oscillations in growth velocity of variable amplitude are observed with a periodicity of approximately 2 years. Seasonal variation in growth rate is also well described.

During childhood, GH and thyroid hormones are the major determinants of growth. It is therefore the time when dysfunction in the GH axis may be recognized. In the ICP model, the childhood component becomes predominant over the waning infancy component by 3 years of age. There is little difference in height between boys and girls before the onset of puberty (Fig. 3.2a).

Clinical recognition of normal growth in childhood

Height or length measurements should be undertaken in a standard manner by trained personnel using calibrated well-maintained equipment. Height should be plotted on a growth chart, on which biological parental heights have also been charted. These should be actual rather than reported. The point at which parental height is plotted is sex dependent. If the index case is male, father's height and (mother's height + 12.5 cm) will be plotted. The reverse holds for a girl. The mid-parental height is defined as the midpoint between these (corrected) heights and the target range is 10 cm (for boys) or 8.5 cm (for girls) either side of this point. If the child's height falls outside the target range, a growth disorder may be present.

Another way to express height (and any other auxological data) controlling for age and sex is to

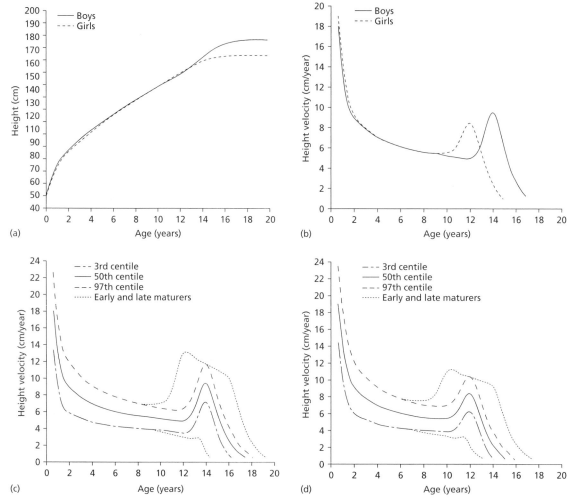

Figure 3.2 (a) Height and (b) mean height velocity for boys and girls according to age. Timing of the pubertal growth spurt for early and late maturers in (c) boys and (d) girls.

derive a standard deviation score (SDS). This requires knowledge of the mean and SD of height at all ages in each sex and is calculated as:

$$SDS = \frac{(\text{observed height} - \text{mean height for age and sex})}{\text{SD for that age and sex.}}$$

Ninety-five percent of normal values would be expected to fall between ± 2 SDS.

Weight is an important parameter for the assessment of infant well-being. In childhood, weight measurements are usually taken coincidentally with height. Their relation to height should be assessed by

calculating body mass index (defined as weight (kg) divided by height (m²)) which can be plotted on a centile chart (Fig. 3.3).

Growth velocity

A single height measurement plotted in relation to parental heights gives useful information but does not reflect the dynamic nature of growth. For this, serial height measurements should be taken. Height velocity (cm/year) is then calculated as (the amount grown (cm) divided by the (decimal) time interval between

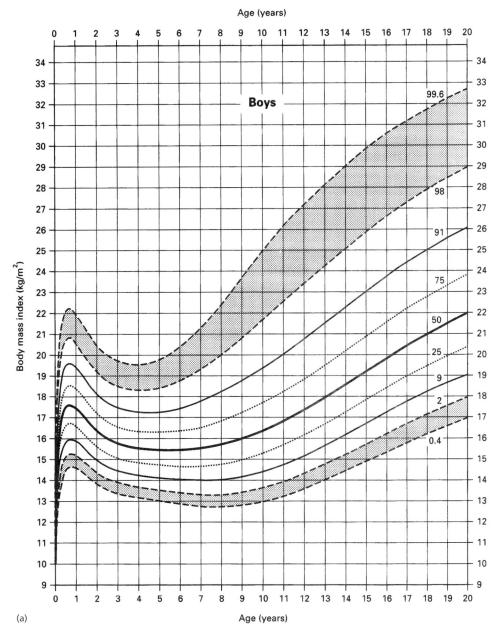

Figure 3.3 Centile charts for body mass index for (a) boys.

measurements). In order to maintain a position close to a given height centile, velocity should not fall below the 25th or above the 75th centile in successive years. Even in experienced hands, the technical error of measurement of height is of the order of 0.15 cm. If velocity is based on measurements taken at short intervals, such as 3 months, measurement error will be magnified four times when extrapolating to an annual growth rate. If this is combined with the non-linearity of growth, an accurate perspective of growth is difficult to obtain. Even if growth is monitored over 12 months, the cycles of growth through the

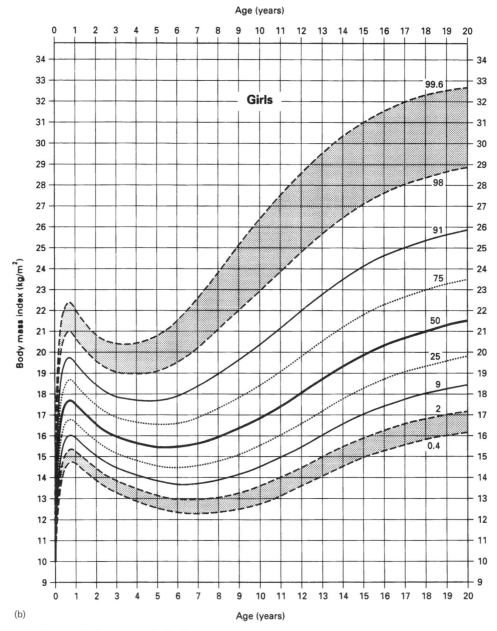

Figure 3.3 Centile charts for body mass index for (b) girls.

prepubertal years could lead to a false impression about growth performance and measurement over longer periods may be required.

The probability that growth velocity over successive years will be inadequate becomes increasingly small. The theoretical chance of annual growth velocities in a child growing normally being below the 25th centile over 2 years (assuming that the velocity in each year is independent) would be 0.25 × 0.25 = 6.25% and below the 10th centile would be 1%.

The degree of physical development and the timing of the pubertal growth spurt complicate assessment of growth velocity around puberty. It is this variation that gives rise to the wide variation in peak height velocity on growth charts (Fig. 3.2 c and d).

Bone age

Bone maturation can be observed directly by visualization of epiphyseal growth plates on X-ray. There is an orderly development of the epiphyseal centers in growing bones of normal children. It has therefore been possible to generate standards for bone maturation in each sex throughout childhood and adolescence, and bone age has evolved as a measure that quantifies physical maturation.

The epiphyseal centers in the non-dominant hand and wrist X-ray can be compared with those found in age-matched representative X-rays from normal boys and girls, as shown in the atlas of Greulich and Pyle (G&P). Alternatively, the maturity of each epiphyseal center can be scored individually by the Tanner–Whitehouse standards (TW-II) to generate an overall bone age. These techniques are in part observer dependent.

Diagnostic information is not obtained from bone age estimation but marked bone age retardation (>3 years) can be associated with hypothyroidism, GH deficiency and hypopituitarism. A diagnosis of constitutional delay in growth and puberty (CDGP) would be supported by bone age delay >2 years in the absence of an endocrine deficit.

Bone age estimates can be used as a means of predicting adult height. For instance, adult height can be predicted using the tables of Bayley and Pinneau and a G&P bone age or using an equation incorporating current age, height and TW-II bone age, each multiplied by a constant defined by age and sex.

Puberty (see Chapter 4)

There is marked variation in the timing of events in puberty. It is therefore important to compare an individual's development with population standards in order to define normality. Once puberty is initiated, the sequence of development should be ordered and completed within the appropriate timeframe. Failure to progress as well as failure to enter puberty could indicate abnormality. The pubertal growth spurt in girls starts early in puberty and later in puberty in boys but the magnitude of the spurt is inversely related to the age at peak height velocity in both sexes.

Thus final height is determined by the height attained at the start of puberty and the amount gained during puberty. Since early puberty entrains a bigger spurt than late puberty, what is gained by growing longer in childhood may be lost by a smaller pubertal growth spurt, all of which reduce the variation in final adult height achieved.

The endocrine control of growth

The principal hormones influencing growth are GH and the IGFs but there are many other hormones that contribute, including thyroid hormones, adrenal androgens, sex steroids, glucocorticoids, vitamin D, leptin and insulin. Often, this contribution is channeled through interaction with the GH–IGF axis.

Hypothalamic control of GH secretion

GH is secreted from the anterior pituitary in discrete pulses every 3–4 h, with very low concentrations of GH present between pulses. This pattern is determined by the interaction between GH-releasing hormone (GHRH), ghrelin and somatostatin (SS). The amplitude of the GH peak is determined by GHRH, which stimulates the pituitary somatotrophs to increase both the secretion of stored GH and GH gene transcription. Ghrelin, a 28-amino-acid peptide, acts in synergy with GHRH to promote GH release. Ghrelin has a potent appetite-stimulating action, indicating a link between nutrition and growth control. SS tone determines the trough concentrations of GH by inhibiting GHRH release from the hypothalamus and GH secretion from the pituitary. Withdrawal of SS is the most important factor in determining the time of a pulse since GH pulsatility is maintained under continuous infusion of GHRH.

Pituitary control of GH secretion

The human GH gene forms part of a cluster of five similar genes found on the long arm of chromosome 17. The main form of GH in the circulation comes from the GH-N (or normal) gene expressed primarily in the pituitary. The full-length transcript from the GH-N gene encodes a 191-amino-acid, 22 kDa protein, which constitutes 80–90% of pituitary GH. Alternative splicing of the mRNA transcripts generates a 20 kDa species that lack amino acids 32–46 and accounts for the remaining 10–20%. Deletion of the GH-N gene in humans leads to severe postnatal growth failure and, in these individuals, treatment with GH generates a short-lived growth response because of the development of anti-GH antibodies.

The homeobox transcription factor Pit-1 binds at sites within the promoter region of the GH-N gene and determines pituitary-specific expression of GH. Pit-1 is also essential for normal pituitary development.

Other factors influencing GH secretion include neuropeptides (e.g. galanin, opioids), metabolites (e.g. glucose, free fatty acids), hormones (e.g. estrogen, testosterone), physical exercise and sleep. GH itself and its downstream effector, IGF-I, are both capable of regulating secretion via negative feedback mediated by SS.

A negative relationship exists between body mass index, a marker of body fatness, and GH secretion in normal prepubertal children as well as in obese children. The fact that GH secretion increases after weight loss or fasting suggests that diminished GH is a result of obesity rather than a cause.

GH in the circulation

GH can be detected in the fetal pituitary from around 8 weeks of gestation and in the serum from 10 weeks. Serum concentrations rise to high concentrations by 24 weeks, decline toward birth and fall further after the first 2 weeks of postnatal life. The high concentrations of GH through gestation are a reflection of the time taken for the neuroendocrine control of GH secretion to develop. In early gestation, GH release from the pituitary is uncontrolled. The decrease in GH after 24 weeks is associated with the development of the inhibitory mechanisms governing GH release.

Few data exist on the changes in GH secretion with age in prepubertal children but cross-sectional data suggest that GH pulse amplitude increases with age. The most profound changes in GH secretion occur through the pubertal years with a marked increase in the amplitude of GH pulses. Androgens and estrogens both increase GH secretion during puberty, although the androgen effect is mediated through the estrogen receptor by aromatization of testosterone to estrogen. Maximal concentrations of GH secretion coincide with the timing of peak height velocity in both sexes and secretion declines thereafter into adulthood.

In prepubertal and pubertal children, episodic GH release generates large peaks of GH lasting 1–2 h separated by periods of low basal secretion. The pattern

of GH secretion is important in generating the diversity of actions mediated by GH. Sexual dimorphism in GH secretion is evident in humans: daily GH output is greater in women compared with men, a difference that disappears when corrected for estrogen concentrations. There are also differences in the profile of 24-h GH secretion between the sexes: in men, there are small pulses in daylight hours with large nocturnal pulses but there is less diurnal variation with more frequent pulses in women. There are associations between the peak and trough attributes of 24-h GH secretion and different endpoints of GH action: trough concentrations of GH are correlated with body composition and metabolic parameters, while peak concentrations correlate with IGF-I production.

Cellular actions of GH

GH exerts its effects on target tissues by binding to a specific GH receptor (GHR), which is expressed in a variety of tissues, particularly the liver. Signal transduction results in the activation of genes involved in mediating the effects of GH. An important target is the IGF-I gene, the product of which mediates many, if not all, its growth-promoting actions *in vivo*.

IGFs and their binding proteins

IGF-I and -II are single-chain polypeptide hormones with structural homology to proinsulin that are expressed in multiple organs and tissues under both endocrine and tissue-specific autocrine and/or paracrine regulation. Both are important in fetal growth and development but only IGF-I appears to be critical for postnatal growth. This may be due to the fact that IGF-II does not appear to be regulated by GH, which is the primary determinant of circulating IGF-I concentrations in postnatal life.

IGFs in the circulation bind to the IGF-binding proteins (IGFBPs), which bind both IGFs with high affinity. The IGFs are present in the circulation at concentrations approximately 1000 times that of insulin and one major role of the IGFBPs is to prevent the insulin-like activity of IGFs. Nearly all IGFs in the circulation are associated with a BP.

The IGFBPs extend the half-life of the IGFs and provide a transport mechanism regulating movement of IGFs across capillary walls. They also play a role in controlling IGF distribution to specific cells or receptors, thereby modulating the paracrine effects of IGFs.

IGFBP-3, the major IGFBP in the circulation, accounts for most of the IGF-I-binding capacity and, like IGF-I, is strongly GH dependent. The main site of production is the liver under GH control, although it is also expressed in most peripheral tissues. When bound to IGF-I, IGFBP-3 associates with another GH-dependent protein, the acid-labile subunit (ALS), to form a ternary complex. In general, the molar concentration of IGFBP-3 in the circulation is equal to the sum of both IGF-I and -II, reflecting the role of IGFBP-3 as the major carrier of IGF. ALS is present in a molar excess, indicating that virtually all IGFBP-3 and IGF exist in the form of the ternary complex.

Two receptors for the IGFs have been identified, the type I or IGF-I receptor, which is homologous to the insulin receptor, and the type II or IGF-II receptor, also known as the mannose-6-phosphate receptor. The mitogenic actions of IGF-I and -II are mediated almost entirely through the IGF-I receptor using a signal transduction cascade similar to that used by insulin. Little is known about the interactions and consequences of IGF-II binding to its receptor but it does not appear to mediate its biological effects through this receptor, acting instead through the IGF-I receptor.

Physiological actions of GH and IGF-I on bone growth

The major role of GH is to promote longitudinal bone growth. Two hypotheses have been generated to explain the mode of action of GH in generating a growth response. The somatomedin hypothesis proposes that GH mediates its effects on its target tissues via stimulation of hepatic IGF-I production, which in turn acts as a classical endocrine hormone. The alternative hypothesis, the dual effector theory, is based on the premise that growth is a result of the differentiation of precursor cells, followed by clonal expansion. According to this hypothesis, GH directly promotes the differentiation of cells and the development of IGF-I responsiveness. Clonal expansion of these differentiated cells is then mediated by local production of IGF-I in response to GH.

Disorders of growth

Short stature and growth failure

Short stature is relative and needs to be defined according to the growth performance of a given population and reference charts relevant to it. Arbitrary cutoffs may be useful when a single measurement is available but do not take into consideration the genetic background of the child nor its growth rate. In addition, children of tall parents may be short but not necessarily have height below the defined cutoff. Short stature may be normal for some children but a feature of disease in others. The probability of organic disease is greater the further below the second or third centile that a child's height is.

Growth failure implies a poor height velocity for age and stage of puberty, irrespective of whether a child is short, normal or tall, and is a sensitive indicator of pathology. After a transient period of growth inhibition, the phenomenon of accelerated linear growth (owing to supranormal height velocity), which allows a child to return to his/her original preretardation growth curve, is called catch-up growth.

Evaluation is recommended for a child with
- height < -2.5 SD (below the 0.4th centile);
- a significant discrepancy between their centile and mid-parental target centile;
- height curve crossing two centile lines, even if the measurements are not below the 0.4th centile or
- in whom there are parental or professional concerns. Children with height between the 0.4th and second centiles or height curve crossing one centile line should have their height velocity monitored.

Epidemiology

The major causes of short stature in children are shown in Table 3.3. In a large population of school-aged children, 1.2% were found have height less than -2 SDS. When these 'short' children were remeasured a year later, less than 50% had height less than third centile and growth rate <5 cm/year. Non-endocrine causes accounted for the growth failure in the majority (familial short stature in 37%, constitutional delay in growth in 27%, familial short stature/constitutional delay in growth in 17%, systemic disease in 9%). Only 5% had an endocrine problem (GH deficiency in 3%, hypothyroidism in <1% and Turner syndrome (TS) in 3% of the girls).

Psychosocial impact

Short stature does not pose significant psychosocial problems for most children or adults but it can have a negative influence on the affected child and parents,

Table 3.3 The major causes of short stature.

No disproportion between trunk and limbs: looks normal			Dysmorphic features and/or disproportionate short stature: looks abnormal	
Normal height velocity	Low height velocity		Dysmorphic features, recognizable syndrome	Disproportion between limbs and trunk
	Underweight	Weight appropriate for height or relatively overweight		
Appropriate for parents Familial short stature *Short for parents* Constitutional delay	*Psychosocial* Child abuse/ neglect anorexia nervosa *Systemic disease* Respiratory (e.g. cystic fibrosis, asthma) Cardiovascular (e.g. congenital heart disease) Gastrointestinal (e.g. celiac disease, Crohn's disease) Nutritional (e.g. rickets, protein calorie malnutrition) Renal (e.g. chronic renal failure, renal tubular acidosis) Infections (e.g. HIV, tuberculosis) Musculoskeletal (e.g. juvenile arthritis) Neurological (e.g. tumor)	*Endocrine disorder* Hypothyroidism Growth hormone deficiency Hypopituitarism Pseudohypopara- thyroidism Cushing syndrome	*Low birthweight* Russell–Silver syndrome Three M slender-boned dwarfism Seckel syndrome *Chromosome* *abnormality* Turner syndrome Prader–Willi syndrome *Autosomal dominant* Noonan syndrome *Autosomal recessive* Bloom syndrome Fanconi pancytopenia Mulibrey Nanism *X-linked dominant* Aarskog syndrome *Rare syndromes* Floating Harbor Kabuki makeup	*Short limbs* Achondroplasia Hypochondroplasia Dyschondrosteosis Metaphyseal chondrodysplasia Multiple epiphyseal dysplasia *Short limbs and trunk* Metatropic dysplasia *Short trunk* Mucopolysaccharidosis Spondyloepiphyseal dysplasia

especially for those presenting to a specialist. Some short children and adolescents feel insecure, have low self-esteem, are introverted, withdrawn, depressed, socially isolated, anxious, aggressive and immature. They may be bullied and have difficulty adjusting at school. These problems need to be recognized so that the child and family can receive appropriate psychological support.

Clinical assessment

The aims of assessment of a short child are to determine whether the child has pathology and to determine the psychosocial impact of appearance on the child. Clinical assessment (Table 3.4), a plot of serial height measurements and determination of height velocity are needed to separate those

Table 3.4 Important aspects of the history and examination in a child with short stature.

History

Reason for referral

  History of growth problem

    Time of first concerns about stature, change in stature over time

    Birth size in relation to gestation: weight, length, head circumference

    Pubertal development: age of onset and progression of secondary sexual characteristics

  Pregnancy and perinatal events

    Clues to growth retardation *in utero* from infections, drugs, smoking, alcohol

    Gestation, vertex or breech presentation, mode of delivery, condition at birth

    Postnatal problems such as hypoglycemia (congenital hypopituitarism), jaundice (congenital hypothyroidism or hypopituitarism), floppiness and feeding difficulty (Prader–Willi syndrome), puffy hands and feet (Turner syndrome)

  Medical history

    Problems associated with specific syndromes such as Turner syndrome

    Symptoms of an endocrine disorder such as hypothyroidism

    Symptoms of tumor around the pituitary gland

    Systemic illness

    Treatments that can impair growth (e.g. corticosteroids, radiotherapy, methylphenidate)

    Developmental problems in specific areas such as speech, hearing, learning, vision

Psychosocial history to determine the impact of short stature on the child

    Self-image and parents' perceptions

    Teasing/bullying at school

    School adjustment

    Personality, emotional and behavioral problems

Family history

    Heights of parents and siblings

    Age of onset of puberty in parents

    Consanguinity, affected family member, known inherited conditions

Examination

Measurements: weight, standing height, sitting height, head circumference

Height in relation to previous heights (height velocity), parents' heights, stage of puberty, weight

Genitalia and pubertal development

Body composition: subcutaneous fat and muscle bulk

Unusual or dysmorphic features in face, eyes, nose, ears, mouth, hairline, neck, upper limbs, hands, palms, fingers, nails, feet or skin

Signs of specific syndromes such as Turner or Noonan syndrome

Signs of specific endocrine disorders such as hypothyroidism, growth hormone deficiency or corticosteroid excess

Signs of a congenital (e.g. septo-optic dysplasia) or acquired (e.g. craniopharyngioma) lesion affecting the hypothalamus, pituitary (and growth hormone secretion) and the optic chiasm: visual fields, fundi, pupils, squint, nystagmus, acuity

Signs of chronic systemic disease

---

who are small but growing normally from those who have an abnormal pattern of growth. Determination of bone age and mid-parental height can be used to estimate height expectation. Physical examination may reveal abnormal body proportions, dysmorphic features and the underlying problem. The clinical impression usually dictates the investigation pathway and, while pathology must not be missed, overly zealous investigation should be avoided.

Endocrine causes of short stature

GH deficiency

GH deficiency may be congenital (e.g. associated with midline congenital abnormalities such as optic nerve

Table 3.5 Causes of GH deficiency (GHD).

GHD can be on a hypothalamic or a pituitary basis

I   GHD resulting from congenital malformations of the hypothalamus/pituitary
    A Septo-optic dysplasia and optic nerve hypoplasia
    B Other midline abnormalities (e.g. holoprosencephaly)
II   GHD resulting from irradiation of the hypothalamus/pituitary
III Trauma to the hypothalamus/pituitary
IV Mutations or gene deletions of transcription factors necessary to pituitary development:
    A HESX1
    B PROP1
    C POUF1 (Pit1)
V   Mutations within the GH gene
VI Mutation of the GHRH receptor
VII GHD of undefined etiology (idiopathic) (including those with abnormal pituitary morphology on MRI – pituitary hypoplasia, interrupted or hypoplastic stalk, ectopically placed posterior pituitary lobe)
VIII Bioinactive GH

hypoplasia/septo-optic dysplasia) or acquired (e.g. secondary to cranial irradiation or, rarely, a tumor in the area of the hypothalamus or pituitary) (Table 3.5). GH deficiency may be isolated or associated with multiple pituitary hormone deficiencies.

Congenital GH deficiency may arise through deletion of the GH gene, in which case no GH molecule can be produced, or by mutations within the gene that result in a dysfunctional GH molecule. The difference between complete absence of the GH gene and relative deficiency is important, since children with the former have no immunological tolerance to the GH molecule and thus develop antibodies when exposed to therapy.

GH deficiency presenting in early childhood without a family history is usually associated with pituitary hypoplasia secondary to a deficiency in the secretion of GHRH from the hypothalamus. Magnetic resonance imaging (MRI) may reveal an absent or attenuated pituitary stalk and/or ectopically positioned pituitary bright spot. These features indicate that other anterior pituitary hormone deficits may evolve but MRI scans can be normal. The etiology of isolated GH deficiency is unclear. There may be a history of birth trauma or prematurity and abnormalities in pituitary development genes may contribute.

If GH deficiency is an isolated pituitary hormone problem, birthweight is characteristically normal and the early postnatal course uneventful. Diminished growth velocity becomes obvious toward the end of the first year as the hormone-dependent childhood phase of growth fails to take over from the nutrition-dependent infant phase.

GH deficiency may not become evident until later in childhood when the pituitary becomes unable to maintain the increase in GH secretion required by increased body size to maintain the peak concentrations of secreted hormone. Lack of sufficient GH causes truncal obesity, poorly developed musculature immature facies and crowding of the facial features from maxillary hypoplasia. Head circumference is normal. Boys may have small genitalia but a very small penis is suggestive of gonadotropin deficiency. Body proportions are normal before puberty. Puberty, if it occurs spontaneously, is usually slightly, but not significantly, delayed. Problems in the newborn period, such as hypoglycemia or conjugated hyperbilirubinemia (secondary to adrenocorticotrophic hormone (ACTH) deficiency), are likely when there are multiple pituitary hormone deficiencies.

Investigations comprise testing the whole hypothalamic–pituitary axis and should be undertaken only in a center properly staffed and equipped for endocrine investigation. Tests include provocation with a variety of stimuli (insulin hypoglycemia, arginine, glucagon, L-dopa, clonidine, pyridostigmine). Peak GH responses are more reproducible when agents that stimulate GHRH secretion and control endogenous SS tone (e.g. arginine, pyridostigmine) are used. Results need to be interpreted in the context of the circumstances, particularly in patients with delayed puberty or obesity. In delayed puberty, GH response can be amplified by the administration of 100 mg of testosterone given intramuscularly 3 days before the test (to a boy) or of 20 μg of ethinylestradiol for 3 days (to a girl).

Many assays for GH are available but values vary widely between assays done on identical samples. Each endocrine unit should therefore be acquainted with the performance of its GH assay. IGF-I should be measured because a low concentration with a low peak GH concentration during a provocation test confirms a diagnosis of GH deficiency, whereas low IGF with normal GH suggests GH insensitivity.

Because of the fallibility of GH tests (suggesting GH deficiency when it is not present), the diagnosis of moderate/partial GH deficiency is difficult. It should be based on clinical and auxological assessment, combined with biochemical tests of the GH–IGF axis and MRI evaluation of the hypothalamic–pituitary axis.

GH deficiency in childhood and adolescence requires pituitary function to be retested at the completion of growth to determine the need for continued GH replacement throughout life or whether another pituitary hormone deficit has evolved. Most patients with isolated GH deficiency in childhood are able to generate normal concentrations of GH when retested after growth ceases and do not require GH replacement in adult life.

GH deficiency is treated with daily injections of recombinant GH (dose 25–50 μg/kg/day or 0.7–1.4 μg/m^2/day). The response to treatment is predictable from the pretreatment growth rate and the dose of GH administered.

GH-insensitive states

The phenotype of GH insensitivity is very similar to GH deficiency but the biochemical hallmark is raised basal and stimulated GH concentrations with low IGF-I and IGFBP-3 concentrations. GH insensitivity may be congenital or acquired. The latter occurs with fasting, poor nutrition and catabolic states. Congenital GH insensitivity (Laron syndrome) is very rare. In the majority, it is a recessive condition caused by mutations of the GHR gene, which results in a truncated nonsense protein. This can be inherited as a dominant trait, thus demonstrating, in a way similar to autosomal-dominant GH deficiency, that genetic short stature may have an endocrine origin.

Other endocrine causes

Congenital hypothyroidism (Chapter 5) is usually detected on a screening program but some inborn errors may present later, as may acquired hypothyroidism, which is usually caused by Hashimoto thyroiditis or iodine deficiency.

Typical features of pseudohypoparathyroidism (Albright's hereditary osteodystrophy) (Chapter 7) include short stocky build, advanced bone age, round face, short thick neck, obesity, short metacarpals (especially the fourth and fifth), short distal phalanx of the thumb and decreased intelligence in 50–70% of cases. Calcification in the subcutaneous tissues, kidneys and brain is common.

Cushing syndrome (Chapter 6) due to excess cortisol secretion (e.g. an adrenal adenoma in early childhood and an ACTH-secreting pituitary adenoma in later childhood) is most frequently associated with corticosteroid treatment. Growth suppression is less with alternate-day oral regimens compared with daily treatment. Corticosteroids suppress GH secretion and have direct inhibitory effects on the growth plate.

Non-endocrine causes of short stature

Idiopathic or 'normal variant' short stature (ISS/NVSS) refers to children with familial/genetic short stature (mid-parental height <10th centile) or CDGP (a disorder of the tempo of growth), who are otherwise healthy. These are diagnoses of exclusion.

Defects in the SHOX (short stature homeobox-containing) gene have been described in some individuals with ISS, as well as Lange mesomelic dwarfism and Leri–Weill dyschondrosteosis.

GH has been used to treat children with ISS to final height. The mean gain in height (the difference between predicted and achieved adult height among treated children compared with those not treated) was 9.2 cm for boys and 5.7 cm for girls.

In short families, autosomal-dominant disorders, such as skeletal dysplasias, need to be excluded because the child is not short compared with parents, has a normal growth rate, normal bone age and a projected adult height within the parental target.

CDGP (Chapter 4) is one of the most common causes. Boys are more likely to present than girls because of greater concerns about short stature and immature physique and because the growth spurt in boys comes later in the sequence of pubertal development than it does in girls. The short stature is temporary and associated with delayed skeletal (bone age delayed >2 years with height appropriate for bone age) and pubertal development. A normal puberty growth spurt can be predicted and eventual height will fall within the target predicted from parents' heights. Nutrition may play a role. The most important aspects of management are explanation and reassurance that the delay in growth and puberty is simply part of the normal variation in maturation.

Treatment with low doses of sex steroids for a brief period of 3–6 months can be offered to activate the pubertal timing mechanism without accelerating bone age and most physicians would consider this if there is no sign of puberty starting by 13 years in a girl or 14 years in a boy. Treatment does not enhance adult height but is safe and does not compromise final height.

IUGR can be considered a prenatal diagnosis; small for gestational age (SGA) describes birth length and/or weight in relation to gestational age and is a post-partum diagnosis. IUGR does not always result in infants being SGA and SGA is not necessarily a consequence of IUGR.

SGA is most widely defined by birth length and/or weight below −2 SDS (or below the third centile) for the reference population mean for gestational age. Low birth length is a stronger predictor of subsequent short stature than weight. Most full-term SGA infants (birth length less than −2 SDS) catch up in the first year and only a minority (<10%) remain short as adults. They are mostly those who failed to catch up by 2 years.

Multiple factors influence growth in SGA children but a relative resistance to GH and IGF-I is also likely. Thus, high doses of GH (dose 35–67 µg/kg/day) may help some children to normalize height during the growing phase, maintain normal growth and attain adult height within the normal range and within parental target. The long-term safety of high doses of GH during childhood and adolescence on glucose metabolism and the consequences of relatively high IGF-I concentrations during this period remain uncertain.

Systemic causes of short stature
A systemic disease should be suspected in short thin children. History and examination generally provide useful clues to the diagnosis. Exceptionally, children who grow slowly for no obvious reason may have an occult condition (e.g. celiac disease, inflammatory bowel disease, renal tubular acidosis). Skeletal maturation is often delayed and there is potential for catch-up growth if the underlying condition can be treated successfully. It is likely that the major factors that impair growth in children with systemic disease, such as chronic inflammation, undernutrition and corticosteroid treatment, do so by attenuating the functional integrity of the GH–IGF-I axis through complex interactions. An interleukin-6-mediated decrease in IGF-I may be an important mechanism by which growth is impaired in chronic inflammatory conditions such as juvenile chronic arthritis independent of nutrition.

Psychosocial and emotional deprivation
Psychosocial and emotional deprivation are uncommon causes of growth failure in infancy and early childhood. Children display behavioral abnormalities (apathy, watchfulness and autoerotic activity) and delayed developmental behavior. The history often reveals rejection or neglect, non-accidental injury or lack of physical handling. The children have poor growth at home but catch-up in hospital or when fostered. They may have high concentrations of fasting GH and also cortisol non-responsiveness with the insulin tolerance test. GH deficiency that is reversible when the caring environment is improved has also been described.

Syndromes with short stature

Children with dysmorphic features may have a recognizable syndrome associated with a chromosomal abnormality, low birthweight and other rare conditions. Inheritance may be autosomal dominant, autosomal recessive or X-linked dominant.

Chromosomal problems
These may include abnormalities of number, structure and imprinting. The common numerical chromosomal abnormalities causing short stature are summarized in Table 3.6.

Turner syndrome
Turner syndrome combines characteristic physical features with complete or partial absence of one of the

Table 3.6 Common numerical chromosome abnormalities associated with short stature.

Chromosomal abnormality	Frequency	Features
Trisomy 21	1:600–1:700	Typical facies (see text), congenital heart disease (50%), macroglossia and tongue protrusion, small hands and feet
Trisomy 18	1:3000–1:7000	Peculiar face, clenched hand, congenital heart disease (80%)
Trisomy 13	1:4000–1:10000	Polydactyly, cleft palate, hypertelorism, scalp defects Dysplastic calvarium, syndactyly 3–4, cystic placenta
Triploidy	Uncertain	
Turner syndrome (45,X syndrome)	1:2500	Webbed neck, short fourth metacarpal, congenital heart disease, broad chest, wide-set nipples

X chromosomes, frequently accompanied by cell mosaicism. It is the most common sex chromosome abnormality, affecting an estimated 2% of all conceptuses. Over 99% of fetuses with the 45,X karyotype are spontaneously aborted, especially in the first trimester, giving a prevalence rate of 1 in 2–2500 live female births. It is thought that only fetuses with the least severe manifestations of the chromosomal abnormality, and probably all of them have chromosomal mosaicism, survive.

In 50% of cases, one entire X chromosome (45,X karyotype) is missing in blood lymphocytes, although probably this does not apply to the whole body. Other patients have a range of karyotypic abnormalities, including partial absence of the second X chromosome and mosaicism. The presence of Y chromosomal material may be associated with the development of gonadoblastoma. The risk for this has been quoted at 30% but is more probably in the range of 7–10%. Gonadectomy is recommended to prevent malignancy.

The short stature of TS may be explained partly by haploinsufficiency of the SHOX gene on the pseudo-autosomal region of the X and Y chromosomes at Xp22.33, which escapes X inactivation. This gene has also been implicated in ISS and the short stature and skeletal abnormalities of the Leri–Weill dyschondrosteosis.

The most common features of TS are short stature and ovarian failure (Fig. 3.4) and the more common phenotypic features are summarized in Table 3.7. These may not be obvious, and any girl with unexplained short stature or ovarian dysfunction should have a karyotype to exclude TS.

Lymphedema in a neonate is a key diagnostic pointer to TS, but it may be a lifelong problem exacerbated by GH or estrogen treatment. Conservative treatments such as diuretics and support stockings may be required. Plastic surgery for neck webbing associated with intrauterine cystic hygroma may be considered, but girls with TS are particularly prone to the formation of keloid scars.

A range of skeletal abnormalities may be found in TS, and there may be overlap in the skeletal phenotypes of the two SHOX haploinsufficiency syndromes, Leri–Weill syndrome (LWS) and TS. Features in common include Madelung deformity (present in 74% of LWS and 7% of TS), high arched palate, skeletal disproportion, increased carrying angle, short fourth metacarpals and scoliosis. In addition, infants with TS have an increased risk of congenital dislocation of the hip.

Low-set ears and mild malformations of the outer ear occur in 30–50% of TS girls. Conductive and sensorineural hearing loss is common, with the sensorineural dip occurring as early as 6 years of age. Hearing loss may be progressive into adult life. The outer, middle and inner ear are affected and hearing problems and ear malformations correlate with the karyotype. Otitis media is extremely common in girls with TS and may progress to mastoiditis and/or cholesteatoma, particularly in very young children. Speech and language problems may occur. Myopia, squint and ptosis are all common and ophthalmological assessment should be performed in childhood.

Congenital cardiac disease occurs in approximately 30% of girls with TS. Left-sided cardiac abnormalities

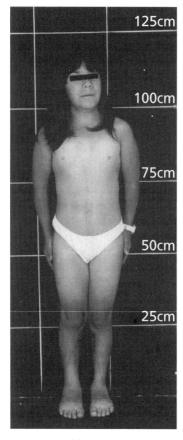

Figure 3.4 An 11-year-old female with TS. Her birthweight was 2 kg at 37 weeks and she presented to the pediatrician at the age of 10 years because of concerns about short stature and slow growth velocity. She had a past history of recurrent ear infections. Her height SDS at presentation was −3.3 and weight SDS was −1.5. Her karyotype was 45XO. Note the rather solid appearance with a broad chest. Mild webbing of the neck was present, as was an increased carrying angle of the elbows and hyperconvex nails. Lymphedema of the fourth and fifth toes was present in the first few months of life.

are most common, with bicuspid aortic valve in 30–50%, coarctation of the aorta in 30% and aortic dilation in 5%. The last is an uncommon but serious complication, particularly if leakage or rupture occurs. It is usually associated with another congenital abnormality such as bicuspid aortic valve, coarctation or hypertension. Because cardiac disease is so common in TS, all patients should have a cardiological assessment, including echocardiography, at diagnosis. Identification of a cardiac lesion requires regular follow-up and prophylaxis for bacterial endocarditis. Monitoring for

aortic root dilation should be performed, particularly if a cardiac lesion (bicuspid aortic valve, coarctation or hypertension), known to be associated with this problem, is present. At adolescence, even in the absence of previous cardiac pathology, repeat assessment of the aortic root possibly including MRI should be performed since aortic dilation may occur in the absence of other cardiac pathology. Aortic root dilation and rupture is a potentially life-threatening complication of TS, particularly during pregnancy.

Hypertension is a particularly common problem for Turner patients and annual blood pressure monitoring is mandatory.

Renal tract malformations, particularly horseshoe kidney and duplex collecting systems, are present in up to 30% of TS girls. Renal disease compounds the likelihood of hypertension; urinary tract infections should be treated promptly. All girls with TS should have renal ultrasound at diagnosis, and ultrasound and urine cultures should be performed routinely every 3–5 years.

Primary hypothyroidism due to Hashimoto thyroiditis occurs in up to 30% of girls with TS. Diabetes mellitus occurs uncommonly in TS but insulin resistance and glucose intolerance may be present and may be exacerbated by treatment with oxandrolone or GH. Obesity is a problem for girls with TS, and short stature and statural disproportion may exacerbate the tendency to obesity.

A range of other problems has been reported in TS, including specific learning difficulties in relation to non-verbal and visuospatial processing tasks. Liver abnormalities have been reported, and TS girls may have a higher risk of developing celiac disease than the general population. Girls with TS may have more dental crowding and malocclusion problems than other girls because of retrognathia.

The diagnosis should be made by obtaining a karyotype counting a sufficient number of cells to exclude the possibility of low-level mosaicism. If TS is strongly suspected on clinical grounds and the blood karyotype is normal, a karyotype should be obtained on a peripheral skin biopsy. If a patient with TS has evidence of virilization or if a marker chromosome suggestive of Y-containing material is located, cytogenetic probing for Y chromosome material should be performed by DNA hybridization or fluorescent *in situ* hybridization (FISH) using a Y-centromeric or short-arm probe.

Table 3.7 Phenotypic features of Turner syndrome (TS) in childhood and adolescence.

Feature	Frequency (%)
Short stature	88–100
Ovarian failure	87–96
Lymphatic abnormalities	
Neck webbing	23–65
Low posterior hairline	40–80
Lymphedema	21–47
Nail convexity/dysplasia	43–83
Skeletal abnormalities	
Micrognathia	60
High arch palate	35–84
Short fourth/fifth metacarpals	35–77
Increased carrying angles	27–82
Madelung deformity	7
Kyphoscoliosis	12–16
Broad chest	33–75
Abnormal upper–lower segment	90
Recurrent middle ear infections	60
Hearing problems	50
Congenital cardiac problems	30
Bicuspid aortic valve	30–50
Coarctation of aorta	30
Aortic root dilation	5 approximately
Renal abnormalities	30
Nevi	22–78
Endocrine	
Thyroiditis	10–30
Glucose intolerance	34

The short stature of TS is characterized by mild IUGR, slow growth during infancy, delayed onset of the childhood component of growth and growth failure during childhood and adolescence without a pubertal growth spurt. This growth failure leads to an adult height approximately 20 cm below the female average for the ethnic-specific population. Mean final heights of women with TS range between 136.7 cm (Japan) and 146.9 cm (Germany). The correlation with mid-parental height for patients with TS is the same as for normal offspring less the constant amount of about 20 cm.

Because of the uniform problem of short stature, many treatments have been tried over the years to improve the final height of TS girls, including estrogen, oxandrolone and GH. It is recommended that GH therapy should be considered when a patient with TS has dropped below the fifth centile of the normal female growth curve, which could be as early as 2 years of age. For girls below 9–12 years of age, therapy can be started with GH alone. In older girls (>9–12 years of age), or in girls above 8 years in whom therapy is started when the individual is already below the fifth percentile of the normal growth curve, consideration should be given to the concomitant administration of oxandrolone. Estrogen to induce puberty should be introduced not later than 13 years of age (see Chapter 4).

The diagnosis of TS at any age may be associated with psychological distress, grief and loss for the family and girl/adolescent. Psychological support should be made available and families and adolescents with

TS should be encouraged to contact their local or national TS support group. The peer and family support provided by such groups is an invaluable educational and emotional assistance for a TS girl and her family. Women with TS need lifelong medical surveillance.

Trisomy 21

Trisomy 21 (Down syndrome) occurs in 1 in 600–700 live births and is the most common single cause of mental retardation. It is associated with malformation of several organs and characterized by short stature. Growth velocity is most reduced between the ages of 6 months and 3 years. Puberty tends to be early but the pubertal growth spurt is impaired. The mean final height for an individual with Down syndrome (DS) is approximately 20 cm below target height. Men with DS are generally infertile, while women with DS are fertile. GH deficiency is not usually present in DS, although suboptimal GH secretion due to hypothalamic dysfunction has been suggested. Subjects with DS often have thyroid disease: the incidence of congenital hypothyroidism is increased, and acquired thyroid dysfunction resulting from autoimmune thyroiditis is common.

GH treatment has been used to treat the short stature of DS. Results vary with some studies showing normalization of growth velocity but the effect of GH on other parameters including metabolic effects, effects on psychomotor and motor function, and predisposition to malignancy requires further study. GH treatment for non-GH-deficient individuals with DS is currently not generally recommended.

Prader–Willi syndrome

Prader–Willi syndrome (PWS) occurs in approximately 1 in 15 000 live births and affects males and females equally in all ethnic groups. Typical clinical features include short stature, muscular hypotonia, hypogonadism, mild to moderate mental retardation and hyperphagia leading to extreme obesity if not controlled. The symptoms vary with age. In neonates and during infancy, muscular hypotonia, feeding problems and underweight are the most prominent symptoms. With increasing age, short stature, hyperphagia and behavioral problems become obvious. Many of the symptoms are non-specific and clinical diagnosis may be difficult.

The majority of individuals with clinical PWS have a chromosomal abnormality, with loss of paternal alleles on the long arm of chromosome 15 in the region 15q11-13. The loss of the same alleles but of maternal origin causes Angelmann syndrome. Of PWS patients, approximately 70% have paternal allele deletion, 25% have maternal disomy and 5% have translocation or other structural abnormalities.

The endocrine and GH/IGF axis in individuals with PWS has been studied extensively, with low spontaneous and stimulated GH secretion and IGF-I concentrations. Evaluation of the true GH status of PWS individuals may be complicated by obesity. GH treatment has been used in children and adults, with benefits demonstrated in growth, body composition and muscular tone and strength. Sudden death in GH-treated children with PWS has been reported; patients with kypho-scoliosis are particularly at risk.

Noonan syndrome

Noonan syndrome (NS) occurs in 1:1000–2500 live births. Clinical features include typical facial features, short stature, congenital heart disease, pectus chest deformity, webbing of the neck, coagulation defects, visual disturbance, hearing impairment, undescended testes and delayed puberty. The facial features include hypertelorism, ptosis, downslanting palpebral fissures and low-set posteriorly rotated ears (Fig. 3.5). Cardiac defects (in decreasing frequency of occurrence) include pulmonary valve stenosis, left ventricular hypertrophic cardiomyopathy and secundum atrial septal defect.

NS is caused by a mutation in the *PTPN11* gene, which encodes the protein tyrosine phosphatase SHP-2 (a protein that controls cardiac semilunar valvulogenesis and has other diverse effects on cell proliferation, differentiation and migration) on the long arm of chromosome 12 (12q24.1).

The mean final height of adults with NS is 162.5 cm in males and 153 cm in females. GH has been used in NS and has shown short- and longer-term benefit but final height analyses are not yet available. NS patients with echocardiographic features of hypertrophic cardiomyopathy may be at risk from GH therapy because of the known effect of GH on cardiac muscle. Such patients should be identified by cardiological

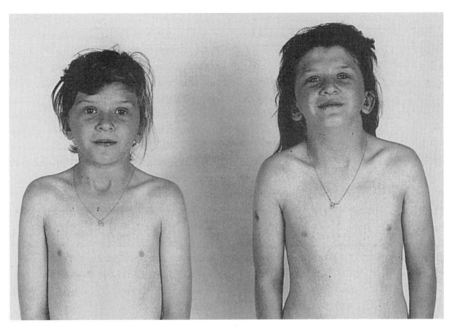

Figure 3.5 Sisters aged 10 and 12 years with NS are shown. Both have short stature, −2.4 SDS, and no evidence of puberty. Phenotypic features include increased carrying angle (not shown in photograph), low-set posteriorly rotated ears and broad chest. The younger girl had mild pulmonary stenosis.

assessment before GH therapy and should be reviewed annually with this issue in mind while on GH.

Silver–Russell syndrome

The Silver–Russell syndrome (SRS) is characterized by intrauterine and postnatal growth restriction with dysmorphic features including a small triangular facies, skeletal asymmetry and fifth finger clinodactyly (Fig. 3.6). The most characteristic feature is feeding difficulty, especially but not exclusively in infancy and early childhood.

The genetic etiology is heterogeneous. Maternal uniparental disomy for chromosome 7 occurs in 7–10% of patients, with strong evidence that disruption of imprinted gene expression, as opposed to mutation of a recessive gene, underlies the SRS phenotype in these cases. Final adult height is generally 3–4 SDS below normal.

Children with SRS are usually included in clinical trials of GH treatment on IUGR, the etiology of which is often not known. In these trials, initial growth response is usual, with some concern regarding excess bone age advancement. Predicted adult height has tended to increase, but final height has shown little

benefit. It is concerning that the catch-up growth seen by some SGA children may be associated with adverse metabolic sequelae such as insulin resistance.

Disproportionate short stature

A skeletal dysplasia should be suspected in patients who are short, are growing normally but have a reduced height prediction, have abnormal body proportions, abnormalities of the limbs and trunk and who fail to have a normal growth spurt despite appropriate pubertal development. Abnormal body proportions may not be clinically apparent but can be discerned from plots of sitting height and subischial leg length. A full skeletal radiographic survey and interpretation by an experienced radiologist are needed to make a diagnosis. Estimates vary but, overall, these disorders occur with an incidence of <1:10 000 live births.

Achondroplasia is caused by a mutation in the transmembrane portion of the FGF receptor-3 (FGFR-3) gene. In 90% of cases, the paternal allele is affected. Most cases are sporadic (90%) and inheritance is autosomal dominant. The typical appearance of patients includes a large head, frontal bossing and

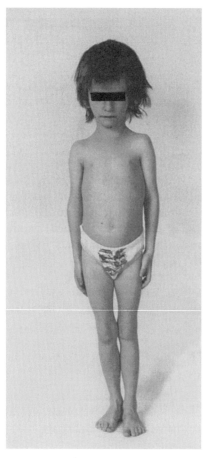

Figure 3.6 Four-year-old male with SRS. His birthweight was 1.68 kg at term and, at age 4 years, his height SDS is −5.3 and weight SDS is −4.5. A triangular face is present with a broad forehead and narrow point to the mandible. There is obvious body asymmetry with the right arm and right leg greater than the left side.

mid-face hypoplasia, severe shortening (rhizomelic) of the extremities but normal trunk length. Mental function is normal. Adult height is severely impaired, generally between 100 and 140 cm. GH corrects spinal shortening, thus making disproportion worse. Limb lengthening surgery is available but expensive in time and complications. Most patients prefer to settle for their condition but parents of newly diagnosed children need a lot of support.

Hypochondroplasia is an autosomal-dominant condition with variable penetrance and a wide spectrum of disease severity. Mutations in the tyrosine kinase domain of the FGFR-3 gene, mapped to chromosome 4p, have been described in some cases. Patients with a severe phenotype have disproportionate short stature and rhizomelic limb shortening in early childhood akin to achondroplasia. In others, the short stature may not become manifest until adolescence, when a reduced pubertal growth spurt results in significant reduction in final height. The characteristic radiological finding is decreased interpedicular distance between lumbar vertebrae L1 and L5 with short pedicles, which may not be evident until the second or third year of life. Final height in males of 145–165 cm and in females of 130–150 cm. The results of GH treatment on final height have not been fully evaluated but do not appear to be impressive. Surgical limb lengthening procedures based on the principle of distraction osteogenesis offer significant gain in length of both lower and upper limbs and allow normalization of body proportions.

Spondyloepiphyseal dysplasia is the term used for a group of skeletal dysplasias that includes spondyloepiphyseal dysplasia congenita, spondylometaphyseal dysplasia and Kneist dysplasia. The disorder is caused by autosomal-dominant mutations of the collagen II gene (COL2A1). The skeletal deformities are severe and include kypho-scoliosis. Adult height is severely impaired (84–132 cm).

Leri–Weill dyschondrosteosis is a form of mesomelic (shortening of forearms and lower legs) short stature with Madelung's deformity caused by haploinsufficiency of the SHOX gene. There is heterogeneity in the clinical expression of this condition in terms of short stature and other skeletal manifestations (e.g. short fourth metacarpals, scoliosis, exostoses). Adult height of males is 156–171 cm and of females is 135–164 cm.

Underweight

Of the various anthropometric methods available (Table 3.8), weight interpreted using available centile charts is the simplest and most reasonable measure of a child's nutritional state. Underweight means weight loss or failure to gain weight at an appropriate rate so that weight falls to lower centiles.

Acute transient weight loss can occur with common childhood illnesses associated with fever, diarrhea and

Table 3.8 Anthropometric measures of a child's nutritional state.

Anthropometric measure	Definitions	
	At risk of malnutrition	Malnutrition
Weight for age	0.4th second centile	<0.4th centile
BMI	0.4th second centile	<0.4th centile
BMI as percentage of population median BMI for age	80–90%	<80%
Actual weight divided by 50th centile weight for age as percentage of the actual height divided by 50th centile height for age	80–90%	<80%

BMI, body mass index.

vomiting. Acute weight loss is also seen in children with endocrine and systemic diseases of recent onset, the most common being diabetes mellitus (Table 3.9).

A prolonged period of poor weight gain in children under 2 years of age is referred to as failure to thrive. Healthy children whose initial weight is between the ninth and 91st centiles often cross one centile space during the first year. A sustained fall through two centile spaces is described as mild to moderate and three centile spaces (=2 SDS) as severe failure to thrive. Linear growth and head growth are not affected with transient periods of being underweight but linear growth may be impaired with long-term failure to thrive.

The causes of failure to thrive or being chronically underweight are predominantly nutritional (Table 3.9). Major organic disease accounts for 5% or less and is generally diagnosed from overt clinical features. Non-organic failure to thrive refers to children with psychosocial deprivation, abuse or neglect and who do not have an organic cause. Abuse or neglect has been reported in 5–10% of children with failure to thrive. Undernutrition owing to poor feeding, inadequate dietary intake and excessive consumption of juice or milk are the commonest causes of failure to thrive in otherwise healthy children. Assessment of a child who is failing to thrive or chronically underweight should include feeding and dietary history (variety and quantity of foods offered and eaten, meal time routines and behavior, drinking pattern, parent's interest in food and cooking), bowel habits and family history. Specific features of endocrine disorders and other organic diseases need to be explored and identified.

Overweight and obesity

Overweight and obesity are defined as body mass index above the 85th and 95th centiles, respectively. The aims of assessment of an overweight child are to determine the cause (Table 3.10) and identify problems associated with it, as well as risk factors for complications. The important aspects of history and examination are presented in Table 3.11.

Tall stature

Children whose height is above the 99.6th centile or who have a significant discrepancy between the child's centile and mid-parental target centile should be evaluated for tall stature.

Causes
There are few pathological causes of tall stature (Table 3.12). Most tall children represent the upper end of the normal distribution of height and have a family history of tallness in one or both parents (i.e. constitutional tall stature). Obese children, especially if the onset of obesity occurred in infancy, are often taller than average for their age and, if skeletal maturity is also advanced, puberty may occur earlier.

Assessment
The assessment of a child with tall stature requires a detailed history, family history of stature and age of onset of puberty, measurements to include sitting height and arm span, determination of height velocity and

Table 3.9 Causes of weight loss, poor weight gain and failure to thrive.

Inadequate calorie intake
Breast-feeding failure
Behavioral problems resulting in poor feeding and excessive consumption of fluids
Psychosocial deprivation
Poverty
Anorexia nervosa, bulimia
Difficulty swallowing due to congenital abnormality (e.g. cleft palate), neurodevelopmental delay or breathing difficulty
  (heart failure or respiratory disease)

Increased losses
Recurrent vomiting (e.g. gastroesophageal reflux)
Diarrhea from malabsorption or other gastrointestinal disorder (e.g. cystic fibrosis, celiac disease, inflammatory
  bowel disease, giardiasis)

Endocrine disorder
Diabetes mellitus
Diabetes insipidus
Thyrotoxicosis
Congenital adrenal hyperplasia (salt wasting)
Adrenal insufficiency
Pheochromocytoma
Idiopathic hypercalcemia of infancy
Congenital lipodystrophy

Other organic causes
Metabolic: galactosemia, urea cycle disorders, organic aciduria, hereditary tyrosinemia
Renal: renal tubular acidosis, cystinosis
Cardiac: large left-to-right shunt
Respiratory: chronic lung disease, bronchiectasis
Chronic inflammation: polyarteritis nodosa, chronic infection (e.g. tuberculosis)
Immunodeficiency: severe combined immunodeficiency, AIDS
Hematological: anemia
Malignancies: renal, brain

Table 3.10 The major causes of obesity.

Height above average and/or normal height velocity	Height low compared with weight and/or low height velocity	
Simple obesity	*Endocrine disorder*	*Hypogonadism, dysmorphic features*
Polycystic ovary syndrome	Hypothyroidism	Prader–Willi syndrome
	Growth hormone deficiency	Laurence–Moon–Biedl syndrome
	Cushing syndrome	Carpenter syndrome
	Pseudohypoparathyroidism	Cohen syndrome
	Hypothalamic lesion	Alstrom syndrome
	Craniopharyngioma	

Table 3.11 The important aspects of assessment of an overweight/obese child.

History
Birthweight
Age of onset of overweight
Diet, quality and quantity of food and drink consumed
Leisure activities and lifestyle, frequency and nature of physical activity
Psychological consequences, bullying
Physical consequences: tiredness, reduced exercise tolerance, joint pain
Family history
Parents' weights and heights
Obesity
Associated problems

Examination
Weight in relation to height
Pubertal status
Distribution of fat
Striae
Hirsutism, acne
Acanthosis nigricans
Blood pressure
Features of endocrine disorder or dysmorphic syndrome

Table 3.12 The major causes of tall stature.

Looks normal			Looks abnormal	
Normal height velocity	**Increased height velocity**		**Abnormal features**	**Disproportion between limbs and trunk**
	Signs of puberty	**No precocious puberty**		
Familial tall stature	*Precocious puberty*	*Endocrine disorder*	*Recognizable syndrome*	*Long limbs*
Obesity	Central	Hyperthyroidism	Cerebral gigantism	Marfan syndrome
	Gonadotropin	Growth hormone	Beckwith–Wiedemann	Homocystinuria
	independent	excess	syndrome	XYY boys
		Familial	Weaver syndrome	*Long limbs and hypogonadism*:
		glucocorticoid		Gonadotropin
		deficiency		deficiency
				Klinefelter syndrome

pubertal status. Tall stature may represent a considerable handicap and parents may be especially concerned if they experienced psychosocial problems during childhood. Adult height prediction using bone age and available equations is essential in the management of tall children.

Management

Treatment with sex steroids (girls 10–50 µg/day ethinylestradiol; boys 50–250 mg of testosterone ester depot at 2–4 weekly intervals) to induce puberty early and accelerate its progress has been used to limit growth. Doses higher than these have not been found to be more effective but are associated with significant side-effects. The reduction in height is greater when treatment is started at a lower bone age (when the remaining growth potential is greater) and is continued until complete fusion of the epiphyses at the knees. Nausea, headaches, weight gain, striae, breast discomfort, abdominal pain, calf cramps and irregular periods are the most commonly observed side-effects of high doses of estrogen. Thromboembolism and hypertension are rare but significant risks of treatment. Potentially serious effects on lipids, glucose tolerance, liver function and development of carcinoma have not been established. The side-effects of high doses of testosterone are acne, fluid retention, hypertension and temporary decrease in testicular size. Surgical damage to knee epiphyses by epiphysiodesis, generally performed to correct limb length inequality, is an alternative treatment option to limit height but the results of this procedure have not been systematically compared with medical treatment.

Endocrine causes of tall stature

The most common endocrine cause of tall stature in childhood is increased sex steroid secretion of either adrenal (e.g. congenital adrenal hyperplasia) or gonadal (e.g. precocious puberty) origin. Testicular volume is small in the former and enlarged in the latter. Less commonly, increased sex steroids may be derived from external sources.

Increased sex steroid secretion is suggested by tall stature associated with increased growth velocity and advanced bone maturation in the preadolescent age group so that final height is likely to be reduced by premature epiphyseal fusion.

Hypogonadism (central or due to gonadal failure) may also give rise to tall stature in adults because of continuing growth into late adolescence and early adulthood but stature in childhood is not affected. As a consequence of continuing growth of the long bones, a eunuchoid habitus in adolescence and early adulthood is characteristic.

Hyperthyroidism

An increase in growth rate associated with advanced bone age is seen in hyperthyroidism and also in hypothyroidism overtreated with thyroxine. Measuring thyroxine, triiodothyronine and thyrotrophin-stimulating hormone (TSH) concentrations makes the diagnosis.

GH excess (gigantism)

GH excess from a GH-secreting tumor in childhood or adolescence is rare. It is characterized by extremely rapid linear growth but bone age is not advanced and overgrowth of soft tissues and metabolic changes are similar to those observed in patients with acromegaly. Concentrations of GH and IGF-I are raised, contrasting with concentrations in constitutional tall stature. The tumor can be diagnosed using cranial MRI. Treatment is aimed at reducing the excessive GH secretion. As for acromegaly, treatment modalities include trans-sphenoidal removal of the tumor, GH antagonist, SS analogs and/or radiotherapy.

Familial glucocorticoid deficiency

Familial glucocorticoid deficiency results from mutations of the ACTH receptor (MC2-R). Inheritance is probably autosomal recessive. Patients are excessively tall for their parents but linear growth is normalized with glucocorticoid replacement. They have hyperpigmentation associated with high ACTH concentrations, increased head circumference and characteristic facial appearance including hypertelorism, epicanthic folds and frontal bossing.

Tall stature associated with an abnormal appearance

Klinefelter syndrome

Klinefelter syndrome (KS) is associated with an additional X chromosome in males due to non-disjunction of the sex chromosomes during the first meiotic division in one of the parents. The most frequent karyotype is 47XXY (93%), but other karyotypes also occur (e.g. 46XY/47XXY, 48XXYY, 49XXXX7) and are associated with a similar phenotype. KS occurs in 1 in 500–1000 live male births. The syndrome is characterized by tall stature with long legs, behavioral and psychological problems, primary hypogonadism with small testes and hyalinization and fibrosis of the seminiferous tubules resulting in infertility and gynecomastia at puberty.

Learning and behavioral problems may occur in KS, although intellectual quotient (IQ) is usually in the normal range. Other problems include mitral valve prolapse, Berry aneurysm, venous ulcers, deep vein thrombosis and pulmonary embolism. There is also an increased risk of carcinoma of the breast, autoimmune disorders (e.g. systemic lupus erythematosus, diabetes, hypothyroidism) and osteoporosis due to androgen insufficiency.

Tall stature is evident before puberty and related to extra leg length. Skeletal maturation is generally appropriate for chronological age throughout childhood. At puberty, testicular size may increase to 10 mL, but progressive hyalinization and fibrosis of the seminiferous tubules result in small adult testes. Despite relatively normal early pubertal androgen concentrations in some males with KS, hypergonadotrophic hypogonadism is evident by mid-puberty in most males with KS and androgen replacement is essential in them to prevent gynecomastia. Testosterone therapy may be introduced from the age of 12 years to induce puberty and prevent physical and psychological effects of hypogonadism. Final mean height is reported as approximately 10 cm taller than in XY males but the correlation with mid-parental height is maintained.

Marfan syndrome

Marfan syndrome (MS) is an autosomal-dominant syndrome of connective tissue. It occurs in 1 in 10 000 births with equal sex prevalence. The underlying defect is caused by a mutation in the fibrillin-I gene located at 15q21.1. Fibrillin is the main component of 1–12 nm extracellular microfibrils that are important for elastogenesis, elasticity and homeostasis of elastic fibers. Patients may arise as a fresh mutation, so a family history is not a prerequisite for diagnosis.

The syndrome consists of the clinical triad of excessively long limbs, ocular abnormalities and cardiovascular problems. Skeletal manifestations include tall stature, long limbs, arachnodactyly, abnormal joint mobility, scoliosis and chest wall deformity. Ocular manifestations can include dislocated lens (upward dislocation), severe myopia, flat cornea, elongated globe and risk of retinal detachment. Cardiovascular manifestations can include dilation of the aortic root, aortic dissection, abdominal aortic aneurysm, and mitral valve prolapse or regurgitation and contribute to decreased lifespan.

Tall stature develops early in infancy and height remains elevated throughout childhood and adult life.

Mean adult height is 177 cm in females and 187 cm in males.

Homocystinuria

Homocystinuria is an autosomal-recessive disorder of amino acid metabolism due to cystathione β-synthase deficiency. The gene is located at 21q22.3, with many mutations found in different kindreds. The physical appearance is similar to MS with tall stature, Marfinoid body habitus, mental retardation and downward lens dislocation. Thromboembolic disease and osteoporosis may complicate the condition. Homocystinuria occurs in 1 in 200 000 live births. Children with homocystinuria appear normal at birth, with the clinical features becoming manifest in the first few years of life.

The diagnosis may be made by newborn screening or as the result of diagnostic testing. Treatment consists of restriction of dietary methionine and supplementation of dietary cysteine. The etiology of the tall stature remains obscure. Good metabolic control is said to ameliorate the excess growth velocity seen in this situation.

Sotos syndrome (cerebral gigantism)

Sotos syndrome (SoS) is a childhood overgrowth syndrome characterized by excessive growth, distinctive craniofacial features, developmental delay and advanced bone age. It occurs in 1 in 10 000–50 000 births. A diagnosis is unlikely if one or more of four criteria (height >97th centile, head circumference >97th centile, bone age >90th centile and developmental delay) are not fulfilled.

Haploinsufficiency of the NSD1 gene has been identified as the major cause of SoS, with intragenic mutations or submicroscopic microdeletions being found in 60–75% of clinically diagnosed patients. Weaver syndrome may resemble SoS, with recent reports of NSD1 mutations in both SoS and Weaver syndromes.

Overgrowth is frequently evident at birth, and the growth velocity is excessive in the first few years of life and then parallels the charts in the high centiles or above the centiles. Bone age is usually advanced by 2–4 years during childhood, and puberty may occur relatively early, although within the normal range. The mean adult height attained is usually in the upper part of the normal range, with reports of mean final height of 172.9 ± 5.7 cm in females and

184.3 ± 6.0 cm in males. Excessive final height is generally not a problem.

Beckwith–Wiedemann syndrome

Beckwith–Wiedemann syndrome (BWS) is a prenatal and postnatal overgrowth syndrome that is characterized by omphalocele and macroglossia. Up to 50% of neonates have persistent neonatal hypoglycemia associated with hyperinsulinism. Other common features are hemihyperplasia, ear anomalies including anterior lobe creases and posterior helical pits, umbilical hernia, visceromegaly, adrenocortical cytomegaly, renal abnormalities and an increased risk of embryonal tumors. The prevalence is reported to be approximately 1 in 14 000, with no gender predilection.

The molecular genetics of BWS are complex and involve a number of growth regulatory genes in an imprinted gene cluster in the chromosome 11p15.5 region. A number of imprinted genes are known to be involved in the pathogenesis of BWS, including the paternally expressed IGF-2 and KvQTI-AS and the maternally expressed H19, p57 KIP2 and KvLQTI.

The overgrowth in BWS can be uniform or regional affecting any part of the body or organs. Infants are born with birthweight and length approximately 2 SD above the mean for gestational age; however, overgrowth may not manifest until the first year of life. Growth velocity is usually above the 90th centile until 4–6 years of age, with skeletal age mildly advanced, and then growth velocity returns to normal through late childhood and puberty. Tall final height is common, but stature is not excessive.

Simpson–Golabi–Behmel syndrome

Simpson–Golabi–Behmel syndrome is an X-linked overgrowth syndrome with prenatal and postnatal overgrowth, craniofacial abnormalities, digital abnormalities (polydactyly, nail hypoplasia) and a wide variety of less common features. There is overlap between the BWS and the Simpson–Golabi–Behmel syndrome, with both syndromes including macroglossia, organomegaly, earlobe creases, hyperinsulinism and hypoglycemia, and risk of embryonal tumors. The syndrome is due to loss of function abnormalities of the glypican-3 (GPC-3) gene on Xq26. The GPC-3 and IGF-2 receptors may be functionally related and may be co-dependent, possibly explaining the relationship with BWS.

4   Problems of Puberty and Adolescence

Learning Points

- Puberty starts in both sexes around 11 years of age but is more evident in girls because of breast development and the onset of the growth spurt
- Male pubertal growth begins about 2 years later at a testicular volume of about 10 mL
- Premature onset of puberty (<8 in girls, <9 in boys) is much more common in girls than boys and is usually idiopathic
- Idiopathic central precocious puberty in a boy is very unusual so early puberty in boys needs extensive investigation which is usually unnecessary in (consonant) early puberty in a girl
- Testicular size distinguishes true puberty from other causes of virilization in boys

- Treatment of precocious puberty stops pubertal development but is not effective in increasing final height
- Delayed onset on puberty (>13 in girls, >14 in boys) is much commoner in boys than girls and is usually idiopathic
- Idiopathic delayed puberty in a girl is unusual and needs thorough investigation which is usually unnecessary in a boy
- Treatment of delayed puberty is psychologically advantageous and does not limit adult height as long as treatment is not excessive, so its institution should be prompt

Puberty marks the transition from childhood through the development of secondary sexual characteristics to the achievement of adult stature. The physical changes of puberty in individuals are defined by the Tanner stages (Fig. 4.1). It is important that the orderly progression of pubertal changes and their consonance is observed. Pubertal arrest or disconsonant features are signs that the process is not going normally.

Physical changes

In boys, an increase in testicular volume to 4 mL is usually the first sign and can easily be assessed

using the Prader orchidometer (Fig. 4.2). Most of the increase is due to enlargement of the Sertoli rather than the Leydig cells. In gonadotropin-independent precocious puberty (GIPP) (testotoxicosis), the testes remain small in relation to the growth of the phallus and pubic hair, since the condition is due to constitutive activation of the luteinizing hormone (LH) receptor with consequent hyperplasia of Leydig rather than Sertoli cells.

Growth of the penis and genitalia in the male correlate well with pubic hair development, since both features are regulated by androgen secretion but stages for pubic hair and genital development should be determined independently since valuable clinical information can be accrued. For example, pubic hair growth without testicular enlargement suggests an adrenal rather than a gonadal source of androgens.

Handbook of Clinical Pediatric Endocrinology, 1st edition. By Charles G. D. Brook and Rosalind S. Brown. Published 2008 by Blackwell Publishing, ISBN: 978-1- 4501-6109-1.

PUBERTAL DEVELOPMENT TIME COURSE – BOYS

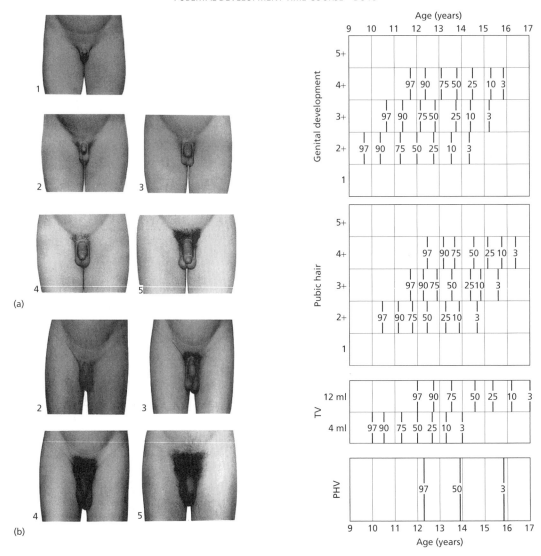

(a)

(b)

Boys: genital development

Stage 1: Preadolescent. The testes, scrotum and penis are of about the same size and proportions as in early childhood.
Stage 2: Enlargement of the scrotum and testes. The skin of the scrotum reddens and changes in texture. Little or no enlargement of the penis.
Stage 3: Lengthening of the penis. Further growth of the testes and scrotum.
Stage 4: Increase in breadth of the penis and development of the glans. The testes and scrotum are larger; the scrotum darkens.
Stage 5: Adult.

Boys: pubic hair

Stage 1: Preadolescent. No pubic hair.
Stage 2: Sparse growth of slightly pigmented downy hair chie y at the base of the penis.
Stage 3: Hair darker, coarser and more curled, spreading sparsely over the junction of the pubes.
Stage 4: Hair adult in type, but covering a considerably smaller area than in the adult. No spread to the medial surface of the thighs.
Stage 5: Adult quantity and type with distribution of a horizontal pattern and spread to the medial surface of the thighs. Spread up linea alba occurs late, in about 80% of men, after adolescence is complete, and is rated Stage 6.

Figure 4.1 Pubertal assessment is an important component of the assessment of gonadal function. Staging of each of the components is separate and should be recorded as such to allow discordance in development to be identified. The figures show the relationship in time of each of the components, and each should be related to other parts of the puberty process. Note that the peak height velocity in girls takes place some 2 years before that in boys.

PUBERTAL DEVELOPMENT TIME COURSE – GIRLS

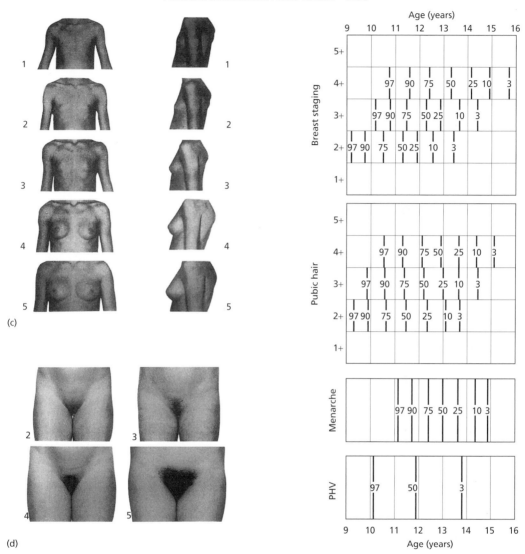

(c)

(d)

Girls: breast development

Stage 1: Preadolescent. Elevation of the papilla only.
Stage 2: Breast bud stage. Elevation of the breast and papilla as a small mound. Enlargement of the areola diameter.
Stage 3: Further enlargement and elevation of the breast and areola, with no separation of their contours.
Stage 4: Projection of the areola and papilla above the level of the breast.
Stage 5: Mature stage, projection of the papilla alone due to recession of the areola.

Girls: pubic hair

Stage 1: Preadolescent. No pubic hair.
Stage 2: Sparse growth of slightly pigmented downy hair chie y along the labia.
Stage 3: Hair darker, coarser and more curled, spreading sparsely over the junction of the pubes.
Stage 4: Hair adult in type, but covering a considerably smaller area than in the adult. No spread to the medial surface of the thighs.
Stage 5: Adult quantity and type with distribution of a horizontal pattern and spread to the medial surface of the thighs. In about 10% of women, after adolescence is complete pubic hair spreads up the linea alba and is rated Stage 6.

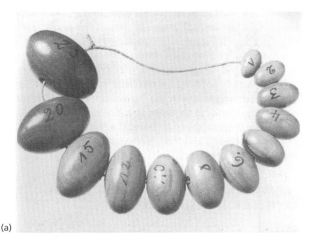

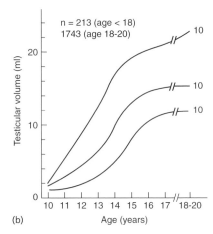

Figure 4.2 (a) Prader orchidometer and (b) standards for testicular volume.

Spermatogenesis can be detected histologically between ages 11 and 15 years and sperm is found in early morning urine samples at a mean age of 13.3 years. Ejaculation occurs by a mean age of 13.5 years without consistent relationship to testicular volume, pubic hair development or phallic enlargement. Adult morphology, motility and concentration of sperm are not found until the bone age advances to 17 years but immature-appearing boys can be fertile.

Breast enlargement occurs to some degree in a majority of boys, usually during the first stages of puberty because of an increase in estrogen production (by aromatization of testosterone) before testosterone secretion achieves concentrations that can oppose the estrogen. In most cases, the tissue regresses within 2 years but, occasionally, in normal, often obese, boys and frequently in pathological conditions such as Klinefelter syndrome or partial androgen resistance, in which the effective amount of bioactive testosterone is reduced, gynecomastia remains permanent. Surgery, usually through a peri-areolar incision, is the only effective mode of therapy at present, although non-aromatizable androgens or aromatase inhibitors are under study as potential treatments.

In girls, breast development is caused by estrogen secreted by the ovaries. Breast development may be unilateral for several months, which can cause concern in girls or their parents. Even though the growth of pubic and axillary hair is mainly under the influence of adrenal androgens, the stage of breast development usually correlates well with the stage of pubic hair

development in normal girls. However, since different endocrine organs control these two processes, the stages of each phenomenon should be classified separately.

Bone mineral density

The most important phases of bone accretion occur during infancy and puberty. Girls reach peak mineralization between 14 and 16 years while boys reach a peak later at 17.5 years. Both are attained after peak height velocity has been achieved in either sex. Bone mineral density (BMD) is influenced not only by sex steroids but also by genetics, exercise and growth hormone (GH) secretion.

There is a poor correlation between calcium intake and BMD during puberty or young adulthood. It seems nonetheless wise to ensure adequate calcium intake in patients with delayed or absent puberty or in those treated with gonadotropin-releasing hormone (GnRH) analogs to hold up puberty.

Body composition

Percentages of lean body mass, skeletal mass and body fat are equal between prepubertal boys and girls but, as boys go through puberty, total body bone mass and fat-free mass (FFM) continue to increase whereas, in girls, only body fat and FFM increase. Using skinfold thickness to derive fat mass (FM), FFM (or lean body mass) and percentage body fat (%BF), boys gain approximately 30 kg in weight from 12 to 18 years, 82% being accounted for by FFM. Girls gain approximately 18.5 kg, 68% being FFM. There are relatively small changes in %BF, 1.7% in boys and 3% in girls. The increase in lean body mass starts at 6 years in girls and at 9.5 years in boys and is the earliest change in body composition in puberty. At maturity, men have 1.5 times the lean body mass and almost 1.5 times the skeletal mass of women, while women have twice as much body fat as men.

Growth in puberty

Growth accelerates as soon as breast development starts and peak height velocity is attained 6–9 months after the appearance of breast stage 2 development. Menarche occurs after peak height velocity has been achieved and rarely before growth velocity has fallen to 4 cm/year.

Peak height velocity occurs relatively late in puberty in boys compared with girls and coincides with a testicular volume of 10–12 mL. Voice changes in boys can be noted at 8 mL testicular volume and become obvious by 12 mL volume.

The mean difference in adult height between men and women of 12.5 cm is due mainly to the taller stature of boys at the onset of the pubertal growth spurt but also to the increased height gained during the pubertal growth spurt in boys compared with girls. A girl who has experienced menarche usually has no more than 2–3% (5–7.5 cm) of her growth remaining since menarche closely accords to a bone age of 13 years, the only event of puberty more closely related to skeletal than chronological age. Post-menarcheal growth exceptionally extends to 11 cm.

The pubertal growth spurt results from many endocrine influences. Sex steroids exert a direct effect on growing cartilage as well as an indirect effect mediated by increasing GH secretion. Increasing sex steroid production at puberty stimulates increased amplitude (but not frequency) of spontaneous GH secretion as well as peak stimulated GH and this in turn stimulates increased production of insulin-like growth factor (IGF)-I.

Estrogen, either from the ovary or aromatized from testicular testosterone, is the factor that mediates the increased GH response during puberty. A prepubertal child given an androgen that can be aromatized to estrogen, such as testosterone, has augmented GH secretion, whereas a non-aromatizable androgen, such as dihydrotestosterone, does not increase GH secretion. An estrogen-blocking agent such as tamoxifen reduces GH secretion.

Thyroid hormone is necessary to allow the pubertal growth spurt to proceed. The rapid growth rate is accompanied by an increase in markers of bone turnover such as serum alkaline phosphatase, serum bone alkaline phosphatase, osteocalcin, Gla protein and the amino-terminal propeptide of type III procollagen; thus, normal adult values of these proteins are lower than concentrations found in puberty.

Estrogen has a biphasic effect on growth; low concentrations stimulate growth while higher concentrations lead to its cessation. Patients with either estrogen receptor deficiency or aromatase deficiency have tall stature; they continue growth into the third decade as a result of lack of fusion of the epiphyses of the long bones and have increased bone turnover, reduced BMD, osteoporosis and absence of a pubertal growth spurt. Estrogen is the main factor that fuses the epiphyses of long bones and stops growth. These observations have raised the possibility of using aromatase inhibitors to allow more time for growth before epiphyseal fusion in short normal individuals.

Endocrine changes in puberty

Gonadotropin-releasing hormone

GnRH, a 10-amino-acid peptide generated from a larger 69-amino-acid prohormone precursor, is localized mainly in the hypothalamus but there is no discrete nucleus that contains all the GnRH neurons, although the arcuate nucleus plays a key role. Gonadotropins are normally released into the bloodstream in a pulsatile manner as a result of the pulsatile nature of GnRH secretion (Fig. 4.3). Variation in the frequency of secretion of GnRH changes the relative concentrations of LH and follicle-stimulating hormone (FSH) released.

The GnRH pulse generator, which is the basis of the central nervous system (CNS) control of puberty and reproductive function, is affected by biogenic amine

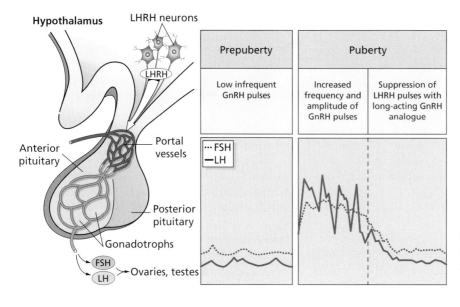

Figure 4.3 Anatomy of the gonadotropin system and the secretory patterns of LH and FSH in puberty.

neurotransmitters, peptidergic neuromodulators, neuroexcitatory amino acids and neural pathways. For example, adrenaline and noradrenaline increase GnRH release whereas dopamine, serotonin and opioids decrease it.

Testosterone and progesterone inhibit GnRH pulse frequency but the suppression of gonadotropin secretion during childhood appears to be mediated by the CNS probably through gamma amino butyric acid (GABA). Damage to the CNS from increased intracranial pressure or tumor may release the inhibition and bring about premature pubertal development.

There appear to be readily releasable pools of LH, which lead to a rise in serum LH within minutes after a bolus of GnRH, as well as pools of LH that take longer to mobilize. While episodic stimulation by GnRH increases gonadotropin secretion, continuous infusion of GnRH decreases LH and FSH secretion and down-regulates the pituitary receptors for GnRH. This phenomenon is used in the treatment of central precocious puberty. Estrogens increase and androgens decrease GnRH receptors. These alterations in the GnRH receptor have an important role in regulating gonadotroph function.

The gene encoding GnRH is located on chromosome 8. Neurons producing GnRH originate in the primitive olfactory placode early in the development of mammals and then migrate to the medial basal hypothalamus. The control of this migration is related to the *KAL* gene located at Xp22.3. The absence of the *KAL* gene or rather of the gene product ANOSMIN-1 causes Kallman syndrome, a decrease in or lack of gonadotropin secretion with hyposmia due to disordered development of the olfactory bulb.

Pituitary gonadotropins (Fig. 4.4)

FSH and LH are glycoproteins composed of two subunits, an α-subunit that is identical for all the pituitary glycoproteins and distinct β-subunits that confer specificity. The β-subunits are 115 amino acids long with two carbohydrate side chains. Human chorionic gonadotropin (hCG) produced by the placenta is almost identical in structure to LH except for an additional 32 amino acids and additional carbohydrate groups.

The same gonadotroph cell produces both LH and FSH. The gonadotrophs are distributed throughout the anterior pituitary gland and abut the capillary basement membranes to allow access to the systemic circulation. Inactive gonadotroph cells that are not stimulated, e.g. as a result of disease affecting GnRH secretion, are small, while the gonadotroph cells of castrate individuals or those with absence of gonads, which are stimulated by large amounts of GnRH, are large and demonstrate prominent rough endoplasmic reticulum.

Serum gonadotropin concentrations change during puberty. Because of the episodic nature of gonadotropin

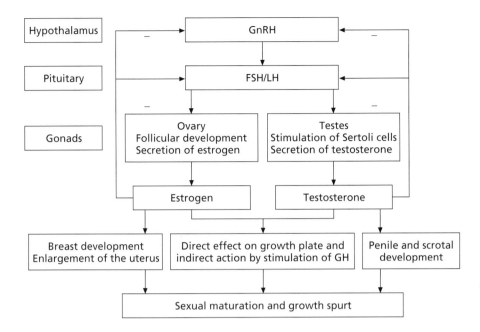

Figure 4.4 Feedforward and feedback loops in the hypothalamo-pituitary–gonadal axis.

secretion, a single gonadotropin determination will not reveal the secretory dynamics of the hormones but current assays are sufficiently sensitive to indicate the onset of puberty in single basal unstimulated samples.

GnRH must stimulate gonadotropin release before any other factors can affect gonadotropin secretion. In the presence of GnRH stimulation, sex steroids and gonadal peptides can change gonadotropin secretion. Negative feedback inhibition is manifest when sex steroids decrease pituitary LH and FSH secretion at the hypothalamic and pituitary levels and is exemplified in individuals with gonadal dysgenesis, who have very high concentrations of LH and FSH during infancy and puberty.

The proteins inhibin, a product of both ovary and testis, and follistatin, an ovarian product, exert direct inhibitory effects upon FSH secretion at the pituitary level. Progesterone slows LH pulse frequency.

Estradiol decreases gonadotropin secretion at low concentrations but causes positive feedback at higher values. Thus a rising concentration of estradiol (>200–300 pg/mL) persisting for more than 48 h triggers the release of a burst of LH from the pituitary gonadotrophs, which stimulates ovulation about 12 h later.

Several steps must prepare the hypothalamo-pituitary–gonadal axis for positive feedback, including a pool of LH large enough to be released to prime the ovary to produce estrogen. Estradiol sensitizes the pituitary to GnRH which, in addition to an increase in GnRH pulse frequency, increases LH secretion. Thus, a follicle must be of adequate size to produce enough estrogen to exert the positive feedback effect, the pituitary gland must have sufficient readily releasable LH to effect a surge of LH release and the hypothalamus must be able to secrete GnRH sufficient to cause the stimulation of pituitary release.

Sex steroids

Testosterone is synthesized by the Leydig cells of the testes and the majority is bound to sex-hormone-binding globulin (SHBG) in the circulation. The remaining free testosterone is the active moiety. At the target cell, testosterone dissociates from the binding protein, diffuses into the cell and may be converted by 5α-reductase type II to dihydrotestosterone or by aromatase to estrogen.

The effects of testosterone are different from those of dihydrotestosterone because a fetus without dihydrotestosterone will not virilize fully. The androgen receptor has a greater affinity for dihydrotestosterone than for testosterone. Testosterone suppresses LH secretion, maintains Wolffian ducts and produces the male body habitus while dihydrotestosterone is responsible for virilization of the external genitalia and for most of the secondary sexual characteristics of puberty, including phallic growth, prostate enlargement androgen-induced hair loss and beard growth. Testosterone itself promotes muscle development, stimulates enzymatic activity in the liver and stimulates hemoglobin synthesis but it must be converted to estrogen to stimulate bone maturation at the epiphyseal plate.

FSH binds to specific receptors on the cell surface of Sertoli cells and causes an increase in the mass of seminiferous tubules and, in an undefined way, supports the development of sperm.

Estrogen is produced mainly by the follicle cells of the ovary utilizing the same initial steps as testosterone production with a final aromatization process. After the onset of ovulation, LH exerts major effects upon the theca of the ovary. FSH binds to its own cell-surface receptors on the glomerulosa cells and stimulates the conversion of testosterone to estrogen.

The main active estrogen in humans is estradiol, which circulates bound to SHBG and affects breast and uterine development, the distribution of adipose tissue and bone mineral accretion. Low concentrations of estradiol are difficult to measure.

Activin and inhibin

Inhibin is produced by Sertoli cells in the male and by ovarian granulosa cells and the placenta in the female. It suppresses FSH secretion from the pituitary gland and provides another explanation for different serum concentrations of LH and FSH with only one hypothalamic peptide (GnRH) stimulating them.

Activin is a subunit of inhibin and has the opposite effect, stimulating the secretion of FSH from the pituitary gland.

Inhibin B secretion rises in early puberty in both boys and girls and reaches a plateau. The infant male has values of inhibin B higher than those achieved in adult males for the first 1–1.5 years after birth, indicating the activity of the testes during this early period. Absence of inhibin due to gonadal failure in pubertal and adult subjects causes a greater rise in serum FSH than LH.

Anti-Müllerian hormone

Anti-Müllerian hormone (AMH) belongs to the same family as inhibin and is produced from the Sertoli

cells of the fetal testes and the granulosa cells of the fetal ovary. In normal males, AMH is high in the fetus and newborn but decreases thereafter, with a further drop at puberty. Girls have low concentrations of AMH in the newborn period.

Patients with dysgenetic testes have decreased serum AMH. Values are elevated in males with Sertoli cell tumors or females with granulosa cell tumors. AMH might differentiate a child with congenital anorchia who has no testicular tissue from one with undescended testes who has testicular tissue.

Ontogeny of endocrine pubertal development

Fetal testosterone secretion in early pregnancy is caused by placental hCG stimulation. The fetal hypothalamus contains GnRH-containing neurons by 14 weeks of gestation and the fetal pituitary gland contains LH and FSH by 20 weeks. Stimulation by GnRH causes gonadotropin secretion to rise to extremely high concentrations in mid-gestation with a decrease in responsivity thereafter. Initially unrestrained GnRH secretion by the hypothalamus comes under restraint from the CNS by mid-gestation and probably also to some degree from increased circulating sex steroid concentrations, which exert a restraining effect upon gonadotropin secretion until after birth.

Gonadotropin concentrations at term are lower than in mid-gestation but still relatively high. Gonadotropin values rise once again in an intermittent pattern after birth with episodic peaks noted up to 2–4 years of age. Estrogen and testosterone from the infantile gonads also rise episodically during this period but mean serum values of gonadotropins and sex steroids during infancy remain much lower than those found in the fetus and the pubertal subject but higher than those found during mid-childhood.

Because sex steroids suppress gonadotropin secretion to a significant degree during the first years after birth, agonadal patients, such as those with Turner syndrome, exhibit high (castrate) serum gonadotropin concentrations while maintaining the same pattern of pulsatile gonadotropin secretion as normal girls but with higher pulse amplitudes.

During childhood, gonadotropin pulsatility and gonadal activity are restrained by the CNS to a low level, which reaches a nadir around 7 years of age. Even in children without gonadal function, such as those with Turner syndrome, serum gonadotropin concentrations are low, demonstrating that the presence of the gonads is not necessary to suppress gonadotropin secretion during this period. Changes in gonadotropin secretion arise as a result of alterations in pulse amplitude with pulse frequency unchanged. Likewise, testosterone and estrogen are measurable in the circulation using sensitive assays, demonstrating low but definite activity of the prepubertal gonads.

Before any physical changes of puberty are evident, gonadotropin secretion increases first at night (Fig. 4.3). As puberty progresses, the secretion of gonadotropins and sex steroids increases during the day until little circadian rhythm remains.

During the peripubertal period, there is also a change in the response of pituitary gonadotrophs to exogenous GnRH administration. The pattern of LH release increases, so that the adult pattern of response to GnRH is achieved during puberty. The release of FSH shows no such change with development, although female subjects have more FSH release than male subjects at all developmental stages.

There is no evidence that leptin is the cause of puberty onset or progression but it does appear to be permissive. Leptin is produced in adipose cells and suppresses appetite by attaching to its receptor in the hypothalamus. It plays a major role in puberty in mice and rats: the leptin-deficient (ob/ob) mouse does not commence puberty until leptin is replaced. Leptin administration will induce puberty in an immature but normal mouse.

The leptin-deficient human has pubertal delay and leptin treatment is associated with the appearance of gonadotropin peaks. These data suggested that leptin might trigger the onset of puberty but clinical studies show that leptin increases in girls during puberty in synchrony with the increase in FM, while leptin decreases in puberty in boys with a decrease in FM and an increase in FFM; leptin varies with body composition only and no sex differences are noted.

Adrenarche

Dehydroepiandrosterone (DHEA) and androstenedione are produced by the zona reticularis and increase two or more years before the increase in the secretion of gonadotropins and sex steroids. This process (adrenarche)

begins by 6–8 years of age in normal subjects and continues until late puberty. Adrenarche occurs as a result of increased adrenal 17, 20-lyase and 17α-hydroxylase activities and causes an increase in height velocity (the mid-childhood growth spurt), secretion of apocrine sweat, the development of pubic and axillary hair and an advance in bone age.

The presence or absence of adrenarche does not seem to influence the onset of puberty. Patients with Addison disease experience puberty and children with premature adrenarche enter gonadarche at a normal age. Thus, adrenarche is usually temporally co-ordinated with gonadarche during pubertal development in normal individuals but appears not to play an important role in the progression of gonadarche.

Abnormal puberty

Limits of normal pubertal development

The limits of the normal timing of puberty in Europe and USA are shown in Tables 4.1 and 4.2. Puberty should be considered precocious when secondary sexual characteristics appear in girls (breast stage 2) under 8 years of age and in boys (genitalia stage 2) under 9 years. Contrary to popular belief, there is no evidence that the age of onset of true puberty is getting earlier; certainly the age of menarche has not changed so reports of widespread early breast development need to be treated with reserve.

There is no controversy about definitions of pubertal delay. Boys should show the earliest signs of pubertal development (testicular volume 4 mL) by 14 years and girls (breast development) by 13 years. Puberty does not often occur spontaneously after 18 years of age. The average time to complete secondary sexual development in girls is 4.2 years (range 1.5–6 years) and 3.5 years (range 2–4.5 years) in boys.

Precocious puberty

Etiology

The causes of early puberty can be divided into those with consonance of puberty and those in which there is a loss of consonance (Fig. 4.5). The former includes central or gonadotropin-dependent precocious puberty (GDPP), in which there is premature

Table 4.1 Age at stage of puberty in girls.

Stage	British girls		Swiss girls		US girls	
	Mean (years)	SD	Mean (years)	SD	Mean (years)	SD
Breast stage 2	11.50	1.10	10.9	1.2	11.2	0.7
Pubic hair stage 2	11.64	1.21	10.4	1.2	11.0	0.5
Breast stage 3	12.15	1.09	12.2	1.2	12.0	1.0
Pubic hair stage 3	12.36	1.10	12.2	1.2	11.8	1.0
Breast stage 4	13.11	1.15	13.2	0.9	12.4	0.8
Pubic hair stage 4	12.95	1.06	13.0	1.1	12.4	0.9
Menarche	13.47	1.12	13.4	1.1	–	–
Breast stage 5	15.33	1.74	14.0	1.2	–	–
Pubic hair stage 5	14.41	1.21	14.0	1.3	13.1	–

Table 4.2 Age at stage of puberty in boys.

Stage	British boys		Swiss boys		US boys	
	Mean (years)	SD	Mean (years)	SD	Mean (years)	SD
Genitalia stage 2	11.64	1.07	11.2	1.5	11.2	0.7
Pubic hair stage 2	13.44	1.09	12.2	1.5	11.2	0.8
Genitalia stage 3	12.85	1.04	12.9	1.2	12.1	0.8
Pubic hair stage 3	13.90	1.04	13.5	1.2	12.1	1.0
Genitalia stage 4	13.77	1.02	13.8	1.1	13.5	0.7
Pubic hair stage 4	14.36	1.08	14.2	1.1	13.4	0.9
Genitalia stage 5	14.92	1.10	14.7	1.1	14.3	1.1
Pubic hair stage 5	15.18	1.07	14.9	1.0	14.3	0.8

activation of the hypothalamo-pituitary-gonadal axis. The latter includes isolated early development of breast tissue (premature thelarche/thelarche variant) or pubic/axillary hair (premature adrenarche, late-onset congenital adrenal hyperplasia (CAH), adrenal tumors). Additionally, there may be activation of the ovaries or testes independently of gonadotropin secretion, so-called GIPP. The causes are listed in Table 4.3.

Precocious puberty is much commoner in girls than in boys. Activation of the hypothalamo-pituitary-gonadal axis requires a lower dose of GnRH in girls than in boys and suppression of sexual precocity with a GnRH analog is more difficult in girls than in boys.

Gonadotropin-dependent precocious puberty (GDPP)

In central or GDPP, the hypothalamo-pituitary-gonadal axis is activated prematurely, the pattern of endocrine change is the same as in normal puberty and pubertal development is consonant. Idiopathic precocious puberty accounts for more than 90% of cases in girls.

In boys, it is a diagnosis of exclusion and neuro-radiological imaging (either computed tomography (CT) or magnetic resonance imaging (MRI)) is mandatory. In girls, in the absence of neurological signs, the diagnostic return is only 15% at all ages with the majority of findings not requiring intervention. Interventional returns are increased in patients under 4 years of age.

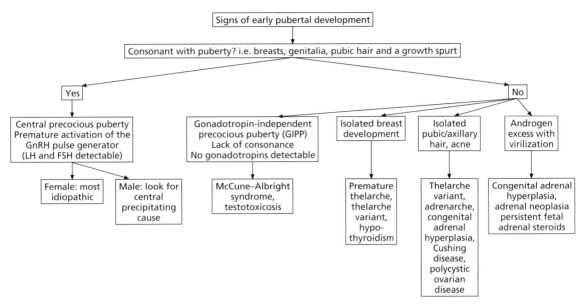

Figure 4.5 Algorithm for evaluating early puberty.

Table 4.3 Causes of premature sexual development.

I	*Gonadotrophin-dependent precocious puberty*	II	*Gonadotrophin-independent precocious puberty*
	Idiopathic central precocious puberty – commonest cause in females		Ovarian cysts
	Secondary central precocious puberty		Defects of LH receptor function: McCune–Albright syndrome, testotoxicosis
	Congenital anomalies (e.g. septo-optic dysplasia)	III	*Abnormal patterns of gonadotrophin secretion*
	Brain neoplasms (e.g. optic nerve gliomas, hamartomas, etc.)		Premature thelarche (isolated breast development)
	Cysts		Thelarche variant and slowly progressing variants of central precocious puberty
	Hydrocephalus		Hypothyroidism
	Post-infection	IV	*Sexual precocity due to adrenal androgens*
	Post-trauma		Steroid secretion by the normal adrenal gland– (adrenarche)
	Post-cranial radiotherapy		Adrenal enzyme defects –(congenital adrenal hyperplasia)
	Neurofibromatosis		Adrenal tumors –(Cushing syndrome and virilizing tumor)
	Adoption	V	*Gonadal tumors secreting sex steroids*
	HCG-producing neoplasms (e.g. choriocarcinoma, hepatoblastoma, germ cell tumors of CNS or mediastinum)	VI	*Exogenous sex steroids*

Secondary GDPP results from CNS lesions that provoke premature activation of the hypothalamo-pituitary–gonadal axis, even if they are not in the region of the hypothalamus. These include tumors, such as optic and hypothalamic gliomas, astrocytomas, ependymomas and pineal tumors, hydrocephalus, trauma, radiotherapy, post-CNS infection and neuro-fibromatosis. Hamartomas of the tuber cinereum are congenital tumors composed of a heterotopic mass of GnRH neurosecretory neurones, fiber bundles and glial cells, which are frequently associated with GDPP, often before 3 years of age. Gelastic epilepsy and developmental delay may be associated and the characteristic appearance on neuroradiological imaging is that of a sessile or pedunculated mass usually attached to the posterior hypothalamus between the tuber cinereum and the mamillary bodies. The tumor is thought to secrete GnRH rather than stimulating secretion from a normal hypothalamus and is associated with very high serum LH concentrations in response to GnRH administration.

The prevalence of GDPP is increased after cranial irradiation for local tumors or leukemia. Low-dose cranial irradiation (18–24 Gy) employed in the CNS prophylactic treatment of acute lymphoblastic leukemia is associated with a downward shift in the distribution of ages at pubertal onset and menarche in girls. Moderate radiation doses (25–47.5 Gy) used for the treatment of brain tumors in children are associated with precocious puberty with a direct relationship between ages at pubertal onset and therapy. Higher doses are usually associated with gonadotropin deficiency.

The clinical picture may be complicated by co-existing GH deficiency (GHD) in children who have received cranial radiotherapy, as well as in children with sexual precocity secondary to congenital anomalies, trauma or CNS infection. GH-deficient children with GDPP grow at a rate between that of children who are GH sufficient with GDPP and that of children who have GHD without sexual precocity. Since children who have received cranial irradiation are often obese and obesity is associated with a reduction in GH secretion, tests of GH secretion can be misleading. Treatment of children with GDPP and true GHD entails the administration of GH and a GnRH agonist (GnRHa).

Children adopted from developing countries and moved to a more affluent environment have an increased incidence of early and precocious puberty.

Sexual abuse has been reported as a precipitating cause of GDPP and, in these cases, the development can regress with a change in environment.

Sex steroid exposure has a direct maturational effect on the hypothalamus and can accelerate the onset of centrally mediated puberty.

Gonadotropin-releasing tumors (usually hCG) leading to sexual precocity are rare tumors, which are usually intracranial, such as pineal germ cell tumors and teratomas, or hepatoblastomas and teratomas. Tumor markers such as α-fetoprotein and pregnancy-specific β1-glycoprotein are often present. Pure gonadotropin-secreting tumors of the pituitary occur but are even rarer.

Gonadotropin-independent precocious puberty (GIPP)

The secretion of sex steroids is independent of the hypothalamic GnRH pulse generator in this condition. There is loss of normal feedback and sex steroid concentrations can be very high with low gonadotropin secretion. The disorder is associated with an abnormally functioning LH receptor.

The LH receptor belongs to the G-protein-coupled receptor superfamily characterized by the presence of seven transmembrane α-helices. The LH receptor is linked to an associated G-protein, which is vital for signal transduction and the intracellular actions of the hormone. LH binds to its receptor and activates the G-protein, which leads to the conversion of guanosine diphosphate (GDP) to guanosine triphosphate (GTP). This causes an increase in intracellular cAMP, which sets off a chain of events culminating in the synthesis and secretion of sex steroids. Phosphorylase activity of the G-protein converts GTP to GDP, which terminates the action of LH.

In boys, familial testotoxicosis (or male-limited GIPP) is associated with premature Leydig and germ cell maturation. It is inherited as an autosomal-dominant condition manifesting only in males. Virilization occurs with very high concentrations of testosterone and enlargement of the testes to the early or mid-pubertal range, although they seem smaller than expected in relation to the stage of penile growth. Premature Leydig and Sertoli cell maturation and spermatogenesis occur. Unstimulated gonadotropin concentrations are prepubertal with a minimal (prepubertal) response to GnRH stimulation. There is a lack of the usual pubertal pattern of LH pulsatility. Fertility and a normal pattern of LH secretion and response to GnRH are demonstrable in adulthood.

Testotoxicosis is associated with a number of constitutively activated mutations of the LH receptor, most of which are in the transmembrane domain of the receptor.

McCune–Albright syndrome (MAS) is a multisystem disorder of both boys and girls characterized by the classical triad of irregularly edged hyperpigmented macules or café-au-lait spots, a slowly progressive bone disorder (polyostotic fibrous dysplasia), which can involve any bone. Facial asymmetry and hyperostosis of the base of the skull are common, especially in girls. There is often a lack of consonance in pubertal development with menses in the presence of minimal breast development.

The sexual precocity in girls with MAS is caused by autonomously functioning luteinized follicular cysts of the ovaries. Multiple follicular cysts with an occasional large solitary cyst may be present. Estrogen production is associated with a prepubertal pattern of LH secretion with an absent LH response to GnRH. Later, GnRH-dependent puberty ensues with ovulatory cycles. Sexual precocity is rare in boys with MAS. When it does occur, it is associated with asymmetric enlargement of the testes in addition to signs of sexual precocity. The seminiferous tubules are enlarged and exhibit spermatogenesis. Leydig cells may be hyperplastic.

Autonomous hyperfunction is most commonly confined to the ovary but other endocrine involvement includes the thyroid (nodular hyperplasia with thyrotoxicosis), the adrenals (multiple hyperplastic nodules with Cushing syndrome), the pituitary (adenoma with gigantism, acromegaly or hyperprolactinemia) and the parathyroids (adenoma or hyperplasia with hyperparathyroidism). At least two of these features should be present for the diagnosis to be made. The condition, which is due to a somatic activating missense mutation in the gene encoding the α-subunit of the G-protein that stimulates cAMP production, is sporadic. The mutation results in a failure of phosphorylation of GTP to GDP and thereby constitutive activation. The mutation is somatic and individuals are chimeric for the condition, hence the variability of the phenotype.

Abnormal patterns of gonadotropin secretion

Premature thelarche

Thelarche means unilateral or bilateral breast development, often with a fluctuating degree of development. Premature thelarche may be present from infancy, usually occurs by the age of 2 years and its

onset is rare after the age of 4 years. It is not accompanied by other signs of puberty. Nipple development is unusual and estrogen-induced thickening and dulling of the vaginal mucosa or enlargement of the uterus on ultrasonography is uncommon. Growth velocity is normal and bone age is not advanced. It is usually benign and self-limiting and most cases regress 6 months to 6 years after diagnosis. Some girls do progress early into puberty.

Premature thelarche is typically associated with FSH secretion, antral follicular development and ovarian function that is greater than that of prepubertal control subjects. Unstimulated and GnRH-stimulated plasma levels of FSH are increased, whereas those of LH are prepubertal.

Thelarche variant

Variations of premature thelarche occur on a spectrum toward precocious puberty. Most cases of premature thelarche present in the first 2 years of life and regress before puberty. Children who present later may demonstrate continuing breast development, which may advance with accompanying growth acceleration and bone age advancement. The name given to this condition is thelarche variant or 'a slowly progressive variant of precocious puberty in girls'. The condition may result from a disorder of ovarian follicular maturation since ovarian volume exceeds the normal prepubertal size. Cyclical breast growth may be seen which does not resolve spontaneously. Pulsatile FSH-predominant gonadotropin secretion is intermediate between premature thelarche and GDPP; LH secretory profiles are more like those observed in normal puberty and, in some girls with a rapid but transient onset of estrogenization, suppress responsiveness to GnRH.

Primary hypothyroidism

In some patients with primary hypothyroidism, FSH concentrations are increased. Thyroid-stimulating hormone (TSH) has weak agonist properties at the human FSH receptor and ovarian stimulation results, with isolated breast development in girls. In boys, testicular enlargement without other secondary sexual characteristics may occur. There is no pubertal progression in the majority of cases, bone age is delayed and growth velocity poor. Sometimes normal gonadotropin-dependent puberty occurs at an inappropriately early age upon starting thyroxine replacement. The prognosis is excellent with reversal of puberty once treatment is commenced but final height may be affected if diagnosis is delayed or if normal puberty progresses at an early age.

Sexual precocity due to adrenal androgens

When signs of adrenarche (pubic and axillary hair, apocrine sweat and rapid growth) occur before the age of 8 years in girls and 9 years in boys, it has been called premature adrenarche or pubarche. The term is misleading in the sense that adrenarche is a physiological process which is not usually revealed by clinical signs other than a small increase in growth rate (the mid-childhood growth spurt).

The fetal adrenal gland secretes DHEA sulphate (DHEAS) which can manifest as pubic hair or clitoromegaly in infancy, especially in premature babies. CAH and virilizing adrenal tumors need to be excluded. Adrenal androgen concentrations diminish as the fetal adrenal zone regresses and appearances return to normal.

Signs of adrenarche are commoner in children from an Asian, Mediterranean or Afro-Caribbean background. An association with low birthweight has been described. In some studies, there appears to be an increased prevalence of minor defects of adrenal steroidogenesis, particularly when genital enlargement is present. In spite of the increase in height velocity and advance in bone age, final height is unaffected but there may be an increased prevalence of polycystic ovarian syndrome (PCOS) in the teenage years.

Congenital adrenal hyperplasia (see Chapter 6)

The classical form of CYP21 deficiency may present with salt loss, labioscrotal fusion and clitoromegaly in girls in the neonatal period. In boys who do not have the salt-losing form and, in some very virilized girls who are not diagnosed at birth and are raised as boys, presentation may be with tall stature, increased height velocity, advanced bone age, clitoromegaly in girls, genital maturation in the absence of testicular enlargement in boys and the development of pubic and axillary hair in both sexes. CYP11A deficiency presents in a similar way but with the additional complication of hypertension. These cases can be eliminated by neonatal screening for CAH.

The non-classical or late-onset form of CAH may present in childhood or adolescence with early pubic hair and acne or in early adulthood with menstrual irregularities, hirsutism or infertility. GDPP and the polycystic ovary syndrome are common sequelae. Final height is usually compromised. Virilization also occurs in undertreated children with CAH.

Approximately 5–10% of children with premature adrenarche are estimated to have late-onset CAH, although this estimate varies depending on the ethnicity of the population sampled. The adrenocorticotrophic hormone (ACTH) stimulation test can differentiate between children with late-onset CAH and precocious pubarche/premature adrenarche. Unstimulated and stimulated concentrations of 17α-hydroxypregnenolone (17PGN) and 17-OHP, DHEA and androstenedione are higher in children with premature adrenarche than in control subjects or those with non-classical 21-hydroxylase deficiency.

Adrenal tumors

The characteristic picture is a short history of virilization, accelerated growth rate and advanced bone age. Cushing syndrome may be present if there is hypersecretion of cortisol. DHEA, DHEAS and androstenedione are secreted in excess and there may be discordance between the first two. CT imaging of the adrenal glands should be performed.

Treatment involves surgical resection of the tumor, with the option of adjuvant chemotherapy. The prognosis is usually guarded and neither operative findings nor histology are of much help. The only factor influencing whether the lesion is likely to behave in a malignant manner or not is tumor size. Tumors less than 5 cm diameter are nearly always benign. An immediate fall in serum or urinary androgens is encouraging and adjuvant chemotherapy or radiotherapy has not been demonstrated to improve long-term prognosis. Adrenal tumors may be associated with syndromes of increased cancer risk (e.g. Li–Fraumeni syndrome).

Gonadal sex steroids

Gonadal tumors are rare tumors leading to sexual precocity. Pubertal development is not consonant and sex steroid concentrations are high, above the normal adult range. Leydig cell tumors of the testis are associated with virilization but conversion of testosterone to estradiol leads to gynecomastia. Granulosa cell and germ cell tumors of the ovary can secrete both androgens and estradiol.

Exogenous sex steroids can occasionally be the cause of sexual precocity. Hormones used in chicken rearing are occasionally implicated as a cause of 'epidemics' of premature thelarche, although the relationship is unproven.

Problems associated with sexual precocity

Growth
When puberty occurs abnormally early, the growth spurt will also take place early. GH concentrations and the increase in growth velocity are similar to those observed in normally timed puberty. Since the growth spurt has occurred early, insufficient childhood growth will have taken place, so the addition of the relatively fixed increment of approximately 30 cm that comes with puberty leads to restricted final height. Sex steroid exposure will result in rapid bone age advance, diminishing adult height potential in turn.

Psychological problems
These are often the major issue for children with sexual precocity and their families since sex steroid exposure in young children may result in disruptive behavior. The child looks older than their chronological age and most patients experience problems at school, which are compounded by the difficulties that teachers and fellow pupils have in understanding them. The child and his/her family may later have problems dealing with normally timed pubertal development and are frequently apprehensive about stopping suppressive treatment. In girls, menstruation at an early age presents practical difficulties.

Additionally, girls may be subject to sexual advances with which they are unable to deal, while boys may have embarrassing erections. Children with special educational needs as a result of a cerebral lesion or hydrocephalus are particularly vulnerable to these problems. Early maturity within the normal range correlates to some extent with an earlier onset of sexual behavior.

Clinical and diagnostic approach to sexual precocity

A careful history and clinical examination should be performed. Bone age should be determined. Most children presenting with sexual precocity do not require extensive investigation but sinister underlying causes for sexual precocity such as tumors should always be considered.

Imaging
All girls with early development of secondary sexual characteristics warrant a transabdominal pelvic ultrasound examination. In GDPP, the ovaries are active with multiple (>6) cysts that are greater than 4 mm in diameter (Fig. 4.6a). Larger cysts are sometimes seen in premature thelarche (<3 cysts), thelarche variant (3–6 cysts) (Fig. 4.6b) and MAS (Fig. 4.6c).

The first signs of estrogenization of the uterus is a change in shape from a tubular structure, where the diameter of the fundus and the cervix are similar, to a pear-shaped structure, where the fundus expands so that its diameter exceeds that of the cervix. In GDPP, the changes resemble those of normal puberty whereas, in premature thelarche or thelarche variant, the uterus remains prepubertal in shape. Endometrial thickening suggests that pubertal concentrations of estrogen have been attained but menarche does not occur until an endometrial thickness of around 6–8 mm has been attained.

When GDPP is treated, the uterus does not return to its prepubertal state, although the endometrium should remain thin. The ovaries may remain large for the child's age but the continuing development of large follicles indicates inadequate suppression. In children in whom an ovarian tumor is suspected, the pelvic ultrasound scan may be highly informative.

Neuroradiological imaging is mandatory if there are neurological signs. All boys with GDPP must have neuroradiological imaging because idiopathic GDPP is extremely uncommon. The need for neuroradiology

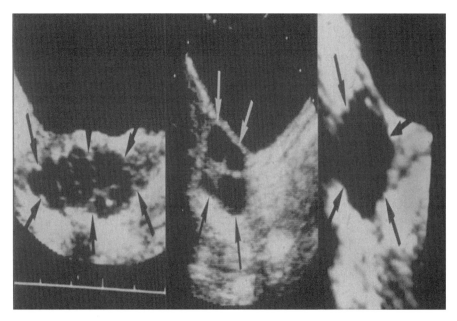

Figure 4.6 Pelvic ultrasound examinations of girls with (a) GDPP showing multicystic ovary characteristic of the effects of pulsatile gonadotropin secretion; (b) the ovary in thelarche variant with several large cysts and (c) the large single cyst present in MAS. Arrows outline ovarian structure. Marker bar depicts 1 cm intervals.

in girls is more contentious but is indicated in girls presenting under the age of 4 years.

If an adrenal tumor is suspected in patients with virilization, a CT or an MRI scan of the adrenal glands is indicated. Ultrasound scan of the adrenal glands is of limited use. In cases where MAS is suspected, a bone scan and skeletal survey are indicated.

Biochemistry

The combination of a GnRH stimulation test and measurement of serum concentrations of sex steroids is a useful start. This entails the administration of a single bolus of GnRH (2.5 mg/kg to a maximum of 100 mg) with measurement of plasma LH and FSH concentrations at 0, 20 and 60 min or leuprolide acetate (20 μg/kg, maximum 500 μg) with measurements of LH and FSH at 0, 60, 120 and 180 min. Normal prepubertal children have an increment of 3–4 IU/L LH and 2–3 IU/L FSH. The increment is greater in puberty, regardless of age, although the cutoffs vary depending upon the assay.

In GDPP, a pubertal LH-dominant response is observed whereas, in GIPP and sexual precocity secondary to gonadal tumors or ovarian cyst formation, gonadotropin concentrations are suppressed by the autonomous sex steroid secretion. The response to GnRH in precocious adrenarche is prepubertal. In premature thelarche, FSH tends to be dominant while, in thelarche variant, response is intermediate between thelarche and GDPP with FSH predominating.

In children with virilization, unstimulated plasma 17-OHP concentrations that are elevated suggest a diagnosis of CAH. The response to ACTH (synacthen or Cortrosyn) with measurement of plasma 17-OHP will confirm the diagnosis. Rapid virilization suggests the presence of an endocrine-secreting neoplasm. Testosterone, dihydrotestosterone, DHEAS and androstenedione are all elevated in adrenal virilizing tumors. Plasma cortisol may also be elevated with a loss of the normal circadian rhythm if Cushing syndrome is a feature. There is a failure of suppression in response to dexamethasone if an adrenal tumor is present, whereas in premature adrenarche and CAH, dexamethasone administration will lead to suppression of adrenal steroids. A urinary steroid profile is also of considerable diagnostic value if an adrenal tumor is suspected.

A raised serum hCG level suggests an hCG-secreting neoplasm. The response to GnRH will be prepubertal. Thyroid function tests to exclude primary hypothyroidism should be undertaken in a girl with premature thelarche or a boy with enlargement of the testes in the face of a lack of virilization combined with short stature, a poor growth velocity and delayed bone age.

Treatment

General

Adrenarche, thelarche and thelarche variant do not require treatment. Hypothyroidism is treated with a cautious introduction of thyroxine with subsequent increase to standard maintenance doses. Non-classical CAH is treated with hydrocortisone and fludrocortisone if indicated by a raised plasma renin concentration. Although some groups suggest that the condition should not be treated, lack of treatment may compromise final height and fertility.

An abnormality underlying GDPP or GIPP needs treatment. The decision to treat precocious puberty *per se* is based on several factors such as the age of onset, the rate of progression of puberty and the emotional impact of experiencing early puberty. Not all children with precocious puberty require treatment to suppress gonadotropin secretion. Indications for therapy include the avoidance or amelioration of the psychological consequences of early puberty, with particular emphasis on menarche in young girls, initial tall stature with its attendant problem of unrealistic expectations by adults and an increased risk of sexual abuse.

In girls with untreated idiopathic GDPP, a mean final height of 151–155 cm is not uncommon, whereas in boys, limited data suggest a greater restriction in final height. Slowly progressive forms of precocious puberty have been described which impact little on final height as the majority of these patients achieve their genetic target heights without intervention.

Treatment will halt pubertal progress and the pubertal growth spurt but significant regression of the signs of sexual precocity does not usually occur, although there may be a reduction of breast size and cessation of menses in girls and of testicular volume in boys. Aggressive behavior is reduced, as is the number of erections in boys. The shape of the uterus does not revert to the prepubertal form.

Gonadotropin-dependent precocious puberty

Progestational agents have been used for the treatment of patients with precocious puberty. Cyproterone acetate is a peripherally acting anti-androgen with some progestogenic and glucocorticoid actions, suppressing both gonadotropin and gonadal steroid secretion.

It was effective in halting the progress of the physical features of puberty and useful in suppressing menstruation but had no effect on final height. Cyproterone is not available in the USA.

More complete suppression of the hypothalamo-pituitary–gonadal axis results from the action of continuous exposure of the GnRH receptor to its ligand. GnRHa are synthetic analogs with a D-tryptophan inserted instead of the naturally occurring L-form to increase the duration of receptor occupancy. This results initially in stimulation followed by receptor downregulation and cessation of gonadotropin secretion. Later in the course of treatment, receptor levels return to normal but desensitization persists because of an uncoupling of the receptor from the intracellular signaling effector pathway. Synthetic depot preparations of GnRHa administered subcutaneously on a once monthly or quarterly basis are available with enhanced activity and a longer half-life than natural GnRH.

Gonadal suppression is observed in most children treated with GnRHa. It has been suggested that the response to treatment is best monitored by measuring basal sex steroid concentrations and peak plasma LH concentrations following a GnRH test but, in clinical practice, because the suppression is so complete, assessment of pubertal stage, height velocity, skeletal maturation and pelvic ultrasound scan is often sufficient for monitoring the response. The depot preparations are more effective in suppressing height velocity and bone maturation than the intranasal preparations, which need to be administered thrice daily. Initial stimulatory effects can be prevented by the use of cyproterone acetate in conjunction with the GnRHa over the first 4–6 weeks at a dose of 50 mg/m^2/day. If the endometrium is thickened, vaginal bleeding may occur at the start of treatment as a result of estrogen withdrawal and can usually (but not always) be prevented by the administration of cyproterone.

Although it has been suggested that treatment with GnRHa improves final adult height, the evidence points more to the age at the onset of treatment as the crucial factor, with a more clearcut effect in younger children. Data on final height suggest that treatment with GnRHa analogs and cyproterone acetate cannot recover lost height potential and children cannot attain their target mid-parental height. This is because of the imposition of pubertal growth on an inadequate childhood stature. Unfortunately, the growth spurt suppressed by treatment does not resume when treatment is stopped.

Children with precocious puberty have higher circulating concentrations of GH and IGF-I than controls of a similar chronological age. Treatment with GnRHa may lead to a fall in circulating GH and IGF-I concentrations with a consequent reduction in growth velocity. It has been suggested that a combination of GH and GnRHa may result in an increase in final height. Although the combination treatment leads to an increase in height velocity and height standard deviation score for bone age and in predicted adult height in girls with precocious puberty, there are limited data to support a similar increase in final height.

There are a number of published studies examining the effects of treatment with cyproterone acetate or GnRHa with or without hGH on final height in children with GDPP. Ideally, the comparison of the final height of a group of treated children with GDPP with that of a well-matched untreated control group in a randomized double-blind study would be the most meaningful method for determining the efficacy of treatment on final height. Most studies are small in size and use final height-predicted height as the arbiter of efficacy.

Using predicted height creates its own problems because there is an increase in height prediction with time in untreated girls with GDPP. Also, the accuracy of final height prediction is poor in children with abnormal growth patterns, including untreated precocious puberty. Bayley–Pinneau predictions are more accurate than other methods in precocious puberty but the Bayley–Pinneau method for height prediction can overestimate final height, particularly in children who have a greatly advanced bone age for chronological age or who have a bone age greater than 7 years. They are not applicable to the younger cohort where any likely effect will be maximal but in whom height predictions are the most inaccurate.

GnRHa treatment is safe and well tolerated but withdrawal of sex steroids due to GnRHa results in a reduction in BMD, although there are no long-term data on how this translates into long-term bone health. Sex steroid withdrawal in children can result in menopausal symptoms, such as hot flushes and mood swings, occasionally necessitating low-dose estrogen therapy. Cyproterone is used less frequently in the treatment of GDPP because of ACTH and adrenal suppression. Additionally, there is a risk of hepatocellular carcinoma.

Gonadotropin-independent precocious puberty

Affected individuals do not exhibit a pubertal LH response to GnRH administration or a pubertal pattern of pulsatile LH secretion so they do not respond to GnRHa. The treatment of GIPP is difficult: testolactone, spironolactone, ketoconazole, flutamide, cyproterone and medroxyprogesterone acetate have been used. Testolactone inhibits those functions of testosterone that are dependent upon its conversion to estrogen by acting as an inhibitor of aromatase. Spironolactone acts as an anti-androgen. Ketoconazole inhibits cytochrome P450c17, which regulates 17-hydroxylation. It therefore suppresses both gonadal and adrenal steroid biosynthesis and is effective in halting pubertal progress, albeit in doses much higher than those used for its antifungal action. It can lead to adrenal insufficiency and, occasionally, to severe hepatic dysfunction. The use of the anti-androgen flutamide is, at best, anecdotal. Cyproterone remains the drug of choice in the majority of cases of GIPP.

Stopping treatment and long-term follow-up

For psychological reasons, treatment should be stopped once the child has reached an age where puberty is acceptable. There is no evidence that longer treatment improves final height. Since hypothalamic maturity is not affected by treatment, pubertal development is recommenced at an advanced stage approximately 3 months later. Gonadotropin secretion recommences approximately 4 months after cessation of depot GnRHa and most girls menstruate within 1 year of stopping treatment. Normal fertility has been documented in girls with both treated and untreated GDPP.

Children with GIPP have been reported to experience centrally mediated puberty at an appropriate time, although the abnormal gonadal activation continues into adult life in MAS and may result in irregular menses and fertility problems.

Delayed puberty

Temporary delay in sexual maturation is not uncommon and resolves with time leading to normal

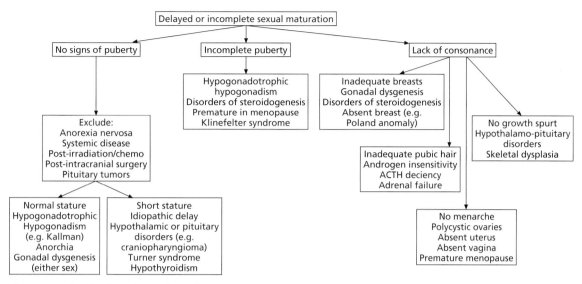

Figure 4.7 Algorithm for evaluating late puberty.

development, optimum final height and fertility. By temporary is meant not much longer than 6 months in any one stage of puberty because, in patients with an underlying organic pathology, early diagnosis and treatment are essential to insure normal pubertal progress and adequate final height. An algorithm is depicted in Fig. 4.7.

Assessment should include a history of symptoms of chronic illness, medications, symptoms suggestive of other hormone deficit or excess, previous treatment or surgery, abnormal eating patterns and a history of the family, including parental heights and ages at onset of puberty. Chronic illness is often associated with delayed puberty, particularly asthma (and/or its treatment), eczema, cystic fibrosis and inflammatory bowel disease.

The majority of those that present with idiopathic delayed puberty are boys, more often because of their short stature than the delay in sexual development. Delay is unusual in girls and should prompt a systematic search especially to include Turner syndrome, eating issues and intense exercise programs.

Examination should include details of present and past heights and weights with pubertal staging. Testicular size should be measured using the Prader orchidometer. Careful documentation for body disproportion with estimation of the upper and lower body segments may suggest Klinefelter syndrome.

Patients with classical XO Turner syndrome are short, have a low hairline, webbing of the neck, prominent ears, broad chest, renal and cardiac abnormalities with streak gonads but presenting features may be more subtle and may be missed, particularly in patients with mosaicism.

Other dysmorphic features may reveal multisystem syndromes, such as CHARGE, Prader–Willi or septo-optic dysplasia. Neurological examination should be performed to include visual field deficits, sense of smell and fundoscopy. Anosmia is suggestive of Kallman syndrome.

Initial investigations should include an estimate of skeletal age in order to calculate a predicted adult height range and its relation to the genetic potential (mid-parental height). Further investigations and management should depend on the skeletal age, stature, symptoms and extent of delay. Laboratory measurement of serum FSH and LH concentrations will help to differentiate patients with hypergonadotrophic hypogonadism (Fig. 4.8).

Serum gonadotropin concentrations are low in all normal children before puberty and caution must be exercised in the interpretation of low serum gonadotropin concentrations especially below the age of 12 years. GnRH stimulation tests rarely clarify whether an individual will progress in puberty or has a permanent defect. Overnight sampling may

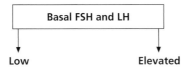

```
                    ┌─────────────────────┐
                    │   Basal FSH and LH  │
                    └─────────────────────┘
                     │                   │
                     ▼                   ▼
                    Low               Elevated
```

Bone age delay
    Constitutional delay of
    growth and puberty
Investigations for reversible conditions
    Thyroid function tests
    Chronic illnesses
    Eating pattern
Evaluate sense of smell
    Kallman syndrome
LHRH test +/− HCG test (males)
MRI scan of pituitary gland
Trial of treatment

Serum autoantibodies
    Autoimmune disease
Karyotype
    Turner syndrome
    Klinefelter syndrome
    XY gonadal dysgenesis
    Androgen insensitivity syndrome

Figure 4.8 Conditions of pubertal delay associated with high and low gonadotropin concentrations.

demonstrate gonadotropin pulsatility but is unhelpful for prognosis. Pelvic ultrasound examination is helpful in girls, where it may reveal the multicystic pattern classical of early puberty.

Differential diagnosis

Constitutional delay in puberty

This is the commonest cause of delayed sexual maturation, especially in boys. In addition to delayed puberty, it is characterized by short stature that is appropriate when skeletal age is taken into account. Growth velocity is normal for a prepubertal individual. As a rule, mean height velocity is 5 cm/year at 12 years of age and declines at a rate of 1 cm/year for every year thereafter that puberty is not entered. The variance on this is ±1 cm/year. Constitutional delay is often familial and has an excellent long-term prognosis. Patients have low serum gonadotropins, as do patients with gonadotropin deficiency.

The rules on growth rate are important and can help to prevent unnecessary investigation of the GH axis. Unless priming of the system is undertaken with sex steroids, low GH secretion may be documented and GH therapy instigated.

Individuals with pubertal delay can experience social difficulties and, in these patients, treatment with oxandrolone, a weak non-aromatizable androgen, in doses of 2.5 mg once daily orally for 3–6 months, improves growth velocity without advancing skeletal maturation or pubertal progress. Sex steroids in small doses for about 6 months will induce puberty that will progress spontaneously, leading to normal sexual development and final height.

Hypogonadotrophic hypogonadism (Table 4.4)

This is defined as a permanent absence of spontaneous pubertal development due to a lack of serum gonadotropin production or action. The deficiency may be isolated or associated with combined pituitary hormone deficiencies, congenital or acquired. Isolated gonadotropin deficiency can be idiopathic or part of X-linked Kallman syndrome associated with anosmia, in association with X-linked adrenal hypoplasia or X-linked ichthyosis.

Acquired gonadotropin deficiency may be due to intracranial trauma, tumors, surgery or radiotherapy. Hemosiderosis associated with transfusion can result in permanent gonadotropin deficiency.

The condition in boys is best diagnosed or rather excluded by a GnRH test in combination with an hCG test to stimulate the testicular release of testosterone. There is no comparable test for girls. In many cases, it is necessary to rule out other pituitary hormone deficiencies and to perform neuroimaging of the hypothalamus and pituitary gland. In some cases, the interpretation of the GnRH test is not straightforward and endocrine reassessment may be necessary at a later time after completion of growth and puberty to ascertain the need for long-term replacement.

Table 4.4 Causes of hypogonadotropic hypogonadism.

Developmental and genetic causes	Pituitary tumors
Kallmann syndrome (HH and anosmia): X-linked (*KAL*), AD, AR	Langerhans cell histiocytosis
Impaired GnRH release and action (e.g. *leptin, leptin R, PC1, GnRHR*)	Post infection
	Granulomatous disorders
Multiple pituitary hormone deficiency (e.g. *HESX1, LHX3, PROP1*)	Vascular malformations
Isolated gonadotrophin defic	Trauma/pituitary stalk transection
iency	Cranial irradiation
Isolated LH deficiency/mutation	
Congenital glycosylation disorders	**Functional causes**
Effects on multiple levels of the HPG axis (e.g. *DAX1, SF1*)	Chronic renal disease
Midline defects	Chronic gastrointestinal disease/malnutrition
	Sickle cell disease/iron overload
Chromosomal abnormalities	Chronic lung disease/cystic fibrosis/asthma
Deletions and rearrangements	Acquired immune deficiency syndrome
	Poorly controlled diabetes mellitus
Syndromic associations	Hypothyroidism
Prader–Willi syndrome	Cushing disease
Laurence–Moon syndrome	Hyperprolactinemia
Gordon–Holmes spinocerebellar ataxia	Metabolic conditions (e.g. Gaucher disease)
CHARGE	Anorexia nervosa
Others	Bulimia nervosa
	Psychogenic/stress
Physical causes	Extreme exercise
CNS tumors	Drugs
Craniopharyngioma, germinoma, hypothalamic glioma, optic nerve glioma	

Hypergonadotrophic hypogonadism (Table 4.5)

Elevated serum gonadotropin concentrations in the absence of pubertal signs may suggest gonadal insufficiency. Radiotherapy, chemotherapy and surgery, particularly orchidopexy for very high placed testes, can all result in gonadal failure.

Turner syndrome (1 in 2500 live female births) should be considered in all short girls, even in the presence of pubertal signs. Patients with Turner syndrome may show markedly elevated serum gonadotropin concentrations from as early as 8–9 years of age due to lack of negative feedback. Pure XX and XY gonadal dysgenesis both present with delayed puberty, raised serum gonadotropins and low sex steroid concentrations. The XY gonadal dysgenesis group reared as females have a high risk of gonadal tumors and need surgery for the removal of the gonads. Gonadal failure in females is also associated with autoimmune ovarian failure, which may be associated with autoimmune polyendocrinopathy syndrome or galactosemia.

In boys, tall stature, pubertal delay and learning difficulties are the classic features associated with Klinefelter syndrome (47XXY). The learning difficulties may be mild and the stature not excessive. Many patients enter puberty but rarely progress beyond 8 mL testicular volumes. The pubertal appearance is discordance between the genital and pubic hair stages and the small testes. The early introduction of testosterone prevents gynecomastia. Other causes in boys include anorchia, torsion or infection.

Treatment

Treatment should be instituted at an appropriate age. There is no advantage in delaying puberty in terms of adult stature because the magnitude of pubertal growth diminishes with advancing age and psychosocial problems are exacerbated by delay. Patients with constitutional delay, chronic illnesses or eating disorders need small amounts of either testosterone or ethinylestradiol for not more than 4–6 months, although a repeat course is sometimes necessary. This results in

Table 4.5 Causes of hypergonadotropic hypogonadism.

Girls

Chromosomal abnormalities
Turner syndrome and variants (e.g. 45,X; 46,XX/45,X; X chromosome abnormalities)
Mixed gonadal dysgenesis (e.g. 46,XY/45,X)
Deletions and rearrangements (e.g. Xq22, Xq26-28)

Abnormalities in gonadal development
Ovarian dysgenesis

Syndromic associations
Perrault, Maximilian, Quayle and Copeland, Pober, Malouf syndromes
Ataxia telangiectasia, Nijmegen, Cockayne, Rothmund–Thompson, Werner syndromes
Bletharophimosis–ptosis–epicanthus syndrome (BPES, *FOXL2*)

Disorders of steroid synthesis and action
LH resistance
FSH resistance
Pseudohypoparathyroidism 1a
SF1, StAR, CYP11a, HSD3B2, Cyp17, aromatase (CYP19) (46,XX karyotype)
HSD17B2, AIS, SRD5A2 (46,XY karyotype)

Other causes of primary ovarian failure
Autoimmune (e.g. AIRE)
Metabolic (e.g. galactosemia, storage disorders)
Hyperandrogenism/polycystic ovarian syndrome

Pelvic/spinal irradiation
Chemotherapy

Boys
Chromosomal causes
Klinefelter syndrome and variants (e.g. 47,XXY; 46,XY/47,XXY)
Mixed gonadal dysgenesis (e.g. 46,XY/45,X)
Deletions and rearrangements

Abnormalities in gonadal development
Testicular dysgenesis (e.g. loss of functional Sry, Sox9, SF1, WT1, DMRT)

Syndromic associations
Noonan syndrome
Robinow syndrome
Others

Disorders of steroid synthesis and action
LH resistance (e.g. *LHR*, *GNAS*)
SF1, StAR, CYP11a, HSD3B2, HSD17B2, PAIS

Other causes of primary testicular (Leydig cell) failure
Anorchia
Cryptorchidism
Sertoli cell only syndrome
Testicular irradiation
Chemotherapy
Infection (e.g. mumps)

triggering endogenous sex steroid production that will sustain further development. Patients with organic causes need lifelong sex steroid replacement but treatment should allow the patient to progress at a normal rate. Suggested dosage schedules are shown in Table 4.6. Patients with Turner syndrome may require GH and/or oxandrolone treatment in addition to achieve adequate final height and bone mass.

Anorchic males and those with hypogonadotrophic states need to be informed about testicular prostheses for cosmetic and psychological reasons. This is best undertaken with silastic implants as a one-stage procedure in the middle to later stages of puberty, when the scrotum is large enough to accommodate the prostheses. Fertility options in both sexes include sperm or ova donation or adoption. Pregnancy rates of *in vitro* fertilization with ovum donation in girls with Turner syndrome have been reported at 20–25%

but adequate uterine growth during a slow induction of puberty plays an important role in success.

Pulsatile subcutaneous GnRH has been used successfully to induce puberty, with a pattern of administration to mimic normal puberty.

Recombinant FSH allows testicular growth and possibly spermatogenesis, although the lack of the postnatal FSH surge may be a key factor in determining success in hypogonadotrophic hypogonadism.

Since delay in puberty is often associated with short stature, it can lead to bullying in school. Although early treatment does not alter long-term effects on height or puberty, a delay in treatment can lead to difficulties in interpersonal relationships and disturbed psychosocial adjustment, especially during the period of delay. The outcome in untreated individuals is not different from those with a normal timing of puberty but most volunteer that they would have preferred earlier intervention.

Table 4.6 Treatment regimens for pubertal induction.

Males	Females
Induction	*Induction*
Depot testosterone (intramuscularly)	Ethinylestradiol (orally)
25–50 mg every 4–6 weeks	2 μg daily for 6 months
100 mg every 4 weeks	5 μg daily for 6 months
200–250 mg every 4 weeks	10 μg daily for 6 months
	15 μg daily for 6 months
Adult replacement	Progesterone
Adult dosage (250 mg every 2–4 weeks) or	Started with the onset of
Transdermal scrotal patches	breakthrough bleeding or
	when ethinylestrogen dosage is 15–20 μg
	Adult replacement
	Ethinylestradiol 20–30 μg daily with cyclic
	progesterone treatment
	Oral contraceptive pill
	Transdermal patches

Poor bone mineralization as a result of suboptimal therapy may result in bone fractures and osteoporosis. There are inconclusive data that delayed puberty can result in permanent loss of bone mass.

Gynecological problems of puberty

Menstrual dysfunction

Menstrual disorders in adolescent girls are thought to be common, but the incidence is unknown because teenagers are loath to present due to embarrassment as well as lack of knowledge of what is normal and of potential treatment options. Presentation with a menstrual disorder may disguise other worries such as contraception, sexually transmitted infection or pregnancy. Vaginal examination should be performed only in consenting adolescents who are sexually active and only when it is likely to add value to the assessment.

Menorrhagia

Troublesome periods may be too frequent, irregular and/or heavy. A menstrual diary may be helpful for reassurance and explanation of the extent of normal variation. In most girls in the early months following menarche, the commonest cause is anovulatory cycles. The menstrual cycle then becomes irregular and late periods may be prolonged. Cystic glandular hyperplasia of the endometrium has been reported, but the incidence is rare. These symptoms can be regarded as normal for the first 2 years while the hypothalamic–pituitary–ovarian axis matures to establish regular cycles. A very small number of girls require hospital admission with severe and profuse bleeding causing cardiovascular compromise and severe anemia.

Acquired and congenital bleeding disorders are relatively common causes of menorrhagia and may account for 10–15% of cases. Conditions such as Von Willebrand disease and immune thrombocytopenic purpura should be excluded in any girl with severe menorrhagia refractory to simple treatments. An ultrasound scan rarely shows pathology.

Treatments include the use of antifibrinolytic drugs such as tranexamic acid, which is effective in reducing blood loss but does not make cycles more regular. Cyclical progestagens are widely used, although their efficacy is poorly established. In order to be effective, progesterone needs to be given for 21 days each month rather than just during the luteal phase, as has been traditional. Disadvantages can include acne and hirsutism with norethisterone, which may interfere with compliance. The mainstay of treatment is the combined oral contraceptive pill, which reduces blood loss and regulates the cycle length.

Dysmenorrhea

Pain during menstruation may have a significant impact on schooling and examination performance. Early periods may often be pain free, and the advent of pain usually coincides with the establishment of regular ovulatory cycles. Pain is attributed to higher levels of prostaglandins, and so anti-prostaglandin drugs such as mefenamic acid can be helpful. Suppression of ovulation with the combined oral contraceptive pill is very effective.

Girls who fail to respond to these measures need further evaluation. Dysmenorrhea can be associated with obstruction of the lower genital tract. A double uterus may have one uterine horn that is non-communicating and becomes obstructed causing worsening pain each month. The girl is usually found to have a large pelvic mass clinically and on ultrasound. The anatomy may be complex, and pelvic MRI is usually required before planning treatment. Treatment is surgical, but removal of an obstructed horn can usually be accomplished laparoscopically.

Endometriosis is a recognized cause of dysmenorrhea and is not a condition restricted to adult women. Some 38% of adolescents presenting with chronic pelvic pain have endometriosis. If pelvic pain is refractory to non-steroidal anti-inflammatory drugs and the oral contraceptive, a diagnostic laparoscopy is indicated. Treatment options are currently as for adult women with a combination of surgical and drug treatment. Psychological support and contact with similarly affected adolescents are thought to be of benefit.

Imperforate vagina

Obstruction to the vagina can prevent the escape of menstrual flow. This causes worsening cyclical pain and a pelvic mass due to hematocolpos. The obstruction most commonly occurs at the junction of the lower third of the vagina, at the level of the hymen. It may be possible to visualize a bulging hymenal membrane, once the labia are gently parted. Ultrasound can confirm the diagnosis. Resection of the obstructing membrane will release the blockage and allow further normal menstruation.

In very rare cases, the obstruction may be due to a transverse vaginal septum. If the septum is thin and low, it may be possible to resect from below, but care must be taken to insure the whole septum is removed to prevent contracture. If the septum is thicker and higher in the vagina, a combined abdominal and perineal approach is needed. It may be possible to remove the septum and anastamose the proximal and distal vagina, but sometimes the distance is too great and must be bridged by a skin graft or section of bowel.

Rokitansky syndrome

Approximately 1 in 5000 girls are born with congenital absence of the uterus and some or all of the vagina, the Rokitansky or Mayer–Rokitansky–Kuster–Hauser (MRKH) syndrome. The clinical spectrum is poorly documented, but patients may frequently have other developmental disorders outside the genital tract; 30–40% of patients have ectopic kidney, renal agenesis, horseshoe kidney and abnormal collecting ducts; 12% have skeletal anomalies, mostly involving the spine. Some fit into other known syndromes such as Müllerian–renal–cervicothoracic somite (MURCS) association, McCusick–Kaufman syndrome, Bardet–Biedl syndrome, Frasier syndrome and Klippel–Feil syndrome.

There is little agreement about the etiology, clinical syndromes and natural history of this syndrome. Its pathogenesis is unknown, and it is unclear whether normal vaginal and Müllerian structures failed to develop, whether development was arrested at some point, or whether destruction of developed structures occurred, e.g. through inappropriate apoptosis. The embryological development of the vagina and Müllerian structures is poorly understood, especially with regard to the proportion of the vagina derived from the urogenital sinus or the Müllerian duct. This leads to difficulty predicting etiological factors in the abnormal development of these structures. At present, there are no well-recognized etiologies for Rokitansky syndrome.

The most common presentation is with primary amenorrhea in the presence of otherwise normal pubertal development. The function of the hypothalamo-pituitary–ovarian axis is normal; FSH, LH and estrogen levels are normal and the karyotype is 46XX. On examination, the vagina will be blind ending and is likely to be short. Ultrasound will confirm the presence of ovaries, but no uterus will be demonstrated. Pelvic ultrasound is not easy in children, and it is not uncommon for a scan to report vestigial uterine tissue with no endometrium when the uterus is actually absent. MRI may add more information. There is no indication for routine laparoscopy or ovarian biopsy in this group of patients.

Treatment options focus on psychology and on the creation of a vagina comfortable for penetrative intercourse. There is currently no treatment available to transplant or create a uterus. Women with MRKH syndrome may have their own genetic children, using retrieval of ova, assisted conception techniques and a surrogate mother. Such a pathway is set with difficulties and may prove too costly in financial and emotional terms for many women.

The discovery of an absent vagina or uterus is a devastating event for a teenage girl and her family. There are few data available looking at the psychological impact of a diagnosis of Rokitansky syndrome. Input from a clinical psychologist experienced in the area is essential. The treatment of choice in creating a vagina sufficient for intercourse consists of using plastic dilator molds to stretch the vaginal area. This is thought to be successful in about 85% of women, although there is little information on compliance or subsequent sexual function. Ideally, dilation should be practiced at least once daily for 3–6 months in order to optimize success. At present, there have been no prospective studies of the impact of vaginal hypoplasia interventions on sexual function. In cases where dilators are unsuccessful or where compliance is difficult, newer techniques such as the laparoscopic Vecchietti or Davidov procedures may be more acceptable and equally as effective as the traditional vaginoplasty with skin grafting or intestinal replacement.

Complete androgen insensitivity syndrome

Intersex conditions such as complete androgen insensitivity syndrome (CAIS) may also present with primary amenorrhea in the presence of normal breast development (see Chapter 2). Treatment of the short vagina is as above.

Polycystic ovary syndrome

PCOS is common and diagnosed with increasing frequency in adolescent girls. Polycystic ovaries are found in about 25% of normal women and are usually asymptomatic but PCOS, which includes hyperandrogenicity, can be responsible for irregular cycles and episodes of secondary (or rarely primary) amenorrhea. Sometimes, but not always, there will be accompanying weight gain, acne and hirsutism.

Classically, the LH will be higher than FSH, with a 3:1 ratio. Testosterone may be at the higher end of normal and, in such a situation, it is worth checking the concentration of 17-hydroxyprogesterone to exclude CAH. Estrogen values are normal. Ultrasound shows a densely thickened ovarian stroma, with a 'chain' of follicles around the edge of the ovary.

Treatment of PCOS is not simple but, at least in adolescence, fertility is not the prime object. In overweight teenagers, weight loss and exercise must be addressed. A change in lifestyle may be all that is needed for symptom improvement. Long-term associations such as diabetes are more common in the obese, and acanthosis nigricans may be a pointer to this. Other treatments depend upon the most troublesome symptoms. Periods may be regulated with the oral contraceptive pill. All combined pills help with skin problems to some extent, but the addition of an anti-androgen is particularly helpful with hirsutism. Yasmin, a newer combined contraceptive pill containing ethinylestradiol and drospirenone, is also useful. Metformin is used in PCOS to increase insulin sensitivity. Several studies have confirmed its efficacy in menstrual regulation and fertility. Metformin is most effective in obese women, but there is little information on its use in adolescent girls. It is appropriate for those unable or unwilling to take the oral contraceptive pill.

5 The Thyroid Gland

Learning Points

- Thyroid diseases are commoner in females than males
- The onset of hypothyroidism is often insidious
- Acquired hypothyroidism is usually autoimmune in nature
- The diagnosis of primary hypothyroidism is made by finding low concentrations of thyroid hormones with (usually) elevated TSH
- In contrast to congenital hypothyroidism, rapid institution of thyroxine replacement is not essential
- Hyperthyroidism is a disabling condition of insidious onset in children

- Diagnosis is made by finding elevated concentrations of thyroid hormones with suppressed TSH
- Treatment modalities are medical, surgical or with radioactive iodine
- Fine-needle aspiration biopsy and ultrasound are useful in the evaluation of thyroid nodules
- Benign thyroid nodules and cysts should be removed
- Thyroid cancer requires total thyroidectomy with or without radioablation

Thyroid dysfunction affects growth and development in infancy and childhood but also results in the metabolic abnormalities found in adults. Because thyroid hormone-dependent effects on tissue maturation are developmentally regulated and organ or tissue specific, the clinical consequences of thyroid dysfunction depend on the age of the infant or child.

Untreated hypothyroidism in the fetus or newborn infant results in permanent abnormalities in intellectual and/or neurological function (see Chapter 2). After the age of 3 years, when most thyroid hormone-dependent brain development is complete, hypothyroidism results in slow growth and delayed skeletal maturation but there is usually no permanent effect on cognitive or neurological development.

Handbook of Clinical Pediatric Endocrinology, 1st edition. By Charles G. D. Brook and Rosalind S. Brown. Published 2008 by Blackwell Publishing, ISBN: 978-1- 4501-6109-1.

Thyroid hormonogenesis

Thyroid hormones are secreted by follicles composed of two types of cells surrounding a central colloid core. The follicular cells are interspersed with calcitonin-secreting parafollicular C-cells. A basal membrane surrounds the follicle and separates it from surrounding blood and lymphatic vessels and nerve terminals. The major constituent of the colloid is thyroglobulin (Tg), a large iodinated, dimeric glycoprotein that functions as a thyroid hormone precursor and permits storage of iodine and iodinated tyrosyl residues.

The synthesis and secretion of thyroid hormone include a series of events, each proceeding simultaneously in the same cell. Dietary iodine is converted to iodide in the gut and concentrated 20–40 times in the thyroid by an active transport mechanism. Iodide transport into the lumen is facilitated by a transporter encoded by pendrin (PDS), a gene on chromosome 7q.

Tg, synthesized at the same time within the follicular cell, undergoes a number of post-translational steps to attain its tertiary and quaternary structure. Tg is transported by exocytosis into the follicular lumen (colloid) to form the backbone for a series of reactions that result in the oxidation of I_2 to an active intermediate and the iodination of tyrosyl residues ('organification') to form monoiodotyrosine (MIT) and diiodotyrosine (DIT). Iodide oxidation and organification are both catalyzed by thyroid peroxidase (TPO), which also catalyzes the coupling of iodotyrosines within the Tg molecule to form triiodothyronine (T_3) and tetraiodothyronine or thyroxine (T_4). T_3 is formed by the coupling of one DIT and one MIT molecule; the coupling of two molecules of DIT results in T_4. Iodination requires hydrogen peroxide, the generation of which is regulated partly by thyroid oxidase.

Thyroid hormones stored in colloid are released into the circulation by a series of steps: initially they are incorporated into the apical surface of the follicular cell by endocytosis. The ingested colloid droplets fuse with apically streaming proteolytic enzyme-containing lysosomes to form phagolysosomes, in which Tg hydrolysis occurs. The freed MIT, DIT, T_3, and T_4 within the phagolysosomes are then released into the follicular cells. T_3 and T_4 released in this way diffuse from the thyroid follicular cell into the thyroid capillary blood. The released MIT and DIT are deiodinated by a deiodinase, the iodide reentering the intracellular iodide pool to be reutilized for new hormone synthesis. Deiodination of T_4 to generate T_3 is a second source of T_3 within the thyroid.

Regulation of thyroid function

Thyrotrophin
The major regulator of thyroid function is thyrotrophin-stimulating hormone (TSH); secretion is under positive feedback control by hypothalamic TSH-releasing hormone (TRH) synthesized in the hypothalamus and transported to the pituitary via the pituitary portal vascular system. TSH secretion is under negative feedback control by thyroid hormone acting at hypothalamic and pituitary levels. Dopamine, somatostatin and high doses of corticosteroids inhibit release of TSH. Decreasing environmental and/or body temperature increases TRH release. TSH stimulates thyroid

gland function and growth by binding to a receptor located on the basal plasma membrane.

Iodide
Adequate dietary iodine is a critical regulator of thyroid gland function through adaptive mechanisms that respond to deficiency or excess. The normal daily requirement of iodine is 150 mg for adults (200 mg for pregnant women), 90 mg for infants and children and 40 mg for premature infants.

In iodine deficiency, there is increased trapping of iodide and increased TSH secretion that stimulates thyrocyte proliferation and hormonogenesis. Tg secretion is increased but, because of the reduced iodine content, there is preferential synthesis and secretion of MIT and T_3 compared with DIT and T_4. Iodine deficiency also results in increased peripheral conversion of T_4 to T_3. The reverse is true in the presence of iodine excess.

Excess iodine inhibits organification of iodide and subsequent hormone synthesis (the Wolff–Chaikoff effect), Tg synthesis, hormone release and thyroid growth. Under normal circumstances, iodide-induced inhibition is transient and normal hormone synthesis resumes.

Thyroid hormone transport

T_4 and T_3 released into the circulation are transported to their target cell with binding proteins produced in the liver. They include thyroxine-binding globulin (TBG), transthyretin and albumin. TBG, although the least abundant, is the most important carrier protein for T_4. Transthyretin binds T_4 but not T_3 and appears to play a role in T_4 transport into the brain. In the euthyroid steady state, almost all circulating thyroid hormone is bound to protein. Transport proteins function as an extrathyroidal storage pool of thyroid hormone that enables the release of free hormone on demand while at the same time protecting tissues from excessive hormone. They are not essential for normal thyroid function.

Thyroid hormone metabolism

Thyroid hormone synthesized and secreted by the thyroid gland is activated and inactivated by a series of monodeiodination steps in target tissues. Sulfation is particularly important in the fetus. By contrast to T_4, the sole source of which is the thyroid gland, only 20% of circulating T_3 is derived by coupling of tyrosyl residues within the thyroid gland itself. The remainder is derived from the peripheral conversion of T_4 to T_3 in liver, kidney, brain and pituitary gland.

T_4 and T_3 are thyronine molecules that consist of an inner (tyrosyl or α) ring and outer (phenolic or β) ring (Fig. 5.1). Monodeiodination of the outer ring of T_4 results in T_3, which is 3 or 4 times more metabolically active than T_4 *in vivo*. Monodeiodination of the inner ring produces reverse T_3 (rT_3), a metabolically inactive metabolite; 98% of rT_3 is derived from peripheral conversion.

Thyroid hormone action

Thyroid hormone stimulates thermogenesis, water and ion transport, acceleration of substrate turnover and amino acid and lipid metabolism. It also potentiates the action of catecholamines, which causes many of the clinical manifestations seen in patients with thyroid overactivity, and stimulates growth and development of various tissues including the brain and skeleton.

Thyroid hormone is transported into cells and initiates its action by binding to receptors in the nucleus. T_3 binding to the thyroid hormone receptor (TR) is 10 times greater than T_4. Thyroid hormone acts as a transcription factor to stimulate or inhibit genes that are tissue dependent and developmentally regulated.

Thyroid gland development

The thyroid gland is derived from the primitive pharynx. Descent of the thyroid anlage into the neck results from the co-ordinate action of a number of transcription factors, including TTF-1, TTF-2 and PAX-8. TTF-1 is important for the development of follicular and C-cells, whereas PAX-8 is involved only in thyroid follicular cell development. Other homeodomain-containing (Hox) genes regulate the expression of PAX-8 and TTF-1, respectively.

Embryogenesis is largely complete by 10–12 weeks of gestation when follicle precursors are first seen, Tg can be detected in follicular spaces and evidence of iodine uptake and organification is first obtained. Low concentrations of T_4 and T_3 are detectable in fetal serum at 10–12 weeks, although it is likely that some of the thyroid hormone measurable at this early stage of the development is maternal in origin.

Tg, first identified in the follicular spaces by 10–11 weeks, can be identified in the human fetal circulation at gestational age 27–28 weeks.

Maturation of the hypothalamo-pituitary–thyroid axis

TSH is detectable in fetal serum at 12 weeks of gestation and increases from 18 weeks to levels of 10 mU/L at term accompanied by a parallel increase in serum concentrations of total and free T_4. Serum TBG concentration also increases during gestation as

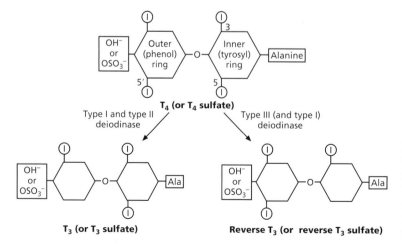

Figure 5.1 Structure of the major thyroid hormones and the action of the monoiodothyronine deiodinase enzymes. The types I and II deiodinases deiodinate the outer (phenol) ring, while the type III (and type I) deiodinases deiodinate the inner (tyrosyl) ring.

a consequence of placental estrogen effects on the fetal liver.

Maturation of hypothalamo-pituitary-thyroid feedback control is observed early in the third trimester, as indicated by an elevated fetal serum TSH in response to hypothyroxinemia and a suppressed TSH in fetuses with hyperthyroidism due to maternal Graves' disease. A fetal TSH response to exogenously administered TRH has been demonstrated as early as 25 weeks' gestation.

Maturation of thyroid hormone metabolism

Circulating T_3 concentrations in the fetus are low while concentrations of rT_3 and the sulfate conjugates of T_4 are markedly elevated. The physiological rationale for the maintenance of reduced circulating T_3 concentrations during fetal life is unknown but it may be to avoid tissue thermogenesis and to potentiate the anabolic state of the rapidly growing fetus.

Fetal brain T_3 levels are 60–80% those of the adult by fetal age 20–26 weeks, despite the low levels of circulating T_3. In the presence of fetal hypothyroidism, T_3 levels are preserved if maternal T_4 levels are normal.

Maturation of thyroid hormone action

Thyroid hormone-mediated effects in the pituitary, brain and bone can be detected prenatally but thyroid hormone-dependent action in brown adipose tissue, liver, heart, skin and carcass is apparent only postnatally.

In the brain, thyroid hormone induces the differentiation and maturation of processes that lead to the establishment of neural circuits during a critical window of brain development. These include neurogenesis and neural cell migration between 5 and 24 weeks, neuronal differentiation, dendritic and axonal growth, synaptogenesis and gliogenesis from late fetal life to 6 months post-partum, myelination from the second trimester to 24 months post-partum and neurotransmitter enzyme synthesis. The absence of thyroid hormone delays rather than eliminates the timing of critical morphological events or gene products, resulting in a disorganization of intercellular communication.

Thyroid hormone-mediated bone maturation involves direct and indirect actions, the latter mediated by regulation of growth hormone gene expression and the insulin-like growth factor (IGF) system. At a direct level, T_3 regulates endochondral ossification and controls chondrocyte differentiation in the growth plate. Both osteoblasts and growth plate chondrocytes express TRs and several T_3-specific target genes have been identified in bone. Longstanding, untreated hypothyroidism in infancy and childhood causes decreased growth velocity and delayed ossification of the epiphyseal growth plate. T_3 also stimulates closure of the skull sutures in vivo, the basis for the enlarged anterior and posterior fontanelle characteristic of infants with congenital hypothyroidism (CH).

Primary hypothyroidism

Chronic lymphocytic thyroiditis
The causes of hypothyroidism after the neonatal period are listed in Table 5.1. The most frequent is chronic lymphocytic thyroiditis (CLT), an auto-immune disease closely related to Graves' disease. In both CLT and Graves' disease, an inherited predisposition to autoimmunity and additional environmental and hormonal factors trigger and modulate the disease process. In CLT, lymphocyte- and cytokine-mediated thyroid destruction predominates whereas, in Graves' disease, antibody-mediated thyroid stimulation occurs but overlap may occur in some patients. Both goitrous (Hashimoto's thyroiditis) and non-goitrous (primary myxedema) variants of thyroiditis have been distinguished. The disease has a striking predilection for females and a family history of autoimmune thyroid disease (both CLT and Graves' disease) is found in 30–40% of patients. The most common age at presentation is adolescence but the disease may occur at any age, even infancy.

Patients with insulin-dependent diabetes mellitus, 20% of whom have positive thyroid antibodies and 5% of whom have an elevated serum TSH level, have an increased prevalence of CLT, which may also occur as part of an autoimmune poly-glandular syndrome (see Chapter 9). The incidence of CLT is increased in patients with Turner, Down and Klinefelter syndromes.

Antibodies to Tg and TPO ('microsomal'), the thyroid antibodies measured in routine clinical practice,

Table 5.1 Differential diagnosis of juvenile hypothyroidism.

Primary hypothyroidism
Chronic lymphocytic thyroiditis
Goitrous (Hashimoto's)
Atrophic (primary myxedema)

Congenital abnormality
Thyroid dysgenesis
Inborn error of thyroid hormonogenesis

Iodine deficiency (endemic goiter)

Drugs or goitrogens
Antithyroid drugs (PTU, MMI, carbimazole)
Anticonvulsants
Other (lithium, thionamides, aminosalicylic acid, aminoglutethimide)
Goitrogens (cassava, water pollutants, cabbage, sweet potatoes, cauliflower, broccoli, soybeans)

Miscellaneous
Cystinosis
Histiocytosis X
Irradiation of the thyroid
   Radioactive iodine
   External irradiation of non-thyroid tumors
Surgery
Mitochondrial disease
Infantile hemangioma

Secondary or tertiary hypothyroidism
Congenital abnormality
Acquired
   Hypothalamic or pituitary tumor (especially craniopharyngioma)
   Treatment of brain and other tumors
Surgery
Radiation

are detectable in over 95% of patients with CLT. They are useful as markers of underlying autoimmune thyroid damage, TPO antibodies being more sensitive and specific. TSH receptor antibodies are also found in a small proportion of patients. When stimulatory TSH receptor antibodies are present, they may give rise to a clinical picture of hyperthyroidism, the coexistence of CLT and Graves' disease being known as hashitoxicosis.

Blocking antibodies, on the other hand, have been postulated to underlie both the hypothyroidism and the absence of goiter in some patients with primary myxedema but are detectable in only a minority of children. In rare instances, the disappearance of blocking antibodies has been associated with normalization of thyroid function in previously hypothyroid patients.

Goiter, which is present in approximately two-thirds of children with CLT, results primarily from lymphocytic infiltration and, in some patients, from a compensatory increase in TSH.

Children with CLT may be euthyroid or may have compensated or overt hypothyroidism. Rarely, they may experience an initial thyrotoxic phase due to the discharge of preformed T_4 and T_3 from the damaged gland. Alternatively, thyrotoxicosis may be due to concomitant thyroid stimulation by TSH receptor stimulatory antibodies (hashitoxicosis).

While most children with CLT who are hypothyroid remain hypothyroid, spontaneous recovery may occur, particularly in those with initially compensated hypothyroidism. On the other hand, some initially euthyroid patients become hypothyroid so, whether or not treatment is initiated, follow-up is necessary.

Thyroid dysgenesis and inborn errors of thyroid hormonogenesis

Occasionally, patients with thyroid dysgenesis escape detection by newborn screening and present later in childhood with non-goitrous hypothyroidism or with an enlarging mass at the base of the tongue or along the course of the thyroglossal duct. Similarly, children with inborn errors of thyroid hormonogenesis may be recognized later in childhood because of a goiter.

Iodine and other micronutrient deficiency: natural goitrogens

Iodine deficiency continues to be a major public health problem in many parts of the world. Endemic cretinism, the most serious consequence, occurs only where iodine deficiency is most severe. Hypothyroidism in older infants, children and adults is seen in regions of moderate iodine deficiency. It develops when adaptive mechanisms fail and may be exacerbated by the coincident ingestion of thiocyanate-containing foods (broccoli, sweet potatoes and cauliflower) which block the trapping and subsequent organification of iodine. Iodine deficiency may also be exacerbated by lack of selenium, a component of the selenocysteine thyroid hormone deiodinases. Iodine deficiency can be due to dietary restriction (for multiple food allergies) or the result of a fad.

Drugs

A number of drugs used in childhood, including antithyroid medication, certain anticonvulsants, lithium, thionamides, aminosalicylic acid and aminoglutethimide, may affect thyroid function.

Secondary or tertiary hypothyroidism

Secondary or tertiary hypothyroidism may be recognized later in childhood as a result of acquired damage to the pituitary or hypothalamus by tumors (particularly craniopharyngioma), granulomatous disease, head irradiation, infection (meningitis), surgery or trauma. Other pituitary hormones are often affected, particularly growth hormone and gonadotropins.

Thyroid hormone resistance

Children with thyroid hormone resistance usually come to attention when thyroid function tests are performed because of poor growth, hyperactivity, a learning disability or other non-specific signs or symptoms. A small goiter may be present. The presentation is highly variable and some individuals may be asymptomatic, whereas others may have symptoms of thyroid hormone deficiency or excess. Thyroid hormone resistance is almost always due to a mutation in the TRβ.

Some individuals have previously been classified as having selective pituitary resistance as distinct from generalized resistance to thyroid hormone because they appeared to have evidence of peripheral hypermetabolism in response to the elevated thyroid hormone levels. However, variable levels of expression of the mutant allele have not been demonstrated. Thus, it has been suggested that the variable clinical manifestations of this syndrome are a result of the genetic heterogeneity of the many cofactors that modulate TR expression.

Miscellaneous causes

The thyroid gland may be involved in generalized infiltrative (cystinosis), granulomatous (histiocytosis X) or infectious disease processes. Hypothyroidism may also occur in patients with mitochondrial disease.

Mantle irradiation for Hodgkin disease or lymphoma and external irradiation of brain tumors may result in hypothyroidism. In the former case, primary hypothyroidism develops; in the latter, hypothyroidism may be primary because of the inclusion of the neck in the radiation field or secondary.

Clinical manifestations

The onset of hypothyroidism in children is insidious. Affected children are usually recognized because of either a goiter or poor growth. Because linear growth is more affected than weight, affected children are relatively overweight for their height, although they are rarely significantly obese (Fig. 5.2). If the hypothyroidism is severe and longstanding, immature facies with an underdeveloped nasal bridge and immature body proportions (increased upper–lower body ratio) may be noted. Dental and skeletal maturation are delayed, the latter often significantly. Patients with

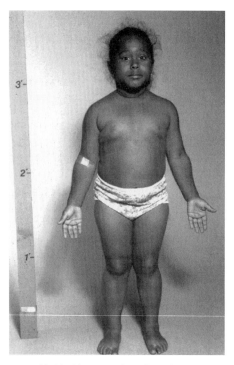 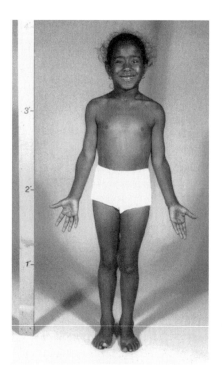

Figure 5.2 Ten-year-old girl with severe l- hypothyroidism due to primary myxedema (a) before and (b) after treatment. Presenting complaint was poor growth. Note the dull facies, relative obesity and immature body proportions prior to treatment. At age 10 years, she had not lost a deciduous tooth. After treatment was initiated, she lost six teeth in 10 months and had striking catch-up growth. Bone age was 5 years at a chronologic age of 10 years. TSH receptor-blocking antibodies were negative.

secondary or tertiary hypothyroidism tend to be less symptomatic than those with primary hypothyroidism.

The classical clinical manifestations include lethargy, cold intolerance, constipation, dry skin or hair texture and periorbital edema. A delayed relaxation time of the deep tendon reflexes may be seen in severe cases. School performance is not usually affected, in contrast to the severe irreversible neuro-intellectual sequelae that occur in inadequately treated babies with CH.

Causes of hypothyroidism associated with a goiter (CLT, inborn errors of thyroid hormonogenesis, thyroid hormone resistance) should be distinguished from non-goitrous causes (primary myxedema, thyroid dysgenesis, secondary or tertiary hypothyroidism).

In patients with severe longstanding hypothyroidism, the sella turcica may be enlarged due to thyrotrope hyperplasia. There is an increased incidence of slipped femoral capital epiphyses. The combination of severe hypothyroidism and muscular hypertrophy, which gives the child a 'Herculean' appearance, is known as the Kocher–Debre–Semelaign syndrome.

Puberty tends to be delayed in hypothyroid children, although sexual precocity has been described in longstanding, severe hypothyroidism. Ovarian cysts may be demonstrated on ultrasonography due to follicle-stimulating hormone (FSH) secretion and females commonly have breast development with little sexual hair and may menstruate. In boys, FSH secretion may cause isolated testicular enlargement. Galactorrhea due to hyperprolactinemia may occur occasionally.

Laboratory evaluation

Measurement of TSH is the best initial screening test for the presence of primary hypothyroidism. If the TSH is elevated, measurement of free T_4 will distinguish whether the child has compensated (normal free T_4) or overt (low free T_4) hypothyroidism.

Measurement of TSH is not helpful in secondary or tertiary hypothyroidism. Hypothyroidism in these cases is demonstrated by the presence of a low free T_4

with a low TSH. In hypopituitarism, there is little or no TSH response to TRH. Occasionally, mild TSH elevation is seen in individuals with hypothalamic hypothyroidism, a consequence of the secretion of a TSH molecule with normal immunoreactivity but impaired bioactivity. A hypothalamic vs. pituitary origin of the hypothyroidism can sometimes be distinguished by TRH testing.

Thyroid hormone resistance is characterized by elevated levels of free T_4 and T_3 and an inappropriately normal or elevated TSH concentration.

CLT is diagnosed by elevated titers of Tg and/or TPO antibodies. Ancillary investigations (thyroid ultrasonography and/or thyroid scintigraphy) may be performed if a nodule is palpable but they are rarely necessary. If thyroid antibody tests are negative and no goiter is present, thyroid ultrasonography and/or scan identify the presence and location of thyroid tissue and thereby distinguish primary myxedema from thyroid dysgenesis. Inborn errors of thyroid hormonogenesis beyond a trapping defect are usually suspected by an increased radioiodine uptake and a large gland on scan.

Therapy

In contrast to CH, rapid replacement of thyroid hormone is not essential, especially in children with longstanding, severe thyroid underactivity in whom rapid normalization may result in unwanted side-effects (deterioration in school performance, short attention span, hyperactivity, insomnia and behavior difficulties). Replacement doses should be increased slowly over several weeks to months. Severely hypothyroid children should also be observed closely for complaints of headache when therapy is initiated because of the rare development of pseudotumor cerebri. Full replacement can be initiated at once in children with mild hypothyroidism without much risk of adverse consequences.

Treatment of children with compensated hypothyroidism, also called mild thyroid failure (normal T_4, elevated TSH), is controversial. Some physicians treat all such patients while others choose to reassess thyroid function in 3–6 months before initiating therapy because of the possibility that the thyroid abnormality will be transient.

Typical replacement doses of thyroxine in childhood are approximately $100 \mu g/m^2$ (4–6 μg/kg for children 1–5 years of age, 3–4 μg/kg for those aged 6–10 years and 2–3 μg/kg for those 11 years of age and older). In patients with a goiter, a somewhat higher thyroxine dose is used to keep TSH in the low normal range (0.3–1.0 mU/L in an ultrasensitive assay) thereby minimizing its goitrogenic effect. Whether and how patients with thyroid hormone resistance should be treated is controversial.

After the child has received the recommended dose for at least 6 weeks, T_4 and TSH should be measured. Once a euthyroid state has been achieved, patients should be monitored every 6–12 months. Close attention is paid to interval growth and bone age as well as to the maintenance of a euthyroid state. Some children with severe, longstanding hypothyroidism at diagnosis may not achieve their adult height potential even with optimal therapy, emphasizing the importance of early diagnosis and treatment. Treatment is usually continued indefinitely.

Asymptomatic goiter

Goiter occurs in 4–6% of schoolchildren in iodine-sufficient areas. Like thyroid disease in general, there is a female preponderance of 2 to 3:1. Patients with goiter may be euthyroid, hypothyroid or hyperthyroid; euthyroid goiters being by far the most common. The most frequent cause of asymptomatic goiter is CLT.

Colloid or simple (non-toxic) goiter

Colloid goiter is a cause of euthyroid thyroid enlargement. There is often a family history of goiter, CLT or Graves' disease, leading to the suggestion that colloid goiter might be an autoimmune disease. Thyroid growth immunoglobulins have been identified in some patients with simple goiter but their etiological role is controversial. It is important to distinguish patients with colloid goiter from CLT because there is a risk of developing hypothyroidism in patients with CLT but not with colloid goiter. Whereas many colloid goiters regress spontaneously, others undergo periods of growth and regression, resulting in the large nodular thyroid glands seen in later life.

Therapy
Thyroid suppression in children with a euthyroid goiter is controversial. There is no evidence of efficacy

91

in CLT and no long-term studies are available in children with colloid goiter. A therapeutic trial may be tried when the goiter is large. In some cases, surgery may be required for cosmesis.

Painful thyroid

Painful thyroid enlargement is rare and suggests either acute (suppurative) or subacute thyroiditis. CLT may sometimes be associated with intermittent pain and be confused with these disorders. In acute thyroiditis, progression to abscess formation may occur rapidly so prompt recognition and antibiotic therapy are essential. Recurrent attacks and involvement of the left lobe suggest a pyriform sinus fistula between the oropharynx and the thyroid as the route of infection. Surgical extirpation of the pyriform sinus will frequently prevent further attacks.

Subacute thyroiditis is characterized by fever, malaise, thyroid enlargement and tenderness. Thyroid function may be normal or elevated, the result of the release of preformed T_4 and T_3 into the circulation. Unlike Graves' disease, radioactive iodine (RAI) uptake is low or absent. A low titer of TPO and Tg antibodies may be found and the sedimentation rate is elevated. The initial thyrotoxic phase characteristically persists for 1–4 weeks and is followed by a period of transient hypothyroidism while the thyroid gland recovers. Treatment is supportive and includes large doses of acetylsalicylic acid or other anti-inflammatory drugs. Corticosteroid medication may be helpful in severe cases. Antithyroid medication is not indicated.

Hyperthyroidism

Graves' disease

The causes of hyperthyroidism in childhood and adolescence are shown in Table 5.2. More than 95% of cases are due to Graves' disease, an autoimmune disorder that, like CLT, occurs in a genetically predisposed population. Genetic predisposition, which has been estimated to account for 70% of the risk, consists of a series of interacting susceptibility alleles of several different genes important in antigen recognition and/or immune modulation. There is a strong female predisposition of 6 to 8:1.

Table 5.2 Causes of thyrotoxicosis in childhood.

Hyperthyroidism
Diffuse toxic goiter (Graves' disease)
Nodular toxic goiter (Plummer disease)

TSH-induced hyperthyroidism
TSH-producing pituitary tumor
'Selective pituitary resistance' to thyroid hormone

Thyrotoxicosis without hyperthyroidism
Chronic lymphocytic thyroiditis
Subacute thyroiditis
Thyroid hormone ingestion

Graves' disease is much less common in children than in adults, although it can occur at any age, especially in adolescence. Prepubertal children, particularly children under 5 years of age, tend to have more severe disease, require longer medical therapy and achieve a lower rate of remission compared with pubertal children.

Graves' disease has been described in children with other autoimmune diseases, both endocrine and non-endocrine, including diabetes mellitus, Addison's disease, vitiligo, systemic lupus erythematosis, rheumatoid arthritis, myasthenia gravis, periodic paralysis, idiopathic thrombocytopenia purpura and pernicious anemia. There is an increased risk of Graves' disease in children with Down syndrome (trisomy 21).

Unlike CLT, in which thyrocyte damage is predominant, the major clinical manifestations of Graves' disease are hyperthyroidism and goiter. Graves' disease is caused by TSH receptor antibodies that mimic the action of TSH. Binding of ligand results in stimulation of adenyl cyclase with subsequent thyroid hormonogenesis and growth.

TSH receptor-blocking antibodies also exist. They inhibit TSH-induced stimulation of adenyl cyclase.

Both stimulatory and blocking TSH receptor antibodies bind to the extracellular domain of the receptor and appear to recognize apparently discrete linear epitopes in the context of a three-dimensional structure but the specific epitope(s) with which they interact is different. Stimulatory antibodies bind to the amino-terminal portion of the extracellular domain, while blocking antibodies bind to the carboxy-terminal domain. In general, blocking antibodies are more potent inhibitors of TSH binding than stimulatory ones.

The clinical assessment of TSH receptor antibodies takes advantage of their ability to bind to the TSH receptor (binding assay, e.g. radioreceptor assay, coated tube chemiluminescent assay or enzyme-linked immunosorbent assay (ELISA)) or to stimulate (or inhibit) TSH-induced stimulation of adenyl cyclase (bioassay). In general, binding assays detect the presence of antibodies interacting at the receptor whatever their biological activity. Most children with Graves' disease also have TPO and/or Tg antibodies in their sera but measurement of the latter is less sensitive and less specific than measurement of TSH receptor antibodies.

Rarer causes of hyperthyroidism

Hyperthyroidism may be caused by a functioning thyroid adenoma, by constitutive activation of the TSH receptor or may be part of the McCune–Albright syndrome. Rarely, hyperthyroidism may be due to inappropriately elevated TSH secretion, the result of either a TSH-secreting pituitary adenoma or pituitary resistance to thyroid hormone.

Miscellaneous causes of thyrotoxicosis without hyperthyroidism include the toxic phase of CLT, subacute thyroiditis and thyroid hormone ingestion (thyrotoxicosis factitia). Thyroxine may be abused by adolescents trying to lose weight or may be eaten inadvertently by toddlers. When the resultant thyrotoxicosis is severe, treatment with iopanoic acid may be effective.

Clinical manifestations

All but a few children with Graves' disease present with some degree of thyroid enlargement and most have symptoms and signs of excessive thyroid activity, such as tremors, inability to fall asleep, weight loss despite an increased appetite, proximal muscle weakness, heat intolerance, headache and tachycardia. If sleep is disturbed, the patient may complain of fatigue. The onset is often insidious.

Shortened attention span and emotional lability may lead to severe behavioral and school difficulties. Some patients complain of polyuria and nocturia, the result of increased glomerular filtration rate. Acceleration in linear growth may occur, often accompanied by advance in bone age but adult height is not affected. Puberty may be delayed and secondary amenorrhea is common.

Physical examination reveals a diffusely enlarged, soft thyroid gland, smooth skin and fine hair texture, excessive activity and a fine tremor of the tongue and fingers. A thyroid bruit may be audible. The finding of a thyroid nodule suggests the possibility of a toxic adenoma. The hands are often warm and moist. Tachycardia, a wide pulse pressure and a hyperactive precordium are common. Café-au-lait spots suggest a possible diagnosis of McCune–Albright syndrome, particularly in association with precocious puberty. If a goiter is absent, factitious thyrotoxicosis should be considered. Severe ophthalmopathy is considerably less common in children than in adults, although a stare, lid lag and mild proptosis are frequently observed.

Laboratory evaluation

The clinical diagnosis of hyperthyroidism is confirmed by the finding of increased concentrations of circulating thyroid hormones and a suppressed TSH, which excludes much rarer causes of thyrotoxicosis, such as TSH-induced hyperthyroidism and pituitary resistance to thyroid hormone in which the TSH is inappropriately 'normal' or slightly elevated.

If the diagnosis of Graves' disease is unclear, TSH receptor antibodies should be measured. This may be particularly useful in distinguishing the toxic phase of CLT and subacute thyroiditis, when TSH receptor antibody is negative, from patients with both CLT and Graves' disease (hashitoxicosis), in whom TSH receptor antibody is positive.

RAI uptake and scan are necessary to confirm the diagnosis of Graves' disease only in atypical cases, for example, if measurement of TSH receptor antibodies is negative and if the thyrotoxic phase of either CLT or subacute thyroiditis or a functioning thyroid nodule is suspected.

Therapy

The choice of medical therapy, RAI or surgery should be individualized and discussed with the patient and his/her family. Each approach has its advantages and disadvantages.

Medical therapy

Thionamides (propyl thiouracil (PTU), methimazole (MMI) and carbimazole (converted to MMI)) are the initial choice of most pediatricians, although radioiodine is gaining increasing acceptance. Thionamides exert their antithyroid effect by inhibiting the organification of iodine and the coupling of iodotyrosine residues on the Tg molecule to generate T_3 and T_4. MMI is often preferred because, for an equivalent dose, it requires taking fewer tablets and has a longer half-life. In addition, MMI is associated with a more rapid resolution of the hyperthyroidism and, with MMI but not PTU, the rate of minor side-effects appears to be dose related and the severe side-effects are seen almost exclusively in patients taking PTU. PTU but not MMI inhibits the conversion of T_4 to the more active isomer T_3, a potential advantage if the thyrotoxicosis is severe.

The usual initial dose of MMI is 0.5–1.0 mg/kg/day (given once or twice daily) and that of PTU is 5–10 mg/kg/day given thrice daily. Carbimazole is best given in a dose of 10–20 mg twice or thrice daily, depending on the concentration of free T_4. In severe cases, a beta-adrenergic blocker (atenolol 25 mg daily or propranolol 0.5–2.0 mg/kg/day given every 8 h) can be added to control cardiovascular overactivity until a euthyroid state is obtained.

Serum concentrations of T_4 and T_3 normalize in 3–6 weeks but the TSH concentration may not return to normal for several months. Therefore, measurement of TSH is useful as a guide to therapy only after it has normalized but not initially. Once the T_4 and T_3 have normalized, the dose of thioamide can be decreased by 30–50%; an alternative is to wait until the TSH begins to rise and add a supplementary dose of L-thyroxine in a block-replacement regimen. Advocates of this regimen cite fewer hospital visits but a larger MMI dose is required, perhaps resulting in a higher incidence of side-effects.

In adults, there does not appear to be advantage in treating patients for more than a year. The optimum duration of therapy in children and adolescents is not known. Approximately 50% of children will go into long-term remission within 4 years, with a continuing remission rate of 25% every 2 years for up to 6 years of treatment. Lack of eye signs, small goiter and, in patients treated with antithyroid drugs alone, a small drug requirement are favorable indicators. Lower initial hyperthyroxinemia ($T_4 < 20 \mu g/dL$ (257.4 nmol/L); T_3/T_4 ratio < 20), body mass index and older age (pubertal vs. prepubertal age) have been associated with increased likelihood of permanent remission. Persistence of TSH receptor antibodies, on the other hand, indicates a high likelihood of relapse.

Toxic drug reactions [erythematous rashes, urticaria, arthralgias, transient granulocytopenia (<1500 granulocytes/mm^3)] have been reported in 5–14% of children. Rarely, hepatitis, a lupus-like syndrome, thrombocytopenia or agranulocytosis (<250 granulocytes/mm^3) may occur. Most reactions are mild and do not contraindicate continued use. In more severe cases, switching to the other thioamide is frequently effective. The risk of hepatitis and agranulocytosis appears to be greater within the first 3 months of therapy. It is important to caution all patients to stop their medication immediately and consult their physician should they develop unexplained fever, sore throat, gingival sores or jaundice. Approximately 10% of children treated medically develop long-term hypothyroidism later in life, a consequence of continuing cell- and cytokine-mediated destruction and/or the development of TSH receptor-blocking antibodies.

Radioactive iodine

Definitive therapy with medical (RAI) or surgical thyroid ablation is usually reserved for patients who have failed drug therapy, developed a toxic drug reaction or are non-compliant. RAI is favored increasingly in some centers, even as the initial approach to therapy, particularly in non-compliant adolescents, in children who are mentally retarded and in those about to leave home (for example to go to college).

The advantages are the ease of administration, the reduced need for medical follow-up and the lack of demonstrable long-term adverse effects. On the other hand, since the goal of therapy is thyroid ablation, daily medication with thyroxine rather than MMI is necessary.

RAI should be used with caution in children under 10 years of age, particularly in those less than 5 years, because of the increased susceptibility of the thyroid gland in the young to the proliferative effects of ionizing radiation. Almost all patients who developed papillary thyroid cancer after the Chernobyl disaster were children aged less than 10 years at the time of the reactor malfunction. Similarly, the risk of benign thyroid nodules following RAI therapy for Graves' disease is greatest in the first decade of life.

Although a dose of 50–200 μCi of ^{131}I/estimated gram of thyroid tissue has been used, the higher dose is recommended, particularly in younger children, in order completely to ablate the thyroid gland and thereby reduce the risk of future neoplasia. Estimation of the size of the thyroid gland is based on the assumption that the normal gland weighs 0.5–1.0 g/year of age up to a maximum 15–20 g. The formula used for the dose of ^{131}I is:

$$\frac{(\text{Estimated thyroid weight in grams} \times 50\text{–}200\ \mu\text{Ci}^{131}\text{I})}{(\text{Fractional }^{131}\text{I 24-h uptake})}$$

Pretreatment with antithyroid drugs prior to RAI therapy is not necessary unless the hyperthyroidism is very severe.

Thyroid hormone concentrations may rise transiently 4–10 days after RAI administration owing to the release of preformed hormone from the damaged gland. Beta blockers may be useful. Analgesics may be necessary for the discomfort of radiation thyroiditis. Other acute complications of RAI therapy (nausea, significant neck swelling) are rare. A therapeutic effect is usually seen within 6 weeks to 3 months.

Worsening of ophthalmopathy, described in adults after RAI, is not common in childhood but, if significant ophthalmopathy is present, RAI therapy should be used with caution and treatment with corticosteroids for 6–8 weeks may be wise. Alternatively, surgery should be considered. There does not appear to be an increased rate of congenital anomalies in offspring nor of thyroid cancer in children with Graves' disease treated with RAI and followed for <5 to >20 years but the numbers of younger children treated with RAI and followed long term are few.

Surgery

Surgery is performed less frequently now than previously. Its major advantage is the rapid resolution of the hyperthyroidism. Near-total or subtotal thyroidectomy is performed depending on whether the goal is to minimize the risk of recurrence or render the patient euthyroid, respectively. Surgery is appropriate for patients who have failed medical management, those who have a markedly enlarged thyroid, those who refuse RAI and for the rare patient with significant eye disease in whom RAI therapy is contraindicated.

Because of the potential complications of transient hypocalcemia, recurrent laryngeal nerve paralysis, hypoparathyroidism and, rarely (as with all forms of surgery), death, this therapy should be performed only by an experienced thyroid surgeon. Occasionally, unsightly keloid formation occurs at the site of the scar.

The child must be euthyroid before surgery. Iodides (Lugol's solution, 5–10 drops twice a day or potassium iodide, 2–10 drops daily) can be added for 7–14 days before surgery in order to decrease the vascularity of the gland.

After medical or surgical thyroid ablation, patients become hypothyroid and require lifelong thyroid replacement therapy. On the other hand, if therapy is inadequate, hyperthyroidism may recur.

Thyroid nodules

Thyroid nodules occur in only 0.05–1.8% of children and adolescents and are rare in the first two decades of life in iodine-sufficient populations. However, in comparison with adults in whom thyroid nodules are much more common (incidence 50% after the sixth decade of life), they are much more likely to be carcinomatous. Follicular adenomas and colloid cysts account for the majority of benign thyroid nodules. Other causes of benign nodular enlargement include CLT and embryological defects, such as intrathyroidal duct cysts or unilateral thyroid agenesis. The most common form of cancer is papillary thyroid carcinoma but other histological types found in the adult, such as follicular and anaplastic carcinomas, may also occur. Thyroid lymphomas are rare.

Clinical evaluation

A high index of suspicion is necessary if the nodule is painless, of firm or hard consistency or if it is fixed to surrounding tissues, especially if it has undergone rapid growth or if there is cervical adenopathy, hoarseness or dysphagia. Children whose thyroids have been exposed to irradiation comprise a particularly high-risk group. Medullary thyroid carcinoma should be considered if there is a family history of thyroid cancer or pheochromocytoma and/or if the child has multiple mucosal neuromas and a marfanoid habitus, findings consistent with multiple endocrine neoplasia (MEN), types IIa and/or IIb, respectively. Extrathyroidal manifestations suspicious of other syndromes associated with nodular thyroid disease (Cowden syndrome, Bannayan–Riley–Ruvalcaba syndrome, familial adenomatous polyposis) should be sought.

Laboratory evaluation

The initial investigation includes evaluation of thyroid function and measurement of anti-TPO and anti-Tg antibodies. A suppressed serum TSH concentration accompanied by an elevation in the circulating T_4 and/or T_3 suggests the possibility of a functioning nodule. Positive antibodies, although indicating the presence of underlying CLT, do not exclude the possibility of co-existent thyroid cancer. Serum calcitonin should be measured if medullary thyroid carcinoma of C-cell origin is a concern, such as in familial cases of thyroid cancer but its routine measurement in the evaluation of thyroid nodules is controversial. Genetic screening for a mutation of the RET proto-oncogene should be performed if MENIIa is suspected.

Ultrasound

Ultrasound examination has replaced thyroid scintiscan as the preferred imaging procedure to confirm and evaluate the morphological characteristics of a thyroid nodule. Nodules that are cystic or homogeneously hyperechoic are reputed to carry a lower risk of malignancy. Conversely, a solid hypoechoic echotexture, calcification, irregular shape or absence of a halo are features associated with malignancy.

Since no sonographic findings reliably predict the likelihood of malignancy, biopsy is indicated for all thyroid nodules ≥ 1 cm. Additional non-palpable nodules may be discovered by ultrasonography and later found to be malignant. Ultrasonography is helpful in the non-invasive monitoring of nodules too small to biopsy or those with benign cytology and in surveillance for local recurrence in patients diagnosed with thyroid carcinoma.

Fine-needle aspiration

Fine-needle aspiration biopsy, popular in the investigation of thyroid carcinoma in adults, has been used increasingly, particularly in older children. Ultrasound guidance improves the diagnostic accuracy and safety of this procedure. This is important, since up to 20% of fine-needle aspirations are insufficient or non-diagnostic. Repeat aspiration of non-diagnostic fine-needle aspirations is usually successful. Papillary thyroid cancer, the most common malignant tumor of the

thyroid in childhood, is readily identifiable on cytology by the presence of characteristic nuclear abnormalities. However, follicular carcinoma is difficult to differentiate from follicular adenoma and so documentation of capsular and/or vascular invasion is required. Benign cytology obviates the need for surgical resection. Conversely, in patients with atypical cytology, the degree and type of cytological abnormality allow a more specific assignment of cancer risk and facilitate the discussion of surgical options. If the child is very young or very anxious, open excisional biopsy is a suitable alternative.

Therapy

Excision of the tumor or lobe is the appropriate treatment for benign tumors and cysts. Total or near-total thyroidectomy with preservation of the parathyroid glands and recurrent laryngeal nerves is the optimal therapy for malignant thyroid tumors since it facilitates radioiodine ablation and subsequent monitoring for recurrence and disease progression.

Bilateral surgery can be reserved for patients at high risk for malignancy, such as those whose cytology predicts a >50% likelihood of differentiated thyroid cancer or who have bilateral nodules with abnormal cytology.

For other patients, thyroid lobectomy can be performed initially, followed by completion thyroidectomy only if lobectomy confirms the diagnosis of cancer. This approach reduces the risk of complications for the majority of patients with benign lesions.

Although unilateral vocal cord paralysis or parathyroid injury may not compromise activities of daily life, these complications increase the risk of permanent morbidity with future surgeries (completion thyroidectomy or neck dissection for local recurrence) in those patients who are found to have cancer at lobectomy.

Children with thyroid nodules <1 cm or with benign cytology should be followed chronically by serial ultrasound every 6–12 months and ultrasound-guided fine-needle aspiration should be repeated if significant interval growth or other concerning sonographic features develop.

Radioactive iodine

Even after total thyroidectomy, radioiodine uptake usually persists in the thyroid bed as a result of residual normal thyroid tissue. Ablation of this thyroid remnant with RAI has been shown to lower recurrence rates and, in some series, to reduce cancer mortality, presumably because of the destruction of malignant or premalignant thyrocytes within the macroscopically normal remnant. Similar to completion thyroidectomy, radioiodine remnant ablation also facilitates disease surveillance by increasing the specificity of Tg measurements and the sensitivity of diagnostic whole body scans. Remnant radioablation, defined as the destruction of residual macroscopically normal thyroid tissue after surgical thyroidectomy, should be distinguished from RAI therapy, the use of higher ^{131}I doses to destroy local or distal differentiated thyroid cancer.

For any given administered dose, the adsorbed radiation dose to normal tissues will be higher in young children due to their smaller organs and increased cross-radiation due to the shorter distances between organs. Formulae for the estimation of relative pediatric doses should be consulted. Both formal quantitative dosimetry and standardized, empiric, fixed dose methods have been used. An interval of at least 12 months between ^{131}I treatments is recommended to minimize the risk of leukemia. Pulmonary fibrosis is another potential consequence of RAI.

The efficacy of radiation therapy is enhanced by clinical interventions that increase thyroidal iodine uptake, such as an elevated circulating TSH concentration and a low iodine diet for 1–2 weeks before the procedure. Thyroxine withdrawal is the standard method of achieving an elevated TSH.

In adults, recombinant TSH avoids the discomfort of hypothyroidism after thyroxine withdrawal and appears to provide equivalent results but similar studies have not been performed in children.

Prepubertal children are more likely to experience nausea and vomiting with ^{131}I therapy so anti-emetic medications should be available.

After RAI therapy, the dose of thyroxine replacement is adjusted to keep the serum TSH concentration suppressed (between 0.05 and 0.1 mU/L in sensitive assays). Measurement of serum Tg, a thyroid follicular cell-specific protein, is used to detect evidence of metastatic disease in differentiated forms of thyroid cancer, such as papillary or follicular cancer. This is best performed after a period of thyroxine withdrawal or after exogenous administration of recombinant TSH.

Follow-up treatment and surveillance

After radioiodine therapy, the dose of thyroxine is adjusted to keep the serum TSH concentration suppressed (± 0.1 mU/L in sensitive assays). The suppression of endogenous TSH secretion reduces cancer recurrence and, in some series, cancer-related death. Measurement of serum Tg, a thyroid follicular cell-specific protein, is used to detect evidence of metastatic disease in differentiated forms of thyroid cancer, such as papillary or follicular cancer. However, it should be noted that Tg is also produced by normal thyroid tissue. Therefore, the utility of this test is best after thyroidectomy and remnant ablation.

Approximately 15–30% of patients with differentiated thyroid cancer possess circulating anti-Tg antibodies that can confound commercially available Tg assays. Accordingly, serum should be screened for the presence of antibodies every time Tg is measured. Serum Tg antibodies may become negative with time after thyroidectomy, so serum Tg should be monitored every 6–12 months even in those children who have interfering antibodies at the time of diagnosis. As with radionuclide scanning, the sensitivity of Tg measurements is greatest when the TSH is elevated, either after a period of thyroxine withdrawal or after exogenous administration of recombinant TSH.

Based upon data in adults, 68% of differentiated thyroid cancer recurrences are local (cervical or mediastinal). Accordingly, surveillance should include annual neck imaging. Thyroid ultrasound is a sensitive and, when coupled with ultrasound-guided fine-needle aspiration, a specific modality to screen for local recurrence. Computed tomography (CT) or magnetic resonance imaging (MRI) is an alternative. Local recurrences that are palpable or easily visualized with ultrasound or CT should be excised surgically rather than treated with RAI.

Thyroxine withdrawals or recombinant TSH-stimulated serum Tg measurements and diagnostic whole body scanning should be performed at yearly intervals throughout childhood. ^{123}I is the preferred agent for diagnostic whole body scanning since it is a pure gamma emitter, which minimizes the patient's radiation exposure.

Prognosis

Based upon the retrospective analyses of large patient cohorts, primary tumor size >1.5 cm, local tumor

6 The Adrenal Gland

Learning Points

- The adrenal cortex produces glucocorticoids, androgens and mineralocorticoids
- These are regulated by the hypothalamo-pituitary axis in the case of the first two and by the renin–angiotensin system for the third
- After congenital adrenal hyperplasia, the commonest cause of endogenous hypoadrenalism in children is autoimmune adrenalitis
- Adrenoleukodystrophy should be considered in any male with hypoadrenalism
- Excessive exposure to glucocorticoids causes Cushing syndrome and causes adrenal suppression after 10 days
- The commonest cause is iatrogenic followed by Cushing disease but, in young children, an adrenal tumor is more common than a pituitary microadenoma
- Steroid withdrawal and the management of stress in hypoadrenal patients require careful attention to detail

The adrenal cortex produces three categories of steroid hormones. *Mineralocorticoids*, principally aldosterone, regulate renal retention of sodium, which influences electrolyte balance, intravascular volume and blood pressure. *Glucocorticoids*, principally cortisol, are named for their carbohydrate-mobilizing activity but influence a wide variety of bodily functions. *Adrenal androgens* modulate the mid-childhood growth spurt and regulate some secondary sexual characteristics in women.

There are three morphologically distinguishable concentric zones within the adrenal cortex: the glomerulosa, the fasciculata and the reticularis (Fig. 6.1). This zonation is functionally important, because aldosterone comes from the zona glomerulosa, cortisol mainly from the zona fasciculata and sex steroids from the zona reticularis.

The outer zone, the zona glomerulosa, lies under a fibrous capsule and makes up 5–10% of the cortex. Its cells are closely packed in small, ill-defined clumps.

The middle cortical zone, the zona fasciculata, forms about 75% of the volume of the adrenal cortex. Its cells are larger than those in the zona glomerulosa and arranged in long cords disposed radially with respect to the medulla; the cords are separated by the straight cortical capillaries.

In the zona reticularis there is an anastomosing network of short cords of cells with interdigitating capillaries. Cell contacts between cortical cells in all the zones involve desmosomes but, in the zona fasciculata and zona reticularis, large and numerous gap junctions are found, functionally coupling the cortical cells.

Cells of the zona glomerulosa migrate continuously centrally through the zona fasciculata to the zona reticularis, which differentiates in children aged 6–8 years. The purpose of this migration is not clear but the secretory product of an individual cell changes as it migrates.

Handbook of Clinical Pediatric Endocrinology, 1st edition. By Charles G. D. Brook and Rosalind S. Brown. Published 2008 by Blackwell Publishing, ISBN: 978-1-4501-6109-1.

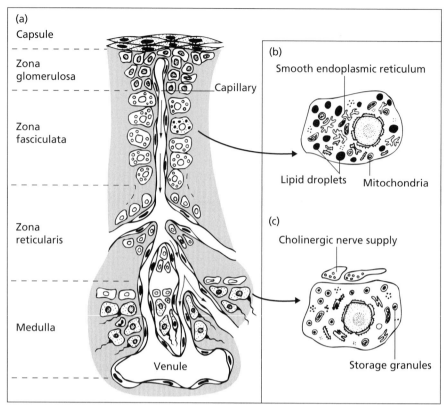

Figure 6.1 (a) A section through the cortex and medulla of the adrenal gland. The capsule surrounds the gland, and capillaries run through the cortex and empty into a medullary venule. The three zones of the cortex are shown: the thin outer zona glomerulosa; the thick central zona fasciculata; and the inner zona reticularis. The medulla consists of chromaffin cells and a cholinergic nerve supply. (b) The cytology of a zona fasciculata cell. Note the large number of lipid droplets and the extensive smooth endoplasmic reticulum associated with mitochondria. (c) The cytology of a medullary chromaffin cell. Note the numerous membrane-bound storage granules of catecholamines and the synaptic terminals of its cholinergic nerve supply.

Embryological development

The adrenal gland is derived from ectodermal neural-crest cells, which form the medulla, and from mesodermal cells, which give rise to the cortex.

Medulla

In the human, cells originating from the neural crest migrate from each side of the neural tube toward the dorsal aorta, where they position themselves laterally and just posterior to it during the fifth week of development. Most of the cells form a bilateral chain of segmentally arranged sympathetic ganglia but some invade the medial aspect of the developing adrenal cortex, position themselves in its center and eventually become the adrenal medulla. These cells do not form

nerve processes, although they are the equivalent of postganglionic neurones. They differentiate into two kinds of chromaffin cells, which synthesize and secrete norepinephrine and epinephrine, respectively. During fetal life, the chromaffin cells secrete only norepinephrine but some cells begin to synthesize epinephrine just before birth.

Cortex

The adrenal cortex originates from mesothelial cells located at the cranial ends of the mesonephros; these lie between the root of the mesentery and the developing urogenital ridge. During the fifth week of development, these cells proliferate and invade the underlying retroperitoneal mesenchyme forming the primitive fetal cortex. A second wave of mesothelial-derived cells proliferate surround the fetal cortex and

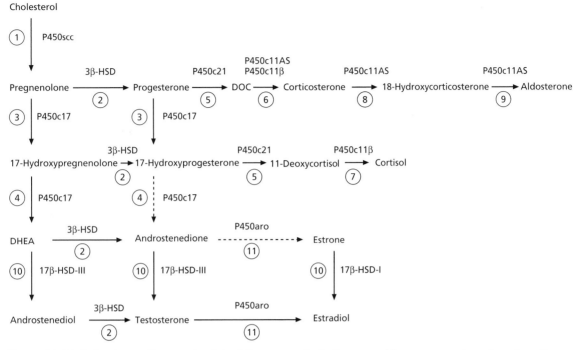

Figure 6.2 Principal pathways of human adrenal steroid hormone synthesis. The names of the enzymes are shown by each reaction, and the traditional names of the enzymatic activities correspond to the circled numbers.

eventually form the cortex of the adult gland. Mesenchymal cells that surround the fetal cortex differentiate into fibroblasts and lay down the collagenous capsule. The blood and nerve supplies of the gland also develop during this period.

The fetal adrenal cortex thus consists of an outer (definitive/adult) zone, the principal site of glucocorticoid and mineralocorticoid synthesis and a much larger (fetal) zone that makes androgenic precursors for the placental synthesis of estriol. The fetal adrenal gland is huge in proportion to other structures. At birth, the adrenals weigh 8–9 g, roughly twice the size of adult adrenals and represent 0.5% of total body weight, compared with 0.0175% in the adult.

The fetal cortex regresses after birth and has usually disappeared by the end of the first year of life. The glands decrease in size by about a third during the first months after birth and do not regain their size at birth until adult life. Complete absence of both glands is rare, as is the existence of true accessory glands consisting of both cortex and medulla. However, ectopic adrenal cortical tissue alone occurs

frequently, as do patches of medullary tissue. These isolated groups of cells may be found in the spleen or retroperitoneally, for example, below the kidneys, along the aorta, in the pelvis or associated with gonadal structures. Ectopic adrenal tissue, whether of cortical or medullary origin, is of no significance unless it becomes hyperplastic or malignant; then its location may become very important.

Differentiation of the cells in the cortex and the development of function in the fetus appear to be under the control of adrenocorticotrophin (ACTH). In the adult, following hypophysectomy or suppressive doses of cortisone, the cells of the zona fasciculata and zona reticularis, which are ACTH dependent, regress but those of the zona glomerulosa do not.

Role of the fetal cortex

The fetal adrenal is capable of steroid production at an early stage of gestation but the function of the gland is not known. Since it does not contain 3β-hydroxysteroid dehydrogenase activity (Fig. 6.2), it produces mainly dehydroepiandrosterone sulfate (DHEAS), which provides the substrate for estrogen synthesis by the placenta. It cannot synthesize progesterone, glucocorticoids or androstenedione. Glucocorticoids obtained from the mother or synthesized from placental progesterone by the fetus are, however, involved in a number of important processes in fetal tissues, which may be due to their interactions with other growth factors. Examples of these development-promoting effects are:

1 Production of surfactant from type II cells of the alveoli of the lung, a lack of which leads to the respiratory distress syndrome in newborn infants.

2 Development of hypothalamic function and of the hypothalamo-pituitary axis.

3 The sequential changes of placental structure and the ionic composition of amniotic and allantoic fluids during development.

4 The initiation of the endocrine changes in the fetus and mother that are responsible for parturition.

5 The development of hepatic enzymes, including those involved in gluconeogenesis.

6 Induction of thymic involution.

Function of the adrenal cortex

Cholesterol is the starting point for all steroid hormone biosynthesis. It is obtained mostly from circulating low-density lipoprotein (LDL) and only very little is synthesized locally from acetate. As Fig. 6.2 shows, cholesterol is modified by a series of hydroxylation reactions. Five of the enzymes (CYP11A, CYP17, CYP21, CYP11B1 and CYP11B2) are members of the cytochrome P450 superfamily of haemoproteins (called P450 because they show a characteristic shift in light absorbance from 420 to 450 nm upon reduction with carbon monoxide). The enzymes of the CYP11 family are located in the mitochondria and the remainder is located in the endoplasmic reticulum, so the substrates have to move around the cell for the process of steroidogenesis to be complete.

The nomenclature of the enzymes and the genes encoding them have been revised, so that the same code shown in Fig. 6.2 applies to the gene when italicized capitals are used (e.g. *CYP11A*) and to the enzyme when ordinary capitals are used (e.g. CYP11A).

Regulation of steroidogenesis

The hypothalamo-pituitary–adrenal axis

Cortisol is secreted in response to adrenocorticotrophic hormone (ACTH); secretion of ACTH is stimulated mainly by corticotrophin-releasing hormone (CRH) from the hypothalamus. CRH is a 41-amino-acid peptide synthesized mainly by neurones in the paraventricular nucleus. These same hypothalamic neurones also produce arginine vasopressin (AVP). Both CRH and AVP are proteolytically derived from larger precursors, with the AVP precursor containing the sequence for neurophysin, which is the AVP-binding protein.

CRH and AVP travel through axons to the median eminence, which releases them into the pituitary portal circulation, although most AVP axons terminate in the posterior pituitary. Both CRH and AVP stimulate the synthesis and release of ACTH but they appear to do so by different mechanisms. CRH functions principally by receptors linked to the protein kinase A pathway, stimulating production of intracellular cAMP, whereas AVP appears to function via protein kinase C and intracellular Ca^{2+}. It is fairly clear that CRH is the more important physiological stimulator of ACTH release, although maximal doses of AVP can elicit a maximal ACTH response. When given together, CRH and AVP act synergistically, as would be expected from their independent mechanisms of action.

ACTH and pro-opiomelanocortin

Pituitary ACTH is a 39-amino-acid peptide derived from pro-opiomelanocortin (POMC), a 241-amino-acid protein. POMC undergoes a series of proteolytic cleavages, yielding several biologically active peptides (Fig. 6.3). The N-terminal glycopeptide (POMC 1–75) can stimulate steroidogenesis and may function as an adrenal mitogen. POMC 112–150 is ACTH 1–39; POMC 112–126; and POMC 191–207 constitute α- and β-MSH (melanocyte-stimulating hormone), respectively. POMC 210–241 is β-endorphin. POMC is produced in small amounts by the brain, testis and placenta but this extrapituitary POMC does not contribute significantly to circulating ACTH. Malignant tumors commonly produce 'ectopic ACTH' in adults, although rarely in children; this ACTH derives from ectopic biosynthesis of the same POMC precursor. Only the first 20–24 amino acids of ACTH are needed for its full biological

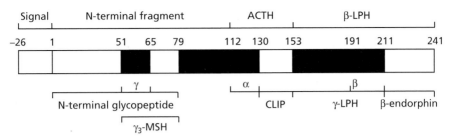

Figure 6.3 Structure of human prepro-opiomelanocortin. The numbers refer to amino acid positions, with No. 1 assigned to the first amino acid of POMC after the 26-amino-acid signal peptide. The a-, b- and g-MSH regions, which characterize the three 'constant' regions, are indicated by diagonal lines; the 'variable' regions are solid. The amino acid numbers shown refer to the N-terminal amino acid of each cleavage site; because these amino acids are removed, the numbers do not correspond exactly to the amino acid numbers of the peptides as used in the text. CLIP, corticotrophin-like intermediate lobe peptide.

activity and synthetic ACTH 1–24 is widely used in diagnostic tests of adrenal function. The shorter forms of ACTH have a shorter half-life than native ACTH 1–39. POMC gene transcription is stimulated by CRH and inhibited by glucocorticoids.

Actions of ACTH

ACTH stimulates steroidogenesis by interacting with receptors that stimulate the production of cAMP, which elicits acute and long-term effects. ACTH stimulates the biosynthesis of LDL receptors and the uptake of LDL, which provides most of the cholesterol used for steroidogenesis.

Diurnal rhythms of ACTH and cortisol

The hypothalamic content of CRH itself shows a diurnal rhythm, with peak content at about 04.00 h. Plasma concentrations of ACTH and cortisol are high in the morning and low in the evening. Peak ACTH levels are usually seen at 04.00–06.00 h and peak cortisol levels follow at about 08.00 h. Both ACTH and cortisol are released episodically in pulses every 30–120 min throughout the day but the frequency and amplitude are greater in the morning. The basis of this diurnal rhythm is complex and incompletely understood.

At least four factors appear to play a role in the rhythm of ACTH and cortisol. They include intrinsic rhythmicity of synthesis and secretion of CRH by the hypothalamus, light–dark cycles, feeding and inherent rhythmicity in the adrenal, possibly mediated by adrenal innervation.

As all parents know, infants do not have a diurnal rhythm of sleep or feeding. They acquire such behavioral rhythms in response to the environment long before they acquire a rhythm of ACTH and cortisol. The diurnal rhythms begin to be established at 6–12 months but are often not well established until after 3 years of age. Once the rhythm is established in the older child or adult, it is changed only with difficulty. When people move time zones, ACTH/cortisol rhythms generally take 15–20 days to adjust.

Physical stress (major surgery, severe trauma, blood loss, high fever or serious illness) increases the secretion of both ACTH and cortisol but minor surgery and minor illnesses (upper respiratory infections) have little effect. Infection, fever and pyrogens can stimulate the release of interleukin-1 (IL-1) and IL-6, which stimulate secretion of CRH and also IL-2 and tumor necrosis factor (TNF), which stimulate release of ACTH, providing further stimulus to cortisol secretion during inflammation.

Adrenal-glucocorticoid feedback

The hypothalamo-pituitary–adrenal axis is a classic example of an endocrine feedback system. ACTH increases the production of cortisol and cortisol decreases the production of CRH and ACTH. Like the acute and chronic phases of the action of ACTH on the adrenal, there are acute and chronic phases of the feedback inhibition of ACTH (and presumably CRH). The acute phase, which occurs within minutes, inhibits release of ACTH (and CRH) from secretory granules. With prolonged exposure, glucocorticoids inhibit ACTH synthesis by directly inhibiting the transcription of the gene for POMC. Some evidence also suggests that glucocorticoids can inhibit steroidogenesis at the level of the adrenal fasciculata cell itself but this appears to be a physiologically minor component of the regulation of cortisol secretion.

Function of the zona fasciculata

The zona fasciculata is the main source of cortisol. There is relatively little cortisol storage and active synthesis is required when the need for hormone increases. Most cortisol is converted in the liver to inactive cortisone; the ratio of cortisol to cortisone in plasma is about 1:2. Cortisol is bound to a binding globulin and in case of need, cortisone can be converted to cortisol and bound cortisol can be freed as required.

The metabolic effects of cortisol generally oppose those of insulin and vary with the target tissue: it is catabolic in muscle, adipose and lymphoid tissue but stimulates the synthesis and storage of glycogen in liver. It increases the concentration of glucose in blood by stimulating gluconeogenesis in the liver and by decreasing the utilization of glucose in other tissues. The increased blood glucose is available for the production of glycogen and is important in maintaining liver glycogen during prolonged fasting.

Enzymes involved in hepatic gluconeogenesis are also stimulated and there is an increased availability of amino acids derived from protein catabolism in several tissues. In the liver, protein anabolism occurs but the net effect is of negative nitrogen balance. The energy required for gluconeogenesis is obtained by breakdown of fats and the release of fatty acids.

Cortisol stimulates appetite, so that when there is excess cortisol, as in Cushing syndrome, there is central obesity with an increase in body fat. The reason for the redistribution of adipose tissue is not understood.

Cortisol acts on body defence mechanisms to suppress tissue response to injury, its anti-inflammatory action, which has been extensively used therapeutically. Cortisol in moderately high concentrations leads to a reduction in the size of lymph nodes and to involution of the thymus. The tissue shrinkage is rapid and dramatic. This situation is an unusual example of a hormone acting as a cytosolic agent, with the cortisol activating a program for apoptosis. It reduces the number of lymphocytes in blood and so decreases antibody production. It thus impairs both cellular and humoral immunity and thereby renders patients susceptible to infection.

Although cortisol is predominantly a glucocorticoid, it does have mineralocorticoid effects when present in large amounts; it can help to maintain extracellular fluid volume and prevent the shift of water into cells and it also supports tissue perfusion, which may be important during stress.

Other effects become apparent only if it is present in excess. It sensitizes arterioles to the action of norepinephrine (resulting in hypertension) and has permissive effects on the action of norepinephrine on carbohydrate metabolism (resulting in hyperglycemia and glucose intolerance). In addition, it can stimulate secretion of acid by the stomach and increase activity in the central nervous system to produce euphoria or even mania.

Transport of circulating cortisol

There is a specific corticosteroid-binding globulin (transcortin) in plasma. About 80% of the circulating cortisol is bound to this protein and serum albumin can bind an additional 15%. If the concentration of cortisol is increased so that the specific binding sites are saturated, much of the surplus is carried by albumin. Transcortin-bound cortisol is protected from metabolism and inactivation in liver. The affinity of transcortin for progesterone is also high but it is much lower for aldosterone so this steroid has a relatively short half-life in the circulation. Transcortin does not bind dexamethasone.

If the concentration of the binding proteins is elevated, the total concentration of the hormone in plasma increases. This happens in pregnancy and following estrogen treatment (e.g. contraception or treatment for cancer of the prostate). Thus, it is necessary to take account of the concentration of binding globulins when considering the physiological significance of a total steroid concentration determined in plasma.

Function of the zona glomerulosa

Aldosterone is produced exclusively in the zona glomerulosa. This is the most potent mineralocorticoid produced by the adrenal.

Cellular actions of aldosterone
Aldosterone binds to specific intracellular mineralocorticoid receptor proteins within its target cells, which

function as hormone-activated transcription factors. The mineralocorticoid receptor binds both cortisol and aldosterone with equal affinities. Despite the higher concentration of cortisol, aldosterone is the dominant mineralocorticoid because aldosterone-responsive cells are protected by the effect of the enzyme 11β-hydroxysteroid dehydrogenase (11β-HSD). This converts cortisol to cortisone, which is not active on the mineralocorticoid receptor. Congenital deficiency of 11β-HSD results in the syndrome of 'apparent mineralocorticoid excess' (AME), a cause of mineralocorticoid hypertension. The consumption of large quantities of liquorice can lead to an acquired deficiency of 11β-HSD, due to the inhibitory effects of glycyrrhetinic acid, which is present in liquorice, on 11β-HSD. The condition manifests as a mineralocorticoid excess state, with hypertension and hypokalaemia.

Effects of aldosterone

The main sites of action of aldosterone are in the distal tubule and the collecting ducts of the kidney, where it increases sodium reabsorption by a cation-exchange mechanism. Aldosterone raises blood pressure partly by increasing plasma volume and partly by increasing the sensitivity of the arteriolar muscle to vasoconstrictor agents. The response of an individual to administered aldosterone is observed only after a lag period of about 1 h, during which there is synthesis of a specific aldosterone-induced protein that promotes sodium transport. If administration of aldosterone is continued, the ability to excrete excess sodium is regained after 1–3 weeks, depending on sodium intake; this 'escape phenomenon' is almost certainly the result of readaptation of the feedback control system that is responsible for the regulation of the rate of reabsorption of filtered sodium in the proximal tubule.

Secretion of aldosterone

Despite the rate of aldosterone secretion being about 100 times lower than that of cortisol, it is responsible for about 80% of the mineralocorticoid activity of the adrenal glandular secretion. Aldosterone is cleared more rapidly from the circulation than cortisol, having a half-life of 20–30 min, as opposed to 100 min for cortisol. This rapid clearance is partly explained by the fact that it is bound only to a limited extent by carrier proteins in the circulation. The circulating concentration

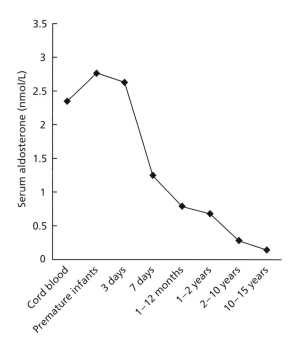

Figure 6.4 Concentrations of aldosterone as a function of age.

of aldosterone is normally about 300 pmol/L (10.8 ng/dL), which is about a thousand times lower than that of cortisol (Fig. 6.4).

Regulation of aldosterone secretion

The renin–angiotensin system is the most important regulator of the secretion of aldosterone. Renin is secreted by special cells in the juxtaglomerular region of the nephrons in the kidney surrounding the afferent arteriole just before it enters the Malpighian corpuscle and breaks up into the glomerular capillaries. They are epithelioid and replace the smooth-muscle cells of the afferent arteriole at this point. They synthesize renin, which is stored intracellularly in granules.

Adjacent to the juxtaglomerular cells are those of the macula densa, which is a specialized part of the distal tubule. The juxtaglomerular cells and the macula densa form the juxtaglomerular apparatus. Release of renin is activated by a fall in plasma fluid volume; it is discharged from the cells by exocytosis and then diffuses into the lumen of the arterioles and thus into the circulation, where it has a half-life of about 20 min.

Renin is a proteolytic enzyme that cleaves a decapeptide from angiotensinogen. The decapeptide is angiotensin I, which is largely biologically inactive but is converted in several tissues to angiotensin II, an octapeptide and the most potent pressor substance known; it raises both systolic and diastolic blood pressures and so pulse pressure does not alter. The lung, the endothelial cells of which contain the appropriate endopeptidase, angiotensin-converting enzyme (ACE), is the primary site of conversion of angiotensin I–II.

Angiotensinogen is normally present in adequate concentrations and the supply of renin is rate limiting for angiotensin II production. For this reason, plasma renin is usually measured to reflect changes in plasma angiotensin II concentration, since the latter is more difficult to measure and its half-life in the circulation is only about 1 min.

Angiotensin II acts directly on the zona glomerulosa cells to stimulate aldosterone secretion. Since it acts also on peripheral arterioles, it helps maintain blood pressure both directly and indirectly. During sodium depletion, angiotensin II has a particularly potent effect on the renal circulation: it reduces the glomerular filtration rate and thereby reduces renal excretion of sodium.

Regulation of the production of renin

Three factors control the secretion of renin. One is neural; the juxtaglomerular apparatus of the kidney is richly supplied by sympathetic neurones and destruction of this nerve supply leads to a blunting of the renin response to sodium depletion.

The second factor is the flux of sodium across the macula densa of the distal tubule. When the flux is high (as, for example, when sodium is plentiful), the secretion of renin is suppressed and it is clear that normally the renin–angiotensin system is not important in maintaining blood pressure in the sodium-replete state. However, when the animal is sodium depleted, renin secretion increases and the effects of sodium on aldosterone production from the adrenal are largely mediated via the renin–angiotensin system. This is essential for maintenance of blood pressure during sodium depletion.

The third factor is the mean transmural pressure (as opposed to the pulse pressure); when the transmural pressure is high, renin secretion is suppressed and when it is low, the secretion of renin is stimulated.

Plasma potassium has only a weak effect on the production of renin which is antagonistic to the direct effect that changes in potassium have on the secretion of aldosterone by the glomerulosa cells. For example, a low concentration of potassium in the plasma sharply reduces aldosterone secretion but at the same time it has a small but definite stimulatory effect on renin production. Because potassium can have a direct action on the adrenal as well as an effect on production of renin, there can be a dissociation between the production of aldosterone and the amount of renin present in some situations.

Interplay of factors regulating the secretion of aldosterone

Angiotensin II, potassium and ACTH can directly stimulate the rate of secretion of aldosterone, as can MSH, while somatostatin and atrial natriuretic peptide can inhibit aldosterone secretion. The effects of potassium can be seen when plasma volume is constant; then, small changes of potassium within the physiological range affect aldosterone secretion. The dependence of the aldosterone secretion rate on plasma volume is mediated by the renin–angiotensin system, which can override any opposing changes in the plasma concentration of potassium and ACTH. For example, the secretion of aldosterone rises during the morning (because of the fall in plasma volume on assuming an upright posture), even though the secretion of ACTH falls during the day. Injection of ACTH can stimulate aldosterone production but this effect lasts only 24–48 h, even if ACTH is administered repeatedly. This is because the aldosterone-producing cells no longer respond to ACTH.

Lack of ACTH as a result of hypophysectomy or disease does not significantly reduce the zona glomerulosa and aldosterone production is maintained, in contrast to the effect on the zona fasciculata or reticularis. Overproduction of aldosterone is not a consequence of prolonged excessive secretion of ACTH.

Adrenal androgen secretion and the regulation of adrenarche

DHEA, DHEAS and androstenedione, which are secreted almost exclusively by the zona reticularis, are referred to as adrenal androgens because they can be converted peripherally to testosterone. These steroids have little if any capacity to bind to and activate androgen receptors and are hence only androgen precursors, not true androgens. The fetal adrenal secretes large amounts of DHEA and DHEAS and these steroids are abundant in the newborn; their concentrations fall rapidly as the fetal zone of the adrenal involutes after birth.

After the first year of life, the adrenals of young children secrete small amounts of DHEA, DHEAS and androstenedione until the onset of adrenarche, usually around age 7–8 years. Adrenarche is independent of puberty, the gonads or gonadotropins and the mechanism by which its onset is triggered remains unknown. The secretion of DHEA and DHEAS continues to increase during and after puberty and reaches maximal values in young adulthood, after which there is a slow, gradual decrease in their secretion ('adrenopause'). Despite the increases in the adrenal secretion of DHEA and DHEAS during adrenarche, circulating concentrations of ACTH and cortisol do not change with age. Thus, ACTH plays a permissive role in adrenarche but does not trigger it. Searches for hypothetical polypeptide hormones that might specifically stimulate the zona reticularis have been unsuccessful.

Steroid catabolism

Only about 1% of circulating plasma cortisol and aldosterone is excreted unchanged in the urine; the remainder is metabolized by the liver. A large number of hepatic metabolites of each steroid is produced, most containing additional hydroxyl groups and linked to a sulfate or glucuronide moiety, rendering them more soluble and readily excretable by the kidney. A great deal is known about the various urinary metabolites of the circulating steroids because their measurement in pooled 24-h urine samples has been an important means of studying adrenal steroids. Although the measurement of urinary steroid metabolites by modern mass spectrometric techniques remains an important research tool, the development of separation techniques and of specific and highly sensitive radioimmunoassays for each of the steroids in plasma has greatly reduced the need to measure their excreted metabolites in clinical practice.

Clinical and laboratory evaluation of adrenal function

Clinical evaluation

Primary adrenal deficiency or hypersecretion is generally evident before performing laboratory tests. Patients with chronic adrenal insufficiency have weakness, fatigue, anorexia, weight loss, hypotension and hyperpigmentation. Patients with acute adrenal insufficiency have hypotension, shock, weakness, apathy, confusion, anorexia, nausea, vomiting, dehydration, abdominal or flank pain, hyperthermia and hypoglycemia.

Early signs of glucocorticoid excess include increased appetite, weight gain and growth arrest without a concomitant delay in bone age. Chronic glucocorticoid excess in children results in typical cushingoid facies but the buffalo hump and centripetal distribution of body fat characteristic of Cushing disease in adults are seen only in long-standing undiagnosed disease.

Mineralocorticoid excess is characterized by hypertension but patients receiving very low-sodium diets (e.g. the newborn) may not be hypertensive, since mineralocorticoids increase blood pressure primarily by retaining sodium and thus increasing intravascular volume.

Deficient adrenal androgen secretion compromises the acquisition of pubic and axillary hair, comedones and axillary odor in female adolescents. Moderate hypersecretion is characterized by mild signs of virilization, whereas substantial hypersecretion of adrenal androgens is characterized by accelerated growth with a disproportionate increase in bone age, increased muscle mass, acne, hirsutism, deepening of the voice and more profound degrees of virilism.

A key feature of any physical examination of a virilized male is careful examination and measurement of the testes. Bilaterally enlarged testes suggest true (central) precocious puberty; unilateral testicular enlargement suggests testicular tumor; prepubertal testes in a virilized male indicate an extratesticular source of androgen, such as the adrenal.

Imaging studies are of limited use in adrenocortical disease. Computed tomography (CT) rarely detects pituitary tumors secreting ACTH, although recent advances in magnetic resonance imaging (MRI) may detect some with gadolinium enhancement. The small size, odd shape and location near other structures compromise the use of imaging techniques for the adrenals. Patients with Cushing disease or congenital adrenal hyperplasia (CAH) have modestly enlarged adrenals but these are often not detectable by imaging with any useful degree of certainty. The gross enlargement of the adrenals in congenital lipoid adrenal hyperplasia, their hypoplasia in adrenal hypoplasia congenita (AHC) or in the hereditary ACTH unresponsiveness syndrome can be imaged, as can many malignant tumors but most adrenal adenomas are too small to be detected. Thus, imaging studies may establish the presence of pituitary or adrenal tumors but never exclude them.

Laboratory evaluation

Steroid measurements

Plasma cortisol is measured by a variety of techniques including radioimmunoassay, immunoradiometric assay and high-performance liquid chromatography (HPLC). It is important to know what procedure one's laboratory is using and what it is measuring, because laboratories have different normal values and most are designed primarily to serve adult, rather than pediatric, patients.

All immunoassays have some degree of cross-reactivity with other steroids and most cortisol immunoassays detect cortisol and cortisone, which are readily distinguished by HPLC. Since the newborn's plasma contains mainly cortisone rather than cortisol during the first few days of life, comparison of newborn data obtained by HPLC with published standards obtained by immunoassays may incorrectly suggest adrenal insufficiency.

With the notable exception of DHEAS, most adrenal steroids exhibit a diurnal variation. Because the stress of illness or hospitalization can increase adrenal steroid secretion and because diurnal rhythms may not be well established in children under 3 years of age, it is best to obtain two or more samples for the measurement of any steroid.

Plasma renin

Immunoassays for renin itself are beginning to enter clinical practice but renin is usually assayed by its enzymatic activity. Plasma renin activity (PRA) is an immunoassay of the amount of angiotensin I generated per milliliter of serum per hour at $37°C$.

PRA is sensitive to dietary sodium intake, posture, diuretic therapy, activity and sex steroids. Because PRA values can vary widely, it is best to measure renin twice, once in the morning after overnight supine posture and then again after maintenance of upright posture for 4 h. A simultaneous 24-h urine for total sodium excretion is generally needed to interpret PRA results.

The greatest use of renin measurements is in the evaluation of hypertension and in the management of CAH. However, several additional situations require assessment of the renin–angiotensin system. Children with simple virilizing adrenal hyperplasia who do not have clinical evidence of urinary salt wasting (hyponatremia, hyperkalemia, acidosis, hypotension, shock) may nonetheless have increased PRA, especially when dietary sodium is restricted. This was an early clinical sign that this form of 21-hydroxylase deficiency (21-OHD) was simply a milder form of the more common, severe, salt-wasting form. Treatment of simple virilizing 21-OHD with mineralocorticoid sufficient to suppress PRA into the normal range will reduce the child's requirement for glucocorticoids, thus maximizing final adult height. All children with CAH need to have their mineralocorticoid replacement therapy monitored routinely by measuring PRA.

Urinary steroid excretion

The measurement of 24-h urinary excretion of steroid metabolites is one of the oldest procedures for assessing adrenal function and is still useful. Examination of the total 24-h excretion of steroids eliminates the fluctuations seen in serum samples. Collection of a 24-h urinary sample can be difficult in the infant or small child and two consecutive complete 24-h collections should be obtained. Because of the diurnal and episodic nature of steroid secretion, one should never obtain 8- or 12-h collections and attempt to infer the 24-h excretory rate from such partial collections.

Measurement of urinary free cortisol avoids non-specificity and drug interference problems. The test is reliable for the diagnosis of Cushing syndrome. The upper limit of normal for urinary free cortisol excretion for children is $80 \, mg/m^2/day$.

Plasma ACTH

Accurate immunoassay of plasma ACTH is more difficult and variable than the assays for most other pituitary hormones. Samples must be drawn into a plastic syringe containing heparin or ethylenediamine tetraacetic acid (EDTA) and transported quickly in plastic tubes on ice, since ACTH adheres to glass and is quickly inactivated. Elevated concentrations can be informative but most assays cannot detect low or low-normal values and such values can be spurious if the samples are handled badly. In adults and older children with well-established diurnal rhythms of ACTH, normal 08.00 h values rarely exceed 50 pg/mL, whereas 20.00 h values are usually undetectable. Patients with Cushing disease often have normal morning values but consistently elevated afternoon and evening ones can suggest the diagnosis. Patients with the ectopic ACTH syndrome have values from 100 to 1000 pg/mL.

Secretory rates

The secretory rates of cortisol and aldosterone (or other steroids) can be measured by administering a small dose of tritiated cortisol or aldosterone and measuring the specific activity of one or more known metabolites in a 24-h urine collection. On the basis of this procedure, most authorities previously concluded that children and adults secrete about 12 mg of cortisol per square meter of body surface area per day but more recent studies indicate a rate of 6–9 mg/m^2 in children and adults. Such differences are of considerable importance in estimating physiological replacement doses of glucocorticoids.

Dexamethasone suppression test

Small doses of dexamethasone suppress secretion of ACTH and cortisol. The dexamethasone suppression test remains the most useful procedure for distinguishing whether glucocorticoid excess is due primarily to pituitary or adrenal disease. Since dexamethasone also suppresses adrenal androgen secretion, the test is useful for distinguishing adrenal from gonadal sources of sex steroids.

A dexamethasone suppression test (see Chapter 13) requires the measurement of basal values and those obtained in response to both low- and high-dose dexamethasone. This is a useful outpatient screening procedure for distinguishing Cushing syndrome from exogenous obesity in adolescents and older children but is of limited value in younger patients. An overnight high-dose dexamethasone suppression test is probably more reliable than the standard 2-day, high-dose test in differentiating adults with Cushing disease from those with the ectopic ACTH syndrome.

Stimulation tests

Direct stimulation of the adrenal with ACTH is a useful way to evaluate adrenocortical function. It diagnoses primary adrenal insufficiency (Addison disease). In secondary adrenal insufficiency, some steroidogenic capacity is present and some cortisol is produced in response to the ACTH.

A single bolus of ACTH (1–24) is administered intravenously and cortisol values are measured at 0 and 60 min. Synthetic ACTH (1–24) (cosyntropin) is preferred since it has a more rapid action and shorter half-life than ACTH (1–39). The usual dose is 0.1 mg in newborns, 0.15 mg in children up to 2 years of age and 0.25 mg for children over the age of 2 years and adults. All these doses are pharmacological.

A very low-dose test may be useful in assessing adrenal recovery from glucocorticoid suppression. Maximal steroidal responses can be achieved after only 30 min but the best available standards are for a 60-min test.

One of the widest uses of intravenous ACTH tests in pediatrics is in diagnosing CAH. Stimulating the adrenal with ACTH increases steroidogenesis, resulting in the accumulation of steroids proximal to the disordered enzyme. Measuring the response of 17-OHP to a 60-min or 6-h challenge with ACTH is the single most powerful and reliable means of diagnosing 21-OHD. Comparing the patient's basal and ACTH-stimulated values of 17-OHP against those from large numbers of well-studied patients usually permits the discrimination of normal persons, heterozygotes, patients with non-classic CAH and patients with classic CAH, although there is inevitably some overlap between groups (Fig. 6.5).

Longer ACTH tests (up to 3 days) are useful in diagnosing the rare syndrome of hereditary unresponsiveness to ACTH.

Insulin-induced hypoglycemia is another commonly used test. The hypoglycemia stimulates the release of counter-regulatory hormones (ACTH and cortisol, growth hormone, epinephrine and glucagon) that have actions to increase plasma glucose concentrations. Most patients experience hunger, irritability, diaphoresis and tachycardia; when these are followed by drowsiness or sleep, blood glucose levels are probably below acceptable limits. If this occurs, a blood sample should

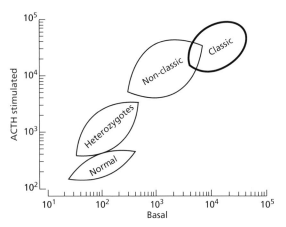

Figure 6.5 17-OHP values before and after stimulation with ACTH in normal subjects, patients with CAH, and heterozygotes.

Table 6.1 Causes of adrenal insufficiency.

Primary adrenal insufficiency
Autoimmune adrenalitis
Autoimmune polyglandular syndromes (types I and II)
Tuberculosis, fungal infections
Sepsis
AIDS
Congenital adrenal hyperplasia
Adrenal hemorrhage or infarction
Congenital adrenal hypoplasia
Adrenoleukodystrophy
Primary xanthomatosis
Unresponsiveness to ACTH

Secondary adrenal insufficiency
Withdrawal from glucocorticoid therapy
Hypopituitarism
Hypothalamic tumors
Irradiation of the CNS

CNS, central nervous system.

be obtained and 2 mL/kg 25% glucose given intravenously to a maximum of 100 mL.

CRH is now generally available as a test of pituitary ACTH reserve. It remains experimental in adults and little experience has been gained from children. It may be useful for distinguishing hypothalamic from pituitary causes of ACTH deficiency and may also be a useful adjunct in establishing the diagnosis of Cushing disease.

Genetic lesions in steroidogenesis

Autosomal-recessive disorders disrupt each of the steps in the pathway shown in Fig. 6.2. Most result in diminished synthesis of cortisol. In response to adrenal insufficiency, the pituitary synthesizes increased amounts of POMC and ACTH, which promotes increased steroidogenesis; ACTH (and possibly other peptides derived from the amino-terminal end of POMC) stimulates adrenal hypertrophy and hyperplasia. Thus, the term CAH refers to a group of diseases traditionally grouped together on the basis of the most prominent finding at autopsy.

In theory, CAH is easy to understand. A genetic lesion in one of the steroidogenic enzymes interferes with normal steroidogenesis. The signs and symptoms of the disease derive from deficiency of the steroidal endproduct and the effects of accumulated steroidal precursors proximal to the blocked step. Thus, reference

to the pathways in Fig. 6.2 and a knowledge of the biological effects of each steroid should permit one to deduce the manifestations of the disease (see Chapter 2 and Table 2.5).

Adrenal insufficiency

Besides CAH, many other conditions cause adrenal insufficiency, including ACTH deficiency and primary adrenal disorders. Primary adrenal insufficiency is commonly termed Addison disease, a vague term that encompasses many disorders (Table 6.1). Up to World War II, most patients with 'Addison disease' had tuberculosis of the adrenal but over 80% of contemporary adult patients have autoimmune adrenalitis and the term *Addison disease* is now widely used to indicate an autoimmune or idiopathic cause.

Chronic primary adrenal insufficiency

Autoimmune adrenalitis
Autoimmune adrenalitis is most commonly seen in 25- to 45-year-old adults, about 70% of whom are women. In children, boys constitute about 75% of patients. Chronic adrenal insufficiency is suggested by poor weight gain or weight loss, weakness, fatigue,

Table 6.2 Signs and symptoms of adrenal insufficiency.

Features shared by acute and chronic insufficiency
Anorexia
Apathy and confusion
Dehydration
Fatigue
Hyperkalemia
Hypoglycemia
Hyponatremia
Hypovolemia and tachycardia
Nausea and vomiting
Postural hypotension
Salt craving
Weakness

Features of acute insufficiency (adrenal crisis)
Abdominal pain
Fever

Features of chronic insufficiency (Addison disease)
Decreased pubic and axillary hair
Diarrhea
Hyperpigmentation
Low-voltage electrocardiogram
Small heart on X-ray
Weight loss

anorexia, hypotension, hyponatremia, hypochloremia, hyperkalemia, frequent illnesses, nausea and vague gastrointestinal complaints (Table 6.2), reflecting chronic deficiency of both glucocorticoids and mineralocorticoids. Early in the course of autoimmune adrenalitis, one may see signs of glucocorticoid deficiency (weakness, fatigue, weight loss, hypoglycemia, anorexia) without signs of mineralocorticoid deficiency (hyponatremia, hyperkalemia, acidosis, tachycardia, hypotension, low voltage on electrocardiogram (ECG), small heart on chest X-ray) or evidence of mineralocorticoid deficiency without glucocorticoid deficiency. Thus, an initial clinical presentation that spares one category of adrenal steroids does not mean it will be spared in the long run. The symptoms listed in Table 6.2 can be seen in primary or secondary chronic adrenal insufficiency.

In primary chronic adrenal insufficiency, the low concentrations of plasma cortisol stimulate the hypersecretion of ACTH and other POMC peptides, including the various forms of MSH, which is characterized by hyperpigmentation of the skin and mucous membranes. Such hyperpigmentation is most prominent in skin exposed to sun and in extensor surfaces such as knees, elbows and knuckles. The diagnosis is suggested by the signs and symptoms, verified by a low morning cortisol level with a high ACTH and confirmed by a minimal response of cortisol to a 60-min intravenous ACTH test.

Associated findings may include the appearance of a small heart on chest X-ray, anemia, azotemia, eosinophilia, lymphocytosis and hypoglycemia. Treatment consists of physiological glucocorticoid and mineralocorticoid replacement therapy.

The diagnosis of an autoimmune cause is based on finding circulating anti-adrenal antibodies. Autopsy studies show lymphocytic infiltration of the adrenal cortex. Thus, it is likely that the primary process is initiated by T lymphocytes and that the antibodies to steroidogenic P450 enzymes are secondary markers, analogous to the antibodies to insulin and glutamic acid decarboxylase seen in type 1 diabetes mellitus.

Autoimmune dysfunction of other endocrine tissues is frequently associated with autoimmune adrenalitis. Approximately half of adult patients with lymphocytic adrenalitis also have disease of another endocrine system and high titers of antibodies specific to the affected tissues (see Chapter 9).

Metabolic causes

Adrenoleukodystrophy (ALDP) (Schilder disease), primary xanthomatosis (Wolman disease), cholesterol ester storage disease, hereditary unresponsiveness to ACTH and AHC cause chronic primary adrenal insufficiency.

ALDP is caused by mutations in a gene on chromosome Xq28. This is an X-linked disorder but a severe autosomal-recessive form occurs in infants. The disease is characterized by high ratios of C_{26} to C_{22} very-long-chain fatty acids in plasma and tissues, permitting diagnosis of carriers and affected fetuses as well as individual patients. Symptoms commonly develop in mid-childhood but a variant of the disorder, adrenomyeloneuropathy, presents in early adulthood. Both ALDP and adrenomyeloneuropathy are caused by mutations in the gene for ALDP. The same mutation causes both forms of the disease, so it is likely that other genetic loci are also involved.

Earliest findings associated with the central nervous system leukodystrophy include behavioral changes, poor school performance, dysarthria and poor memory, progressing to severe dementia. Symptoms of adrenal insufficiency usually appear after symptoms of white-matter disease but adrenal insufficiency may be the initial finding in some children. Adrenomyeloneuropathy begins with adrenal insufficiency in childhood and adolescence and signs of neurological disease follow 10–15 years later. Dietary therapy with the so-called Lorenzo's oil has not been effective.

Wolman disease and cholesterol ester storage disease appear to be two allelic variants in the secreted form of lysosomal acid lipase (cholesterol esterase) that mobilizes cholesterol esters from adrenal lipid droplets. The gene for this enzyme is on chromosome 10q. Because insufficient free cholesterol is available to P450scc, there is adrenal insufficiency. The disease is less severe than congenital lipoid adrenal hyperplasia with respect to steroidogenesis and patients may survive for several months after birth. However, the disease affects all cells, not just steroidogenic cells, since all cells must store and use cholesterol; hence, the disorder is relentless and fatal.

Vomiting, steatorrhea, failure to thrive, hepatosplenomegaly and adrenal calcification are the usual presenting findings. The diagnosis is established by bone marrow aspiration yielding foam cells containing large lysosomal vacuoles engorged with cholesterol esters and is confirmed by finding absent cholesterol esterase activity in fibroblasts, leukocytes or marrow cells. Cholesterol ester storage disease appears to be a milder defect in the same enzyme.

Hereditary unresponsiveness to ACTH (familial glucocorticoid deficiency) can present as an acute adrenal crisis precipitated by an intercurrent illness in an infant or with the signs and symptoms of chronic adrenal insufficiency in childhood. Unlike patients with autoimmune adrenalitis or other forms of destruction of adrenal tissue, patients with hereditary unresponsiveness to ACTH continue to produce mineralocorticoids normally because production of aldosterone by the adrenal zona glomerulosa is regulated principally by the renin–angiotensin system. Thus, the presenting picture consists of failure to thrive, lethargy, pallor, hyperpigmentation, delayed milestones and hypoglycemia (often associated with seizures) but serum electrolytes are normal and dehydration is seen only as part of the precipitating intercurrent illness. The disorder is transmitted as an autosomal-recessive trait.

Some but not all affected patients have mutations of the gene encoding the ACTH receptor (melanocortin-2 receptor, MC2R) on chromosome 18p11, indicating the heterogeneous nature of the defect.

Triple A (Allgrove) syndrome consists of ACTH-resistant adrenal (glucocorticoid) deficiency, achalasia of the cardia and alacrima. The disorder appears to be autosomal dominant and resembles ACTH resistance but mutations in the ACTH receptor have been excluded. Many patients also have progressive neurological symptoms, including intellectual impairment, sensorineural deafness, peripheral neuropathies and autonomic dysfunction. The disorder is caused by mutations in a gene called ALADIN.

Adrenal hypoplasia congenita (AHC) generally affects males because the principal form is caused by mutations of the DAX-1 gene on chromosome Xp21. This gene encodes a nuclear transcription factor that participates at various steps in the differentiation of adrenal and gonadal tissues, as well as in gonadotropin expression, so that successfully treated children may not enter puberty.

In this disorder, the definitive zone of the fetal adrenal does not develop and the fetal zone is vacuolated and cytomegalic. Poor function of the fetal zone results in low maternal estriol concentrations during pregnancy but parturition is normal.

Neonatal glucocorticoid and mineralocorticoid deficiencies manifest with a typical salt-wasting crisis and respond well to replacement therapy.

Deletions of the *DAX-1* gene may also encompass adjacent genes, causing glycerol kinase deficiency, Duchenne muscular dystrophy and mental retardation. Genetic 46,XY males with adrenal hypoplasia have normal male external genitalia but the distinction between AHC and congenital lipoid adrenal hyperplasia cannot be made hormonally in 46,XX females and requires imaging of the adrenals, which are small in adrenal hypoplasia and large in lipoid CAH. A much rarer miniature form has autosomal-recessive inheritance but the gene responsible has not been identified.

Other causes

Chronic adrenal insufficiency may result from causes other than these. Adrenal hypoplasia, hemorrhage and infections are causes of acute primary adrenal insufficiency but some adrenal tissue may be spared, leaving severely compromised, rather than totally absent, adrenal function. The result is a chronic disorder with insidious onset of the broad range of non-specific findings described above. Tuberculosis, fungal infections and amyloidosis may cause a similar clinical picture.

Acute primary adrenal insufficiency

Acute adrenal crisis occurs most commonly in children with undiagnosed chronic adrenal insufficiency who are subjected to an additional stress such as major illness, trauma or surgery. The major presenting symptoms and signs include abdominal pain, fever, hypoglycemia with seizures, weakness, apathy, nausea, vomiting, anorexia, hyponatremia, hypochloremia, acidemia, hyperkalemia, hypotension, shock, cardiovascular collapse and death. Treatment consists of fluid and electrolyte resuscitation, ample doses of glucocorticoids, chronic glucocorticoid and mineralocorticoid replacement and treatment of the precipitating illness.

Massive adrenal hemorrhage with shock due to blood loss can occur in large infants who have had a traumatic delivery. A flank mass is usually palpable and can be distinguished from renal vein thrombosis by microscopic rather than gross hematuria. The diagnosis is confirmed by CT or ultrasonography.

Massive adrenal hemorrhage is more commonly associated with meningococcemia (Waterhouse–Friederi-chsen syndrome). Meningitis is often but not always, present. The characteristic petechial rash of meningococcemia can progress rapidly to large ecchymoses; the blood pressure drops and respirations become labored, frequently leading rapidly to coma and death. Immediate intervention with intravenous fluids, antibiotics and glucocorticoids is not always successful. A similar adrenal crisis may also occur rarely with septicemia from streptococcus, pneumococcus or diphtheria.

Secondary adrenal insufficiency

Chronic adrenal insufficiency may result from insufficient trophic stimulation of the adrenal and tissue insensitivity to adrenal steroids. Insufficient trophic stimulation of the adrenal can be due to idiopathic hypopituitarism, central nervous system tumors that damage the cells producing CRH and/or POMC or chronic suppression of these cells by long-term glucocorticoid therapy.

Idiopathic hypopituitarism (multiple anterior pituitary hormone deficiency) is a hypothalamic rather than a pituitary disorder. The deficient secretion of growth hormone, gonadotropins, thyroid-stimulating hormone (TSH) and ACTH is due to insufficient stimulation of the pituitary by the corresponding hypothalamic hormones. Isolated growth hormone deficiency, a common disorder, and isolated ACTH deficiency, a rare disorder, are variants of this theme.

In hypopituitarism from most causes, growth hormone secretion is generally lost first, followed in order by gonadotropins, TSH and ACTH. Combined deficiency of growth hormone and ACTH predispose the patient to hypoglycemia, since both hormones act to raise plasma glucose. Patients with ACTH deficiency, either with or without deficiency of other anterior pituitary hormones, have a relatively mild form of adrenal insufficiency. Mineralocorticoid secretion is normal, whereas cortisol secretion is reduced but not absent. However, adrenal reserve is severely compromised by the chronic understimulation of biosynthesis of the steroidogenic enzymes.

Because some cortisol synthesis continues, the diagnosis may not be apparent unless a CRH or metyrapone test of pituitary ACTH production capacity and an intravenous ACTH test of adrenal reserve are performed. This can be especially true when TSH deficiency is a component of hypopituitarism. The hypothyroidism resulting from TSH deficiency will result in slowed metabolism of the small amount of cortisol produced, which therefore protects the patient from the symptoms of adrenal insufficiency. Treatment of the hypothyroidism with thyroxine will accelerate metabolism of the small amounts of cortisol, thus unmasking adrenal insufficiency due to ACTH deficiency sometimes precipitating an acute adrenal crisis. Careful evaluation of the pituitary–adrenal axis is required in hypopituitarism with secondary hypothyroidism. Many clinicians will choose to 'cover' a patient with small doses of glucocorticoids (one-quarter to one-half of physiological replacement) during initial treatment of such secondary hypothyroidism.

Hypothalamic and pituitary tumors, such as craniopharyngioma, are associated with ACTH deficiency in about 25% of patients, perhaps more in tumors such as germinoma and astrocytoma. Adrenal insufficiency is rarely the presenting complaint but may contribute to the clinical picture. After surgery and radiotherapy, the great majority of these patients have ACTH deficiency as part of their pituitary damage and all patients should receive glucocorticoid coverage during treatment, irrespective of the status of the hypothalamo-pituitary–adrenal axis at the time the tumor is identified. Cortisol is required for the kidney to excrete free water. Treatment of secondary adrenal insufficiency in some central nervous system tumors can unmask a previously unapparent deficiency of antidiuretic hormone (ADH) and thus precipitate diabetes insipidus.

Long-term glucocorticoid therapy can suppress POMC gene transcription and the synthesis and storage of ACTH. Furthermore, long-term therapy apparently decreases the synthesis and storage of CRH and diminishes the abundance of receptors for CRH in the pituitary. Therefore, recovery of the hypothalamo-pituitary axis from long-term glucocorticoid therapy entails recovery of multiple components in a sequential cascade and often requires considerable time. Patients successfully withdrawn from glucocorticoid therapy or successfully treated for Cushing disease may exhibit a fairly rapid normalization of plasma cortisol values while continuing to have diminished adrenal reserve for over 6 months.

Glucocorticoid therapy of pregnant women can suppress the fetal adrenal. Treatment of pregnant women with cortisone or prednisone will result in minimal suppression of the fetal adrenal, because placental 11β-HSD converts the biologically active form of these steroids, cortisol and prednisolone, back to their biologically inactive parent compounds. Thus, when radiolabeled cortisol or prednisolone is administered to a pregnant woman, the equilibrium concentrations in maternal plasma are 10 times higher than those in cord plasma. However, dexamethasone is a poor substrate for 11β-HSD, so that administration of low doses to a pregnant woman can affect fetal adrenal steroidogenesis.

Adrenal excess

Cushing syndrome

The term *Cushing syndrome* describes any form of glucocorticoid excess. *Cushing disease* designates hypercortisolism due to pituitary overproduction of ACTH. The related disorder caused by ACTH of non-pituitary origin is termed the *ectopic ACTH syndrome*. Other causes of Cushing syndrome include adrenal adenoma, adrenal carcinoma and multinodular adrenal hyperplasia. All these are distinct from *iatrogenic Cushing syndrome*, which is the clinical result of administration of supraphysiological quantities of ACTH or glucocorticoids.

Cushing disease is rare in adults but 25% of patients referred to large centers are children, so it is clear that the disorder is relatively more common in children. Many patients first seen as adults actually experienced the onset of symptoms in childhood or adolescence. In adults and children over 7 years of age, the most common cause of Cushing syndrome is Cushing disease. In infants and children under 7 years, adrenal tumors predominate.

Clinical findings

Central obesity, 'moon facies,' hirsutism and facial flushing are seen in over 80% of adults. Striae, hypertension, muscular weakness, back pain, buffalo hump fat distribution, psychological disturbances, acne and easy bruising are also commonly described. These are the signs of advanced Cushing disease. When photographs of such patients are available, it is often apparent that the features can take 5 or more years to develop. Thus, the classic cushingoid appearance will usually not be the initial picture seen in the child with Cushing syndrome.

The earliest, most reliable indicators of hypercortisolism in children are weight gain and growth arrest (Table 6.3); any overweight child who stops growing should be evaluated for Cushing syndrome (and hypothyroidism). The obesity of Cushing disease in children is initially generalized rather than centripetal and a buffalo hump is evidence of long-standing disease. Psychological disturbances, especially compulsive overachieving behavior, are seen in about 40% of children and adolescents. An underappreciated aspect is the substantial degree of bone loss and undermineralization in these patients. It is likely that Cushing disease is generally regarded as a disease of young adults because the diagnosis was missed, rather than absent, during adolescence. Rarely, Cushing syndrome caused by adrenal carcinoma and the ectopic ACTH syndrome can produce a fulminant course.

Cushing disease

The development of trans-sphenoidal surgical approaches has led to pituitary exploration in large

Table 6.3 Findings in 39 children with Cushing disease.

Sign/symptom	Number of patients	%
Weight gain	36/39	92
Growth failure	31/37	84
Ostopenia	14/19	74
Fatigue	26/39	67
Hypertension	22/35	63
Delayed or arrested puberty	21/35	60
Plethora	18/39	46
Acne	18/39	46
Hirsutism	18/39	46
Compulsive behavior	17/39	44
Striae	14/39	36
Bruising	11/39	28
Buffalo hump	11/39	28
Headache	10/39	26
Delayed bone age	2/23	13
Nocturia	3/39	8

numbers of patients with Cushing disease. Among adults, over 90% of such patients have identifiable pituitary microadenomas, which are generally 2–10 mm in diameter, are not encapsulated, have ill-defined boundaries and are frequently detectable with a contrast-enhanced pituitary MRI. They are often identifiable only by minor differences in their appearance and texture from surrounding tissue, so the frequency of surgical cure is correlated with the technical skill of the surgeon. Although histological techniques may not distinguish the tumor from normal tissue, molecular biological techniques confirm increased synthesis of POMC in these tissues.

Among children and adolescents, about 80–85% of those with Cushing disease have surgically identifiable microadenomas. Although removal of the tumor usually appears to be curative, 20% of patients relapse within about 5 years, so that the net cure rate is 70–75%. Trans-sphenoidal surgery offers the best initial approach for rapid and complete cure of most patients, thus maximizing final height, which is typically reduced by 1.5–2.0 SD by the long-term hypercortisolism.

The high cure rate of trans-sphenoidal microadenomectomy in Cushing disease indicates that the majority of patients have primary disease of the pituitary itself, rather than secondary hyperpituitarism resulting from hyperstimulation by CRH or other agents. In most post-operative patients, the circadian rhythms of ACTH and cortisol return to normal, ACTH and cortisol respond appropriately to hypoglycemia, cortisol is easily suppressed by low doses of dexamethasone and the other hypothalamo-pituitary systems return to normal. Some patients with Cushing disease have no identifiable microadenoma, which suggests that this smaller population of patients may have a primary hypothalamic disorder.

Thus, Cushing disease is usually caused by a primary pituitary adenoma but sometimes it is caused by hypothalamic dysfunction. Microsurgery can be curative in the former but not in the latter. Unfortunately, no diagnostic maneuver is available to distinguish the two possibilities, so trans-sphenoidal exploration remains the preferred initial therapeutic approach to the patient with Cushing disease.

Other therapeutic options include hypophysectomy, pituitary irradiation, cyproheptidine, adrenalectomy and drugs that inhibit adrenal function. All have significant disadvantages, especially in children.

Laparascopic adrenalectomy is the preferred approach when two trans-sphenoidal procedures fail. In addition to the obvious effects of eliminating normal production of glucocorticoids and mineralocorticoids, removal of the adrenal eliminates the physiological feedback inhibition of the pituitary. This can result in the development of pituitary macroadenomas, producing large quantities of ACTH which can expand and impinge on the optic nerves, producing POMC sufficient to yield enough MSH to darken the skin (Nelson syndrome).

Ketoconazole and other drugs that inhibit steroidogenesis may provide a useful form of therapy for selected patients but metyrapone is not useful for long-term therapy. *Ortho-*, *para*-DDD (mitotane), an adrenolytic agent, may be used to effect a chemical adrenalectomy but its side-effects of nausea, anorexia and vomiting are severe.

Other causes of Cushing syndrome

The ectopic ACTH syndrome is commonly seen in adults with oat cell carcinoma of the lung, carcinoid tumors, pancreatic islet cell carcinoma and thymoma. Ectopically produced POMC and ACTH are derived from the same gene that produces pituitary POMC but it is not sensitive to glucocorticoid feedback in the malignant cells. This phenomenon permits distinction between pituitary and ectopic ACTH by suppressibility of the former by high doses of dexamethasone. Although the ectopic ACTH syndrome is rare in children, it has been described in infants younger than 1 year of age. Associated tumors include neuroblastoma, pheochromocytoma and islet cell carcinoma of the pancreas. The ectopic ACTH syndrome is associated typically with ACTH concentrations 10–100 times higher than those seen in Cushing disease.

Adults and children with this disorder may show little or no clinical evidence of hypercortisolism, probably because of the rapid onset of the disease and the general catabolism associated with malignancy. Unlike patients with Cushing disease, patients frequently have hypokalemic alkalosis, presumably because the extremely high levels of ACTH stimulate the production of DOC by the adrenal fasciculata and may also stimulate the adrenal glomerulosa in the absence of hyper-reninemia.

Adrenal tumors, especially adrenal carcinomas, are the more typical cause of Cushing syndrome in infants and small children. They occur with much greater frequency in girls. Adrenal adenomas almost always secrete cortisol with minimal secretion of mineralocorticoids or sex steroids. Adrenal carcinomas tend to secrete cortisol with androgens. Congenital bodily asymmetry (hemihypertrophy) may be associated with adrenal adenoma or carcinoma, with or without association with the Beckwith–Wiedemann syndrome. CT and MRI are useful in the diagnosis of adrenal tumors. The treatment is surgical, although the prognosis for adrenal carcinoma is generally poor. A few patients have done well with adjunctive therapy with *ortho-*,*para*-DDD. Size is the best guide to differentiating adenoma (<10 cm) from carcinoma.

ACTH-independent multinodular adrenal hyperplasia, a rare entity characterized by the secretion of both cortisol and adrenal androgens, is seen in infants, children and young adults, with females affected more frequently. Familial instances have been seen and many have an autosomal-dominant disorder (Carney complex), consisting of pigmented lentigines and blue nevi on the face, lips and conjunctivae, atrial myxomas and a variety of other tumors including schwannomas and Sertoli cell tumors. Adrenalectomy is usually indicated, although some successes have been reported with subtotal resections. A form of multinodular adrenal hyperplasia is occasionally seen in the McCune–Albright syndrome, suggesting that this form of adrenal hyperfunction may be associated with a G-protein defect.

Differential diagnosis

The suspicion of Cushing syndrome in children is usually raised by weight gain, growth arrest, mood change and change in facial appearance (plethora, acne, hirsutism). The diagnosis may be subtle and difficult when it is sought early in the natural history of the disease. Absolute elevations of concentrations of plasma ACTH and cortisol are often absent. Rather than finding morning concentrations of cortisol >25 μg/dL (700 nmol/L) or of ACTH >50 pg/mL (11 pmol/L), it is more typical to find mild, often equivocal elevations in the afternoon and evening values. This loss of diurnal rhythm, evidenced by continued secretion of ACTH and cortisol throughout the afternoon, evening and night, is usually the earliest reliable laboratory index of Cushing disease. Values for ACTH and cortisol are typically extremely high in the ectopic ACTH syndrome, whereas cortisol is elevated but ACTH suppressed in adrenal tumors and in multinodular adrenal hyperplasia (Table 6.4).

The performance of low- and high-dose dexamethasone suppression tests can be useful. Two days of baseline (control) data should be obtained. Low-dose dexamethasone (20 μg/kg/day) should be given, divided into equal doses given every 6 h for 2 days followed by high-dose dexamethasone (80 μg/kg/day) given in the same fashion. Values at 08.00 and 20.00 h for ACTH and cortisol and 24-h urine collections for free cortisol and creatinine should be obtained on each of the 6 days of the test.

Because of variations due to episodic secretion of ACTH, 08.00 and 20.00 h blood values should be drawn in triplicate: on the hour and 15 and 30 min after. In patients with exogenous obesity or other non-Cushing disorders, cortisol, ACTH and urinary steroids will be suppressed readily by low-dose dexamethasone.

Patients with adrenal adenoma, adrenal carcinoma or the ectopic ACTH syndrome will have values relatively insensitive to both low- and high-dose dexamethasone, although some patients with multinodular adrenal hyperplasia may respond to high-dose suppression.

Table 6.4 Diagnostic values in various causes of Cushing syndrome.

Test	Values	Normal	Adrenal carcinoma	Nodular adrenal adenoma	Adrenal hyperplasia	Cushing disease	Ectopic ACTH syndrome
Plasma cortisol	AM	>14	↑	↑	↑	±	↑↑
concentration	PM	<8	↑	↑	↑	↑	↑↑
Plasma ACTH	AM	<100	↓	↓	↓	↑	↑↑
concentration	PM	<50	↓	↓	↓	↑	↑↑
Low-dose dex	Cortisol	<3	No Δ	No Δ	No Δ	—[a]	No Δ
suppression	ACTH	<30	No Δ	No Δ	No Δ	—[a]	No Δ
	17-OHCS	<2	No Δ	No Δ	No Δ	—[a]	No Δ
High-dose dex	Cortisol	↓↓	No Δ	No Δ	—[b]	↓	No Δ
suppression	ACTH	↓↓	No Δ	No Δ	—[b]	↓	No Δ
	17-OHCS	↓↓	No Δ	No Δ	—[b]	↓	No Δ
Intravenous ACTH test	Cortisol	>20	No Δ	±↑	±↑	↑	No Δ
Metyrapone test	Cortisol	↓	±↓	No Δ	±↓	↓	±↓
	11-Deoxycortisol	↑	±↑	No Δ	±↑	↑	±↑
	ACTH	↑	No Δ	No Δ	±↑	↑	No Δ
	17-OHCS	↑	No Δ	No Δ	±	↑	No Δ
24-h urinary	17-OHCS		↑↑	↑	↑	↑	↑ (basal)
excretion	17-Ketosteroids		↑↑	±↑	↑	↑	↑
Plasma concentration	DHEA or DHEAS		↑↑	↓	±↑	↑	↑

Dex, dexamethasone.
Cortisol concentration in mg/dL. ACTH concentration in pg/mL. 17-OHCS in mg/24 h.
[a]Incomplete response (i.e. ±).
[b]Usually no Δ.

Patients with Cushing disease classically respond with suppression of ACTH, cortisol and urinary steroids during the high-dose treatment but not during the low-dose treatment. However, some children, especially those early in the course of their illness, may exhibit partial suppression in response to low-dose dexamethasone. Thus, if the low dose that is given exceeds 20 μg/kg/day or if the assays used are insufficiently sensitive to distinguish partial from complete suppression, false-negative tests may result. In general, the diagnosis of Cushing disease is considerably more difficult to establish in children than in adults.

Virilizing and feminizing adrenal tumors

Most virilizing adrenal tumors are carcinomas producing a mixed array of androgens and glucocorticoids. Virilizing and feminizing adrenal adenomas are rare. Virilizing tumors in boys have a presentation similar to that of simple virilizing CAH with phallic enlargement, erections, pubic and axillary hair, increased muscle mass, deepening of the voice, acne and scrotal thinning; testicular size will be prepubertal. Elevated concentrations of testosterone in young boys alter behavior, with increased irritability, rambunctiousness, hyperactivity and rough play without evidence of libido. Diagnosis is based on hyperandrogenemia that is insuppressible by glucocorticoids. The treatment is surgical; all such tumors should be handled as if they are malignant, with care exerted not to cut the capsule and seed cells on to the peritoneum. The pathological distinction between adrenal adenoma and carcinoma is difficult.

Feminizing adrenal tumors are extremely rare. P450aro, the enzyme aromatizing androgenic precursors to estrogens, is not normally found in the adrenals but is found in peripheral tissues such as fat. It is not known whether most feminizing adrenal tumors exhibit ectopic adrenal production of this enzyme, whether some other enzyme mediates aromatization in the tumor or whether these are truly androgen producing, virilizing tumors occurring in a setting where there is unusually effective peripheral aromatization of adrenal androgens.

Feminizing adrenal (or extra-adrenal) tumors can be distinguished from true (central) precocious puberty in girls by the absence of increased circulating concentrations of gonadotropins and by a prepubertal response of luteinizing hormone to an intravenous challenge of gonadotropin-releasing hormone (GnRH).

In boys, such tumors will cause gynecomastia, which will resemble the benign gynecomastia that often accompanies puberty. However, as with virilizing adrenal tumors, testicular size and the gonadotropin response to GnRH testing will be prepubertal. The diagnosis of a feminizing tumor in a pubertal boy can be extremely difficult but is usually suggested by an arrest in pubertal progression and can be proved by the persistence of circulating plasma estrogens after the administration of testosterone.

Conn syndrome

Conn syndrome, characterized by hypertension, polyuria, hypokalemic alkalosis and low PRA due to an aldosterone-producing adrenal adenoma, is well described in adults but is extremely rare in children. The diagnostic task is to differentiate primary aldosteronism from physiological secondary hyperaldosteronism. Loss of sodium, retention of potassium or decrease in blood volume will result in hyper-reninemic secondary hyperaldosteronism. Renal tubular acidosis, treatment with diuretics, salt-wasting nephritis or hypovolemia due to nephrosis, ascites or blood loss are typical settings for physiological secondary hyperaldosteronism. Primary aldosteronism is characterized by hypertension and hypokalemic alkalosis. The cause is a small adrenal adenoma, usually confined to one adrenal. Both adrenals need to be explored surgically because adrenal vein catheterization is not possible in children and is difficult in adults.

Glucocorticoid therapy and withdrawal

Glucocorticoids have been used to treat virtually every known disease. Their rational use falls into two broad categories, replacement in adrenal insufficiency and pharmacotherapeutic use. The latter is largely related to the anti-inflammatory properties of glucocorticoids but also includes their actions to lyze leukemic leukocytes, lower plasma calcium concentrations and reduce increased intracranial pressure through glucocorticoid receptors, which are found in most cells. Glucocorticoids increase glucose by inducing genes encoding enzymes that result in increased plasma concentrations of glucose, obesity and muscle wasting.

Because there appears to be only one major type of glucocorticoid receptor, all glucocorticoids affect all tissues containing such receptors. Thus, with the exception of the distinction between glucocorticoids and mineralocorticoids, tissue-, disease- or response-specific analogs of naturally occurring glucocorticoids cannot be produced. The only differences among the various glucocorticoid preparations are their ratio of glucocorticoid to mineralocorticoid activity, their capacity to bind to various binding proteins, their molar potency and their biological half-life. Dexamethasone is commonly used in reducing increased intracranial pressure and brain edema. Neurosurgical experience indicates that the optimal doses are 10–100 times those that would thoroughly saturate all available receptors, suggesting that this action of dexamethasone may not be mediated through the glucocorticoid receptor.

Replacement therapy

Glucocorticoid replacement is complicated by undesirable side-effects with even minor degrees of overtreatment or undertreatment. Overtreatment can cause the signs and symptoms of Cushing syndrome and even minimal overtreatment can impair growth. Undertreatment causes signs and symptoms of adrenal insufficiency only if the extent of undertreatment (dose and duration) is considerable but undertreatment may impair the capacity to respond to stress.

To optimize glucocorticoid replacement in children, physicians have aimed to mimic the endogenous secretory rate of cortisol, generally reckoned to be 12.5 (9.5–15.5) mg/m^2/day. This time-honored value may be too high and appropriate replacement may be as low as 6 mg/m^2 in younger children and 9 mg/m^2 in older children and adolescents but there is considerable variation in the normal cortisol secretory rate among different children of the same size.

The specific form of adrenal insufficiency influences therapy. When treating Addison disease, it is prudent to err slightly on the side of undertreatment. This eliminates iatrogenic growth retardation and permits the pituitary to continue to produce normal to slightly elevated concentrations of ACTH which stimulates the remaining functional adrenal steroidogenic machinery and provides a convenient means of monitoring the effects of therapy.

When treating CAH, the adrenal should be suppressed more completely, since any adrenal steroidogenesis will result in the production of unwanted androgens, with their consequent virilization and rate of advancement of bony maturation that is more rapid than the rate of advancement of height.

The presence or absence of associated mineralocorticoid deficiency is important. Children with mild degrees of mineralocorticoid insufficiency, such as those with simple virilizing CAH, may continue to have mildly elevated ACTH values, suggesting insufficient glucocorticoid replacement in association with elevated PRA. Chronic hypovolemia itself leads to elevated ACTH in an attempt to stimulate the adrenal to produce more mineralocorticoid. In this situation, children may not manifest signs and symptoms of mineralocorticoid insufficiency but treatment with mineralocorticoid replacement may permit a decrease the amount of glucocorticoid replacement needed to suppress plasma ACTH, which reduces the likelihood that adult height will be compromised.

The specific formulation of glucocorticoid is of great importance. Long-acting glucocorticoids, such as dexa-methasone or prednisone, are preferred in the treatment of adults but are rarely appropriate for children. Small, incremental dose changes are more easily carried out with weaker glucocorticoids. It is easy to change from 25 to 30 mg of hydrocortisone but virtually impossible to change from an equivalent 0.5 to 0.6 mg of dexamethasone. The efficacy of attempting to mimic the physiological diurnal variation in steroid hormone secretion remains controversial. Since ACTH and cortisol concentrations are high in the morning and low in the evening, it is intellectually and logically appealing to attempt to duplicate this circadian rhythm in replacement therapy. However, the results do not indicate clearly that better growth is achieved by giving relatively larger doses in the morning and lower doses at night.

Dose equivalents among various glucocorticoids can be misleading (Table 6.5) because most preparations of glucocorticoids are intended for therapeutic use rather than replacement therapy and because the most common indication for pharmacological doses of glucocorticoids is for their anti-inflammatory properties.

All these variables explain why there is little unanimity in recommendations for designing a glucocorticoid replacement regimen. An understanding of them will permit appropriate monitoring of the patient and encourage the physician to vary the treatment according to the responses and needs of the individual child.

Commonly used glucocorticoid preparations

Numerous steroid preparations are commercially available. Choosing the appropriate product can be simplified by considering only the most widely used steroids listed in Table 6.5. There are four relevant considerations.

Firstly, the glucocorticoid potency of the various drugs is generally calculated and described according to the anti-inflammatory potency.

Secondly, the growth-suppressant effect of a glucocorticoid preparation may be significantly different from its anti-inflammatory effect.

Thirdly, the mineralocorticoid activity of various glucocorticoid preparations varies widely.

Fourthly, the plasma and biological half-lives of preparations may be discordant and vary widely.

In addition to these chemical considerations, the route of administration is critical and each preparation is designed to deliver the maximal concentration of steroid to the desired tissue while delivering less steroid systemically. All preparations are absorbed to varying extents, so that the inhaled preparations used to treat asthma can cause growth retardation and other signs of Cushing syndrome.

Orally administered steroids are absorbed rapidly but incompletely, whereas intramuscularly administered steroids are absorbed slowly but completely. Thus, if the secretory rate of cortisol is $8 \, mg/m^2$ body surface area, the intramuscular or intravenous replacement dose of cortisol (hydrocortisone) would be $8 \, mg/m^2$. However, because only about half of an oral dose is absorbed intact, the oral equivalent would be about 15–20 mg of hydrocortisone. The efficiency of absorption of glucocorticoids can vary considerably depending on diet, gastric acidity, bowel transit time and other

Table 6.5 Potency of various therapeutic steroids (set relative to the potency of cortisol).

Steroid	Anti-inflammatory glucocorticoid effect	Growth-retarding glucocorticoid effect	Salt-retaining mineralocorticoid effect	Plasma half-life (min)	Biological half-life (h)
Cortisol (hydrocortisone)	1.0	1.0	1.0	80–120	8
Cortisone acetate (oral)	0.8	0.8	0.8	80–120	8
Cortisone acetate (IM)	0.8	1.3	0.8		18
Prednisone	3.5–4	5	0.8	200	16–36
Prednisolone	4		0.8	120–300	16–36
Methyl prednisolone	5	7.5	0.5		
Betamethasone	25–30		0	130–330	
Triamcinolone	5		0		
Dexamethasone	30	80	0	150–300	36–54
9α-fluorocortisone	15		200		
DOC acetate	0		20		
Aldosterone	0.3		200–1000		

individual factors. Thus, the dose equivalents listed in Table 6.5 are only general approximations.

ACTH can be used for glucocorticoid therapy by its action to stimulate endogenous adrenal steroidogenesis but this is no longer generally favored, principally because it will stimulate synthesis of mineralocorticoids and adrenal androgens as well as glucocorticoids.

Pharmacological steroid therapy

Pharmacological doses of glucocorticoids administered for more than 1 or 2 weeks will cause signs and symptoms of iatrogenic Cushing syndrome. These are similar to the glucocorticoid-induced findings in Cushing disease but may be more severe because of the high doses involved (Table 6.6). Iatrogenic Cushing syndrome is not associated with adrenal androgen effects and mineralocorticoid effects are rare.

Alternate-day therapy can decrease the toxicity of pharmacological glucocorticoid therapy, especially suppression of the hypothalamo-pituitary–adrenal axis and growth. The basic premise of alternate-day therapy is that the disease state can be suppressed with intermittent therapy, while there is significant recovery of the hypothalamo-pituitary–adrenal axis during the 'off' day. Alternate-day therapy requires the use of a short-acting glucocorticoid administered once in the morning of each therapeutic day to ensure that the 'off' day is truly 'off'. Long-acting glucocorticoids, such as dexamethasone, should not be used for

Table 6.6 Complications of high-dose glucocorticoid therapy.

Short-term therapy	Long-term therapy
Gastritis	Gastric ulcers
Growth arrest	Short stature
Increased appetite	Weight gain
Hypercalciuria	Osteoporosis, fractures
Glycosuria	Slipped epiphyses
Immune suppression	Ischemic bone necrosis
Masked symptoms of infection, especially fever and inflammation	Poor wound healing
	Catabolism
Toxic psychoses	Cataracts
	Bruising (capillary fragility)
	Adrenal/pituitary suppression
	Toxic psychosis

alternate-day therapy; results are best with oral prednisone or methyl prednisolone.

Withdrawal of glucocorticoid therapy

Withdrawal of glucocorticoid therapy can lead to symptoms of glucocorticoid insufficiency. When glucocorticoid therapy has been used for up to 10 days, therapy can be discontinued abruptly, even if high doses have been used, because the hypothalamo-pituitary–adrenal axis recovers very rapidly from short-term suppression.

When therapy has persisted for 2 weeks or longer, recovery of hypothalamo-pituitary–adrenal function is slower and tapered doses of glucocorticoids are indicated. Acute discontinuation of therapy in such patients will lead to symptoms of glucocorticoid insufficiency, the so-called steroid withdrawal syndrome. This symptom complex does not include salt loss, since mineralocorticoids are regulated by the renin–angiotensin system, which remains normal. However, blood pressure can fall abruptly, since glucocorticoids are required for the action of catecholamines in maintaining vascular tone.

Symptoms of the steroid withdrawal syndrome include malaise, anorexia, headache, lethargy, nausea and fever. Reducing pharmacological doses to physiological replacement doses is rarely successful and occasionally disastrous. Even when given physiological replacement, patients who have been receiving pharmacological doses of glucocorticoids experience steroid withdrawal probably because long-term pharmacological glucocorticoid therapy inhibits transcription of the gene(s) for glucocorticoid receptors, thereby reducing the number of receptors per cell.

The duration of glucocorticoid therapy is a critical consideration in designing a glucocorticoid withdrawal program. Therapy for a couple of months will completely suppress the hypothalamo-pituitary–adrenal axis but will not cause adrenal atrophy. Therapy of years' duration may result in almost total atrophy of the adrenal fasciculate and reticularis, which may require a withdrawal regimen that takes months.

Procedures for tapering steroids are empirical. In patients on long-standing therapy, a 25% reduction in the previous level of therapy is generally recommended weekly. When withdrawal is done with steroids other than cortisone or cortisol, measurement of morning cortisol values can be a useful adjunct. Morning cortisol values of 10 µg/dL (250 nmol/L) or more indicate that the dose can be reduced safely.

Even after the successful discontinuation of therapy, the hypothalamo-pituitary–adrenal axis is not normal and may be incapable of responding to stress for 6–12 months. Evaluation of the hypothalamus and pituitary by a CRH or metyrapone test and evaluation of adrenal responsiveness to pituitary stimulation with an intravenous ACTH test should be done at the conclusion of a withdrawal program and 6 months thereafter. The results of these tests will indicate if there is a need for steroid cover in acute surgical stress or illness.

Stress doses of glucocorticoids

The cortisol secretory rate increases significantly during stress such as trauma, surgery or severe illness. Patients receiving glucocorticoid replacement therapy or those recently withdrawn from pharmacological therapy need cover with stress doses.

It is generally said that doses 3–10 times physiological replacement are needed for the stress of surgery but it is probably not necessary to give more than 3 times physiological requirements. It is not necessary to triple a child's physiological replacement regimen during simple colds, upper respiratory infection, otitis media or after immunizations.

The preparation of the hypoadrenal patient on replacement therapy for surgery is simple if planned in advance. Although stress doses of steroids can be administered intravenously by the anesthetist during surgery, this may be suboptimal. Doses administered as an intravenous bolus are short acting and may not provide cover throughout the procedure. The transition from ward to operating room to recovery room usually involves a transition among three or more teams of personnel, increasing the risk for error. Because intramuscularly administered cortisone acetate has a biological half-life of about 18 h, intramuscular administration of twice the day's physiological requirement at 18 h and again at 8 h before surgery is recommended. This provides the patient with a body reservoir of glucocorticoid throughout the surgical and immediate post-operative period. Regular therapy at 2–3 times physiological requirements can then be reinstituted on the day after the surgical procedure.

Mineralocorticoid replacement

Replacement therapy with mineralocorticoids is indicated in salt-losing CAH and in syndromes of adrenal insufficiency that affect the zona glomerulosa. Only one mineralocorticoid, 9α-fluorocortisol (Fluorinef), is currently available. There is no parenteral mineralocorticoid preparation, so hydrocortisone and salt must be used.

Mineralocorticoid doses used are essentially the same irrespective of the size or age of the patient. Newborns are quite insensitive to mineralocorticoids and may require larger doses than adults. The replacement dose of 9α-fluorocortisol is usually 50–100 mg daily; sodium must be available to the nephrons for mineralocorticoids to promote reabsorption of sodium.

Cortisol has significant mineralocorticoid activity and, when given in stress doses, provides adequate mineralocorticoid activity so that mineralocorticoid replacement can be interrupted. Because 9α-fluorocortisol can be administered only orally and because this may not be possible in the post-operative period, the appropriate drug for glucocorticoid replacement is cortisol or cortisone, which have mineralocorticoid activity, rather than a synthetic steroid such as prednisone or dexamethasone, which have little mineralocorticoid activity.

7 Disorders of Calcium and Bone Metabolism

Learning Points

- Calcium homeostasis is maintained principally by parathyroid hormone (PTH) and vitamin D
- Calcium is important for bone and neuromuscular function
- Hypocalcemia may be associated with hypoparathyroidism, PTH resistance, or causes of rickets
- Rickets due to vitamin D deficiency is more common in exclusively breast fed, dark-skinned infants who do not receive adequate sun exposure or vitamin D supplementation

- Hypoparathyroidism may be the presenting feature of autoimmune polyglandular syndrome type 1
- Activating or inactivating mutations of G-proteins cause McCune–Albright syndrome or pseudohypoparathyroidism and may cause dysfunction of other G-protein receptors
- Activating or inactivating mutations of the calcium-sensing receptor cause hypo- or hypercalcemia, respectively
- Hyperparathyroidism is less common than hypoparathyroidism in children and may be associated with multiple endocrine neoplasia

---

Calcium has an important role in maintaining normal neuromuscular function but it also has a structural role as a component of bone. The mechanisms that exist to juggle these two processes can be disrupted by a wide variety of causes.

Physiology of calcium metabolism

Calcium

Calcium circulates in plasma in three fractions. The most important is the ionized fraction, which constitutes about 50% of the total and is maintained at a concentration of between 1.1 and 1.3 mmol/L. This

determines optimal neuromuscular function and is maintained by various endocrine factors. Most of the remainder, approximately 40%, circulates bound to albumin and conditions associated with hypoalbuminemia may reduce the total circulating concentration without affecting the ionized calcium. The remainder of the total calcium circulates complexed to other molecules such as citrate and sulfate.

It is possible to measure ionized calcium directly, although this is not routine in most laboratories, which usually measure total calcium and albumin, often making an adjustment to allow for the albumin concentration. In practice, these adjustments have little clinical relevance unless severe hypoalbuminemia is present.

Calcium is absorbed in the upper small bowel via an active transcellular transport mechanism, which is stimulated by the action of $1\alpha,25$-dihydroxyvitamin D ($1\alpha,25(OH)_2D$) and is saturable, and a smaller passive

Handbook of Clinical Pediatric Endocrinology, 1st edition. By Charles G. D. Brook and Rosalind S. Brown. Published 2008 by Blackwell Publishing, ISBN: 978-1-4501-6109-1.

paracellular mechanism. Absorption of calcium may be reduced in the presence of calcium-binding agents such as phytate or oxalate.

Excretion is mainly via the kidney and is influenced by a number of dietary factors including sodium, protein, and acid load, all of which increase calcium excretion. Most reabsorption occurs in the proximal tubule (70%) with a further 20% in the ascending loop of Henle. Only 5–10% is reabsorbed in the distal tubule but it is this that is mainly under hormonal control.

During childhood, particularly during the phases of rapid growth in infancy and adolescence, calcium absorption exceeds excretion sufficiently to allow for bone mineralization and it is at these times that the highest proportion of ingested calcium is absorbed.

Urinary calcium excretion is most easily measured by assessing the ratio of calcium to creatinine (Ca/Cr) in a mid-morning urine specimen, which should not normally exceed 0.7 mmol/mmol (0.25 mg/mg). Excess calcium excretion occurs in hypercalcemic conditions associated with hyperparathyroidism and vitamin D excess, as well as in those not associated with hypercalcemia such as activating mutations of the calcium-sensing receptor (CaSR) and distal renal tubular acidosis, all of which may cause nephrocalcinosis. Hypercalcemia associated with inactivating mutations of the CaSR or hypocalcemia caused by hypoparathyroidism results in low urinary calcium excretion.

Phosphate

Phosphate circulates in plasma in the form of phospholipids, phosphate esters, and free inorganic phosphate (P_i). Plasma P_i concentrations are not tightly controlled and reflect the fluxes of phosphate entering and leaving the extracellular pool. Phosphate concentrations vary considerably during life, being highest during phases of rapid growth. Thus, phosphate concentrations in premature infants are normally above 2.0 mmol/L (6 mg/dL), falling to 1.3–2.0 mmol/L (3.9–6 mg/dL) during infancy and childhood and to 0.7–1.3 mmol/L (2.1–3.9 mg/dL) in young adults.

Phosphate is absorbed throughout the small bowel by passive and active mechanisms. The total amount absorbed is largely dependent on dietary phosphate but may be inhibited by phosphate-binding agents such as calcium carbonate. This is of value in hyperphosphatemic states, such as chronic renal failure, when phosphate absorption needs to be limited.

Regulation of plasma phosphate occurs principally in the renal tubule. Between 85% and 98% of the filtered load of phosphate is reabsorbed, mainly by the proximal renal tubule. This represents about 10 times the amount absorbed via the intestine. The tubular reabsorption of phosphate (TRP) by the renal tubule is a saturable process determined both by the filtered load, which is itself determined by glomerular filtration rate (GFR) and plasma concentration, and by hormonal factors, particularly parathyroid hormone (PTH), which increases phosphate excretion.

Control of phosphate excretion is determined by two genes, PHEX and FGF23. The PHEX (phosphate-regulating gene with homology to endopeptidases on the X chromosome) gene encodes a 749-amino-acid membrane glycoprotein and is present in several tissues but not kidney. It is located on the X chromosome and mutations cause classical autosomal-dominant X-linked hypophosphatemic rickets (XLH).

The FGF23 gene is located on chromosome 12p13 and encodes a 251-amino-acid peptide that is further processed to amino- and carboxy-terminal fragments. Mutations in this gene are thought to prevent this processing, and the presence of FGF23 appears responsible for the excess phosphate wasting seen in autosomal-dominant hypophosphatemic rickets (ADHR).

Excess phosphate excretion is seen in renal tubular abnormalities, such as the Fanconi syndrome (whatever the cause) and in hereditary hypophosphatemic rickets with hypercalciuria (HHRH), the cause of which is unknown. Some cases of McCune–Albright polyostotic fibrous dysplasia also have excess phosphate excretion.

Alkaline phosphatase

This enzyme exists in three main isoforms, intestinal (IAP), placental (PLAP), and tissue non-specific (TNAP). Different post-translational modifications of TNAP enzyme result in three tissue-specific forms in bone, liver, and kidney.

Magnesium

This cation circulates in plasma in a concentration of 0.7–1.2 mmol/L (1.4–2.4 mEq/L) and is important because adequate magnesium is required for normal PTH secretion.

It is absorbed in the small intestine via a specific active transport mechanism. Excretion occurs along several sites in the nephron, particularly the ascending loop of Henle and distal convoluted tubule. Renal tubular transport occurs by both paracellular and transcellular mechanisms and defects in these mechanisms can lead to excessive urinary losses.

Calcium homeostasis

Four factors maintain normal calcium physiology, PTH, vitamin D and its metabolites, PTH-related protein (PTHrP), and calcitonin. The first two are the most important outside fetal life. Magnesium has an important part to play since deficiency interferes with PTH secretion.

The concentration of plasma ionized calcium is controlled by a cascade of events (Fig. 7.1). The calcium concentration is detected by a CaSR located on the surface of the parathyroid glands. This is linked to secretion of PTH via an adenylate cyclase system. PTH acts via receptors on the various target organs. These actions are effected mainly via adenylate cyclase, to which it is linked by G-proteins. Defects in any part of this cascade can give rise to hyper- or hypocalcemia. Other factors (vitamin D, magnesium, and PTHrP) have an impact on the cascade and interact with it.

Calcium-sensing receptor (CaSR)

A CaSR is present in the PT glands, renal tubule, bone, cartilage, and other tissues. PTH secretion changes in a sigmoidal fashion in response to acute changes in plasma calcium and there is a continuous tonic secretion of PTH, which maintains plasma-ionized calcium at whatever level is 'set' by the CaSR. Magnesium also binds to the CaSR and influences PTH secretion in a fashion similar to that of calcium. However, severe magnesium deficiency inhibits PTH secretion, probably because the adenylate cyclase coupled to the G-protein is itself magnesium dependent.

Mutations within the CaSR gene result in either inactivation or activation of the receptor, which result in hyper- and hypocalcemia, respectively. Inactivating mutations cause insensitivity to calcium so PTH secretion is switched off at a higher concentration than normal and hypercalcemia results. The receptors are also present in the renal tubule and renal calcium excretion is thereby reduced. The resulting condition is known as familial benign hypercalcemia (FBH) or familial hypocalciuric hypercalcemia (FHH).

Activating mutations of the receptor cause chronic hypocalcemia and hypercalciuria, a condition known as autosomal-dominant hypocalcemia (ADH).

Parathyroid glands

The four parathyroid glands are derived from the third (lower glands) and fourth (upper glands) branchial arches. Several transcription factors are involved in their development. Mutations within the genes responsible for these factors result in congenital hypoparathyroidism, which may be isolated or associated with other conditions such as the hypopara-thyroidism, deafness, renal anomalies (HDR) syndrome, and the CATCH 22 complex, of which the DiGeorge syndrome (DGS) is part. Destruction of the glands may occur as a result of surgery, autoantibodies, or infiltration (e.g. with iron).

Parathyroid hormone

PTH is a single-chain, 84-amino-acid, polypeptide hormone encoded by a gene on chromosome 11. It is synthesized by the parathyroid glands from prepro-PTH, which has an additional 31 amino acids. Synthesis occurs in the ribosomes, where the initial 25-amino-acid 'pre' sequence acts as a signal peptide to aid transport through the rough endoplasmic reticulum. The 'pre' sequence is cleaved and pro-PTH then travels to the Golgi apparatus where the 6-amino-acid 'pro' sequence is cleaved to yield the mature hormone, which is stored in secretory vesicles that fuse with the plasma membrane prior to secretion. Very little PTH is stored so most secreted hormone is newly synthesized.

Only the first 34 N-terminal amino acids are required for full activity and the function of the remainder of the molecule is not understood. The half-life of PTH in the circulation is 1–2 min. The molecule is cleaved at various sites, which results in a number of fragments that can be identified in the circulation. Assays of PTH measure 'intact' 1–34 PTH, which correlates well with bioactivity.

PTH has two principal target organs, bone, and kidney. In bone, PTH promotes bone mineralization by an action on osteoblasts when present in physiological concentrations. During phases of hypocalcemia, when PTH concentrations rise, its main target cell is the osteoclast, where it activates bone resorption.

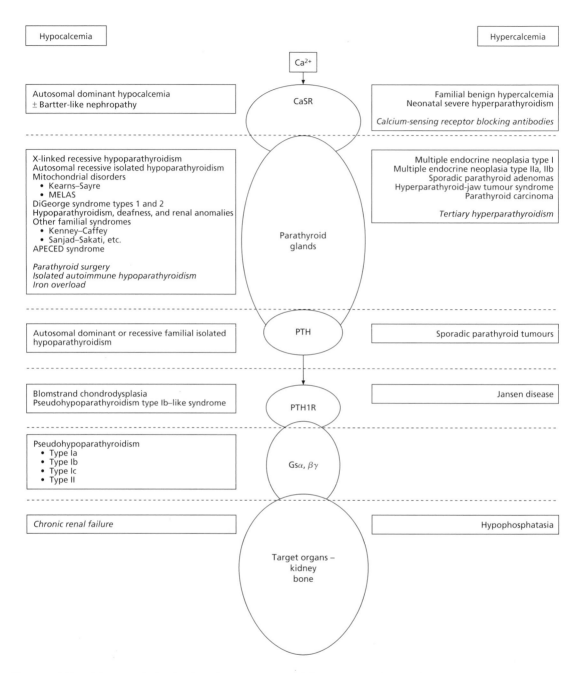

Figure 7.1 The calcium cascade showing the various components and the points along the cascade at which abnormalities can occur. Genetic conditions are shown in normal type and acquired conditions in italics.

In the nephron, most of the filtered calcium is reabsorbed passively in the proximal tubule, where PTH stimulates the action of 1α-hydroxylase, the enzyme that converts vitamin D to its active metabolite, 1α,25(OH)$_2$D. PTH also promotes calcium and magnesium transcellular reabsorption in the distal nephron. Phosphate excretion increases in response to PTH, which allows excess phosphate (removed from

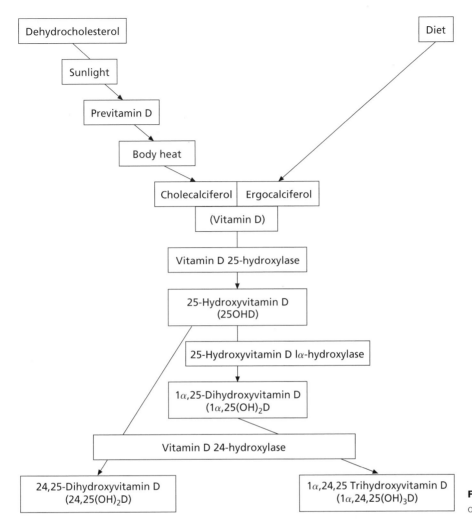

Figure 7.2 Principal steps of vitamin D metabolism.

bone with calcium following PTH-stimulated bone resorption) to be excreted. PTH also stimulates renal excretion of bicarbonate and amino acids. Thus, hyperparathyroidism results in a mild acquired form of the Fanconi syndrome.

Vitamin D

Vitamin D exists in two forms. Cholecalciferol is synthesized as a result of the action of ultraviolet (UV) light on 7-dehydrocholesterol. Ergocalciferol is synthesized by plants and is equipotent with cholecalciferol and metabolized in a similar fashion. The generic term vitamin D is used to include both compounds.

Under normal circumstances, about 80% of vitamin D consists of cholecalciferol synthesized in skin, the remainder being acquired from dietary sources as both chole- and ergocalciferols. The amount of vitamin D synthesized in skin is dependent upon skin color and exposure. Following synthesis, it becomes bound to a specific vitamin D-binding protein (DBP) and passes to adipose tissue and the liver for storage and further metabolism.

Vitamin D does not have significant biological activity. Its activity requires hydroxylation at the 25 and 1 positions (Fig. 7.2). The first step is catalyzed by vitamin D 25-hydroxylase.

25-Hydroxyvitamin D (25(OH)D) circulates in plasma bound to the DBP in nanomolar concentrations. Assay

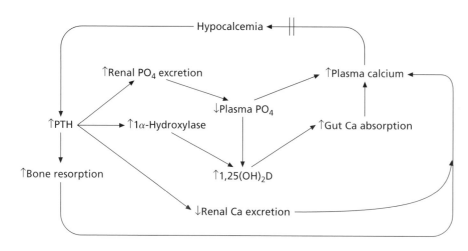

Figure 7.3 Principal responses to a hypocalcemic stimulus.

gives a measure of vitamin D status. Its level varies depending on the supply of vitamin D and shows a considerable annual variation with a peak about 6 weeks after maximal exposure to sunlight. It has some weak activity, which is not normally of clinical significance but may become so in the presence of vitamin D excess. Vitamin D 25-hydroxylase also catalyzes the conversion of the synthetic vitamin D analog, 1α-hydroxy-cholecalciferol (alfacalcidol), to 1α,25(OH)$_2$D.

25(OH)D is metabolized to 1α,25(OH)$_2$D by 25(OH)D 1α-hydroxylase, which is active only against metabolites that are already hydroxylated at position 25. A single enzyme has been identified in the proximal renal tubule. Activity is also present in osteoblasts, keratinocytes, and lymphohematopoietic cells, where 1α,25(OH)$_2$D may have an autocrine or paracrine role. Activity of 1α-hydroxylase is stimulated by PTH.

1α,25(OH)$_2$D is a highly potent compound that circulates in picomolar concentrations. Its synthesis is tightly controlled by the plasma calcium concentration. In order to ensure that changes in 1α,25(OH)$_2$D can occur rapidly, a second enzyme, 25(OH)D 24-hydroxylase, exists to divert metabolism of 25(OH)D away from 1α,25(OH)$_2$D synthesis when this is not needed, and to participate in the degradation of existing 1α,25(OH)$_2$D. It is inhibited by PTH and stimulated by 1α,25(OH)$_2$D.

1α,25(OH)$_2$D acts via a specific vitamin D receptor (VDR) widely distributed in gut, PT glands, chondrocytes, osteoblasts, and osteoclast precursors. It promotes calcium absorption in the small intestine,

suppresses PTH secretion from the PT, influences growth plate mineralization, and stimulates differentiation of osteoclasts.

Calcitonin

Calcitonin is secreted in response to hypercalcemia and acts via specific receptors to counteract the effects of PTH in osteoclasts.

Interactions between calciotropic agents

The primary aim of interactions between the various influences on calcium metabolism is to maintain plasma-ionized calcium within narrow limits. At the same time, bone metabolism must be allowed to proceed satisfactorily so that adequate calcium and phosphate accumulation and bone remodeling can occur during growth.

The hormone factors responsible for calcium homeostasis are summarized in Fig. 7.3.

Disorders of calcium metabolism

Hypocalcemia

Symptoms of hypocalcemia include muscle twitching and spasms, which can be very painful, apnea, stridor, carpopedal spasms, and focal or generalized seizures. A measurement of plasma calcium should always be part of the investigation of unexplained fits to avoid confusion with epilepsy. It is unusual for symptoms to occur until total calcium falls below 1.8 mmol/L (7.2 mg/dL) and some patients remain

Table 7.1 Table of investigations that are indicated when a patient presents with a disorder of calcium metabolism. Not all investigations are indicated in all patients.

Blood – initial investigations	**Urine – initial investigations**
Calcium	Calcium
Phosphate	Phosphate
Albumin	Creatinine
Alkaline phosphatase	
Creatinine	**Calculate**
25(OH)D	Calcium/creatinine ratio
Intact PTH	Fe_{PO4} and TRP
Save serum for $1\alpha,25(OH)_2D$	T_mPO_4/GFR
Subsequent investigations as necessary	**Subsequent investigations as necessary**
Blood gases	Glucose and amino acids
$1\alpha,25(OH)_2D$	Bone turnover and markers
DNA analysis for genetic abnormalities	
PTHrP	
Bone turnover markers	
Radiology and nuclear medicine	
Hand and knee for rickets	
Skeletal survey for bone abnormalities	
Renal ultrasound for parathyroid tumors	
CT scan for intracranial calcification	
SestaMIBI scan for PT gland localization	

asymptomatic with a plasma calcium as low as 1.2 mmol/L (4.8 mg/dL).

Clinical examination may reveal positive Chvostek or Trousseau signs and chronic hypocalcemia may cause calcification of the lens of the eye. Signs of rickets may be present in some instances. Soft tissue calcification is sometimes present in conditions such as pseudohypoparathyroidism (PHP) and computed tomographic (CT) scanning of the brain may reveal the presence of basal ganglion and frontal lobe calcification.

Investigation of disorders of calcium metabolism is summarized in Table 7.1. First-line investigations should include measurement of total (and, if available, ionized) calcium, phosphate, albumin, magnesium, alkaline phosphatase, creatinine, PTH, and 25(OH)D in blood, a sample of which should also be stored for future measurement of $1\alpha,25(OH)_2D$ later if this becomes relevant, particularly if rickets is also present. Urine should be taken for measurement of calcium, phosphate, and creatinine.

X-rays may reveal the presence of rickets, skeletal dysplasias (e.g. in PHP), hyperparathyroid bone disease,

or soft tissue calcification. They are relatively insensitive in detecting intracranial calcification, for which CT scanning is most appropriate. Early nephrocalcinosis can best be detected by ultrasonography. X-rays are less sensitive but, if nephrocalcinosis is demonstrated, this may require further investigation and management of renal function.

Childhood hypocalcemia

Hypocalcemia results from defects in any part of the calcium metabolic cascade. Causes of hypocalcemia that affect the early part of the cascade are generally associated with low PTH and those affecting the latter part with high PTH. The reverse is true of hypercalcemic conditions.

Disorders of the CaSR

Autosomal-dominant hypocalcemia (ADH) is caused by an activating mutation of the CaSR gene. Calcium is sensed as being normal at subphysio-logical levels and PTH secretion is therefore switched off, inappropriately causing hypoparathyroidism. The extent of the resulting hypoparathyroidism is determined by how much the mutation shifts the calcium response curve. Patients may or may not be symptomatic. Several mutations have been described and, although there is no genotype–phenotype correlation, symptoms are related to the degree of hypocalcemia, which remains fairly constant within individuals. Inheritance is usually autosomal dominant but sporadic cases have been described.

It can be difficult to distinguish ADH from isolated hypoparathyroidism in the absence of a family history, and germline mosaicism in an apparently unaffected parent can confuse the issue further and make prediction of recurrence difficult. Diagnosis depends on demonstrating hypocalcemia with normal PTH levels. In contrast to hypoparathyroidism, urinary calcium excretion is relatively high and these patients are susceptible to nephrocalcinosis, especially if treated to prevent symptoms.

The need for treatment largely depends on whether or not symptoms are present. In patients whose plasma calcium is above 1.95 mmol/L (7.8 mg/dL), treatment is unnecessary and, in those with a lower level of calcium, treatment is required only if symptoms are present. 1αOHCC should be used cautiously and in the smallest dose required to prevent symptoms. It is not necessary to restore plasma calcium to normal. Urinary calcium excretion should be monitored to avoid nephrocalcinosis and regular renal ultrasonography can be helpful in detecting early changes. If it proves difficult to prevent symptomatic hypocalcemia without causing nephrocalcinosis, thiazide diuretics may be used. Selective CaSR blocking agents may become available in the future.

Disorders of the parathyroid glands

X-linked recessive familial isolated hypoparathyroidism (FIH), autosomal-recessive isolated hypoparathyroidism and autosomal-dominant hypoparathyroidism, deafness and renal anomalies (HDR) have been described presenting with severe hypoparathyroidism at an early age.

The Kearns–Sayre syndrome (KSS) comprises hypoparathyroidism with progressive external ophthalmoplegia, pigmentary retinopathy, heart block or cardiomyopathy, and proximal myopathy. It may also be associated with diabetes mellitus. It overlaps with the mitochondrial encephalopathy, lactic acidosis, and stroke (MELAS) syndrome in which hypoparathyroidism is associated with a childhood onset of MELAS-like episodes. Proximal myopathy and diabetes mellitus have also been described with this condition.

The DiGeorge syndrome (DGS) consists of PT gland hypoplasia, thymic immunodeficiency, congenital heart disease and facial anomalies, structures all derived from the third and fourth branchial pouches. It is related to the velocardiofacial syndrome (VCFS) and conotruncal anomaly facial syndrome (CTAFS) and a number of non-syndromic cardiac conditions, such as pulmonary atresia with ventricular septal defect, Fallot' s tetralogy, truncus arteriosus, and interrupted aortic arch. Only the DGS includes hypoparathyroidism but they are all linked under the umbrella of the CATCH 22 (*c*ardiac anomalies, *a*bnormal facies, *t*hymic hypoplasia, *c*left palate, and *h*ypocalcemia associated with microdeletions in the long arm of chromosome *22*) syndrome.

The autosomal-recessive Kenny–Caffey and Sanjad–Sakati syndromes as well as that described by Richardson and Kirk are probably all variants of the same condition where hypoparathyroidism is associated with short stature and developmental delay. They have been described mainly in consanguineous families from Saudi Arabia and Kuwait.

The autoimmune polyendocrinopathy–candidiasis–ectodermal dystrophy (APECED) syndrome, also known as the polyglandular autoimmune type 1 syndrome, is an evolving association between mucocutaneous candidiasis and hypoparathyroidism that usually develops in mid-childhood (see Chapter 9).

Other acquired non-genetic forms of hypoparathyroidism include PT gland destruction during thyroid surgery or following parathyroidectomy. Isolated autoimmune hypoparathyroidism may also occur and destruction of the PT glands can occur following iron overload with multiple transfusions in β-thalassemia major.

Disorders of the PTH/PTHrP receptor

Blomstrand's chondrodysplasia is a rare autosomal-recessive condition that results in advanced bone maturation, accelerated chondrocyte maturation, increased density of the skeleton, increased ossification, and poor bone modeling, particularly of the long bones. It is rapidly lethal.

Treatment of hypoparathyroidism

Treatment is aimed at maintaining plasma calcium levels within the lower part of the normal range without causing hypercalciuria. The mainstay of treatment is vitamin D either in its active form, $1\alpha,25(OH)_2D$ (calcitriol), or the analog 1α-hydroxy-cholecalciferol (alfacalcidol). The dose of calcitriol is usually 15–30 ng/kg/day to maintain normocalcemia but requires twice-daily dosage. Alfacalcidol usually requires about twice the dose but, because it has to be metabolized first, it has a longer half-life and needs to be given only once daily. Calcium supplements are usually required, which may enable the dose of alfacalcidol to be reduced. This is a particular advantage in hypoparathyroid disorders in which the renal tubular reabsorptive effects of PTH are lacking and hypercalciuria may supervene. In those patients in whom cardiac failure is also present (e.g. DGS), loop diuretics such as frusemide/furosamide should be used with caution since the hypercalciuric effects of these agents may precipitate symptomatic hypocalcemia. Ultrasound examinations are useful in detecting early nephrocalcinosis.

Hypomagnesemia

Magnesium is a ligand for the CaSR and, if plasma magnesium levels fall, PTH secretion is stimulated in a manner similar to that of hypocalcemia. Hypomagnesemia (<0.5 mmol/L, 1.0 mEq/L) inhibits PTH secretion in response to hypocalcemia. This inhibition is incomplete initially and PTH remains elevated but not as high as would be expected from the degree of hypocalcemia. As levels fall to 0.2–0.3 mmol/L (0.4–0.6 mEq/L), PTH secretion is completely inhibited and a state of hypoparathyroidism then exists. During the initial phase of mild hypomagnesemia, when PTH levels are still elevated, resistance to the action of PTH worsens the hypocalcemia. Thus, hypocalcemia secondary to hypomagnesemia is resistant to treatment until magnesium levels have been restored to normal.

Hypomagnesemia is rare in childhood. It usually arises as a result of impaired intestinal absorption or increased urinary losses, which may occur as a primary defect of renal tubular function or secondary to renal tubular damage.

Treatment of hypomagnesemia is aimed at restoring plasma magnesium concentrations to normal to prevent inhibition of PTH secretion. In the acute state, intramuscular magnesium may be given as a 50% solution of $MgSO_4 \cdot 7H_2O$, which contains 2 mmol (4 mEq)/mL. This may be repeated until magnesium levels are satisfactory. Intravenous infusion should be avoided since magnesium is an intense vasodilator and can cause cardiac arrhythmias. Normal magnesium levels can usually be maintained by oral supplementation, although this may need to be given several times a day. Magnesium glycerophosphate is a useful preparation since it does not cause as much diarrhea as some other preparations.

Parathyroid hormone resistance

This group of conditions, which occurs as a result of defects toward the end of the calcium cascade, is characterized by hypocalcemia, usually but not always accompanied by hyperphosphatemia and raised PTH. The two most important are PHP and deficiencies in the supply or metabolism of vitamin D.

Pseudohypoparathyroidism type Ia (PHP-Ia) is an autosomal-dominant condition characterized by the biochemical features of hypoparathyroidism (hypocalcemia and hyperphosphatemia) with raised levels of PTH. Resistance to the action of PTH can be confirmed by demonstrating lack of cAMP or phosphaturic responses to PTH infusion. A characteristic set of features includes short stature, round facies, shortening of the metacarpals, and meta-tarsals, particularly the fourth and fifth and obesity (collectively termed Albright's hereditary osteodystrophy (AHO)) (Fig. 7.4). Other features include intra-cranial calcification, sensorineural deafness, and a poor sense of smell. Resistance to other cAMP-dependent hormones, especially thyroid-stimulating hormone (TSH) and gonadotropins, may be present, leading to mild hypothyroidism and menstrual irregularity. This syndrome is referred to as PHP-Ia. Following the discovery of the $Gs\alpha$ subunit of the G-protein, it was recognized that inactivating mutations within the gene are responsible for the PTH resistance.

Ten years after the original description of PHP, a second syndrome was described in which AHO was present without an abnormality of calcium metabolism. This was termed *pseudopseudohypoparathyroidism* (PPHP). It subsequently became apparent that both conditions can occur within the same family but not within the same sibship. While both conditions are associated with the skeletal manifestations, it emerged

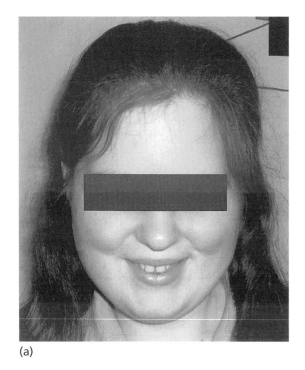

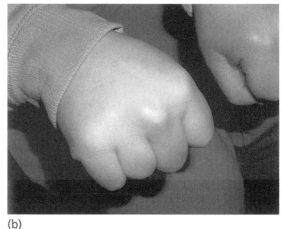

(b)

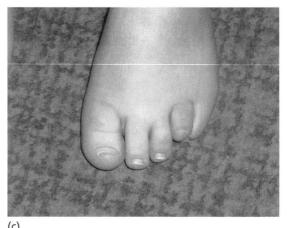

(a)

(c)

Figure 7.4 Photographs of the face (a), showing the typical rounded facies, and of the right hand (b) and left foot (c) of a patient with PHP type Ia showing the typical shortening of the metacarpals and metatarsals seen as part of AHO. She had presented with short stature.

that, when hypocalcemia was present, the gene had been inherited from an affected mother; paternal transmission of the gene did not result in PTH resistance, despite the fact that identical mutations could be demonstrated within families. Gene imprinting was suspected and subsequently confirmed.

In *Pseudohypoparathyroidism type Ib* (PHP-Ib), features of AHO are absent but PTH resistance is present. Renal resistance to PTH can be demonstrated by impaired cAMP and phosphaturic responses. Some patients exhibit hyperparathyroid bone disease, indicating that some measure of bone sensitivity to PTH is retained. These patients have been variously referred

to as pseudohypohyperpara-thyroidism or PHP with raised alkaline phosphatase. The term PHP-Ib is preferred. The etiology is not clear.

Pseudohypoparathyroidism type Ic (PHP-Ic) is characterized by multiple hormone resistance, including PTH, together with features of AHO. No defect in Gsα has been demonstrated and the genetic defect is not known.

Pseudohypoparathyroidism type II (PHP-II) is reserved for a small group of patients who have PTH resistance without features of AHO. The PTH resistance is confined to the phosphaturic response, whereas cAMP responses are normal. The defect has not been identified.

Table 7.2 Biochemical findings in calciopenic vs. phosphopenic rickets.

	Serum						Urine	
	Calcium	Phosphorus	PTH	Alkaline phosphatase	25(OH)D	1,25(OH)$_2$D	TRP	Amino acids
Calciopenic rickets								
Vitamin D deficiency	Normal	Normal or low	High or low	High	Low	Low, normal or high	Low	Negative
Vitamin D 1α-hydroxylase deficiency	Low	Normal or low	High	High	Normal	Low	Low	Negative
Hereditary 1,25(OH)$_2$D-resistant rickets	Low	Low	High	High	Normal	Very high	Low	Negative
Phosphopenic rickets								
Familial hypophosphatemic rickets	Normal	Low	Normal	High	Normal	Normal	Low	Negative
Hereditary hypophosphatemic rickets with hypercalciuria	Normal	Low	Normal	High	Normal	High	Low	Negative
Fanconi syndrome	Normal	Low	Normal	High	Normal	High	Low	High

Treatment of PHP

The principles of treatment of PHP are similar to those of hypoparathyroidism. Alfacalcidol (1–3 mg/day) is usually sufficient to maintain normocalcemia. Hypercalciuria is less likely to occur than in primary hypoparathyroidism and the plasma calcium concentration can usually be kept well within the normal range. Patients with PHP-Ia or PHP-Ic may have resistance to other hormones. TSH is frequently slightly raised and thyroxine is required to suppress this and ensure optimum thyroid function. Menstrual irregularities may require estrogen therapy. The role of growth hormone for short stature is controversial but has been used in some patients with variable effect. If resistance to GHRH can be demonstrated, there is some logic to this therapy. No treatment has a significant effect on the osteodystrophy.

Rickets

Rickets is a disorder of the growth plate defined by a decrease in the endochondral calcification at the growth plate, which results in growth plate deformities, decreased growth rate, and skeletal deformities. Rickets can occur only in growing children; in adults, osteomalacia occurs. Osteomalacia is defined by a decrease in the mineralization of osteoid on the trabecular and cortical surfaces at sites of bone turnover. Children may also develop osteomalacia.

Rickets can be broadly classified into calciopenic and phosphopenic rickets (Table 7.2). *Calciopenic rickets* is characterized by osteopenia and hypocalcemia leading to secondary hyperparathyroidism, which results in excessive bone resorption and decreased bone mass. Symptoms result from hypocalcemia and include irritability, tetany, and seizures. *Phosphopenic rickets* is characterized by increased undermineralized osteoid. Osteopenia does not occur and thus secondary hyperparathyroidism is not a feature; as a result, there is no excessive resorption of bone and bone mass is not decreased. Hypophosphatemia is associated with few symptoms, other than bone pain sometimes, and patients are generally less symptomatic than those who have calciopenic rickets.

There is another group of disorders that are not considered classic forms of rickets but in which mineralization is inhibited and thus rachitic features occur. Examples include hypophosphatasia and fluoride toxicity.

Manifestations of rickets

Clinical

The manifestations of rickets result from the hypocalcemia or hypophosphatemia, the resulting osteomalacia and the effects of the underlying etiology (e.g. vitamin D deficiency) on other organ systems. The age of the child and the bones that sustain the most stress also determine the presentation.

Presenting complaints include decreased growth rate, skeletal deformities, and delayed standing or walking. Young children often do not present with rickets until they start walking and the weight bearing on the legs leads to bowing. In the case of hypocalcemia, muscle weakness, lethargy, irritability, tetany, and seizures may be present.

The physical manifestations of rickets are age dependent. The most common findings are due to swelling around growth plates, especially at wrists and ankle, since these are the sites where growth velocity is greatest. The linear growth rate decreases. The skeletal deformities that occur are due to mechanical stresses on undermineralized bone. Genu varum (bowlegs) and tibial and femoral torsion are common and develop with ambulation in young children with rickets, often leading to a waddling gait. In older children, in whom physiological bowing has disappeared, genu valgum (knock-knees) or a windswept deformity (genu varum on one leg and genu valgum on the other) can occur. In children with severe rickets, coxa vara of the femoral neck can occur and lead to pelvic deformities that may persist into adult life.

Chest deformities include rachitic rosary due to swelling of the costrochondral junction of ribs, which appears as beading along the anterolateral aspect of the ribs. Harrison sulci (grooves) represent indentations where the muscular diaphragm attaches to and pulls on the lower ribs. Eventually, with longstanding rickets, as the ribs become softer, the chest narrows because of negative intrathoracic pressure. Combined with muscle weakness, there can be significant respiratory distress. Scoliosis, kyphosis, and lordosis can occur as a result of muscle weakness and are especially common in adolescents with rickets.

In young children, closure of the fontanelles may be delayed. Craniotabes occurs when there is softening of the skull in the occipital region behind the ears. There may be delayed eruption of primary teeth.

Additional manifestations include muscle weakness, presenting as hypotonia and a delay in the acquisition of gross motor skills in young children, and a proximal myopathy in older patients. This is thought to be due to the effects of vitamin D on muscle, in which there are $1,25(OH)_2D$ receptors, and not of hypocalcemia *per se*. Electrocardiographic changes and left ventricular dysfunction are probably directly related to hypocalcemia.

In children with vitamin D-deficient rickets, there can be manifestations related to the effects of vitamin D on immune function. There may be an increase in respiratory infections due to this, exacerbated by muscle weakness and a small chest size, resulting in poor lung function. In addition, there appears to be an increase in gastrointestinal infections in children with vitamin D deficiency.

Radiographic findings

The radiographic features of rickets are due to lack of endochondral calcification at the growth plate (rickets), decreased mineralization of osteoid at sites of bone turnover (osteomalacia) and secondary hyperparathyroidism.

The first radiographic sign is loss of the demarcation between the growth plate and the distal end of metaphysis as a result of loss of the provisional zone of calcification at the distal metaphysis. The growth plate widens and the distance from epiphyseal center to metaphysis increases. Widening of the growth plate is evident as widening of the ends of the long bones (especially the wrist) and at the costrochondral junctions (rachitic rosary). As the disease progresses, the metaphyses become flared, cupped and widened with irregular outlines and the epiphyses become indistinct or invisible. Because the growth plates of the long bones are most affected, the wrist in young children and knees in older children are the best sites for obtaining radiographs.

The findings of osteomalacia are more difficult to detect. Generalized demineralization or osteopenia is seen. Looser zones (pseudofractures) are not as common in children with osteomalacia as in adults but pathological fractures can occur, as can vertebral compression fractures. Genu varum (bowlegs) and genu valgum (knock-knees) are due to a combination of osteomalacia of the shaft of the long bones and deformation occurring at the unmineralized growth plate.

Secondary hyperparathyroidism contributes to osteopenia but the pathognomonic features of hyperparathyroidism are much less commonly seen in rickets. A coarse trabecular pattern can be seen at the ends of the long bones.

A transverse line of calcification at the end of the metaphysic, usually seen within 1 month of starting treatment, signals the healing of rickets. The metaphyses mineralize, the coarse trabecular pattern fills in and the osteoid mineralizes, appearing as periosteal new bone. The entire healing process takes several months but the skeletal deformities may take years to normalize.

Calciopenic rickets

Calciopenic rickets results from deficiency in calcium or in vitamin D intake or action (Fig. 7.3). Calcium deficiency can be due to inadequate calcium intake or to the use of calcium chelators. Alterations in vitamin D can be due to lack of dietary vitamin D and/or lack of exposure to the sun. Secondary vitamin D deficiency can be due to fat malabsorption from gastrointestinal or hepatobiliary diseases. Decreased production of $1,25(OH)_2D$ can occur as a result of renal osteodystrophy or $25(OH)D$-1α-hydroxylase deficiency. Increased turnover of vitamin D occurs with anticonvulsant use. Nephrotic syndrome leads to increased loss of vitamin D in urine with protein. Finally, there can be resistance to $1,25(OH)_2D$, termed vitamin D-resistant rickets.

Nutritional rickets

Nutritional rickets spans a spectrum from vitamin D deficiency to calcium deficiency, with combinations of relative vitamin D insufficiency and reduced intake of calcium in the middle. Vitamin D deficiency is by far the most common cause of nutritional rickets in developed countries.

Causes of nutritional rickets

Vitamin D-deficient rickets results from a combination of lack of vitamin D formation in the skin and inadequate vitamin D intake. The amount of UV-B radiation that reaches the skin influences the amount of vitamin D made there. In the winter months, at latitudes far from the equator, little vitamin D is synthesized in the skin. For example, in Boston in the winter (42° N), there is insufficient UV-B radiation to convert 7-dehydrocholesterol to pre-vitamin D. Air pollution, the amount of skin exposed and the time it is exposed also influences the amount of vitamin D made. Sunscreens interfere with absorption, as do greater amounts of skin melanin.

Vitamin D-deficient rickets is most common in children between 3 and 18 months of age. Breastfed infants are at high risk because breast milk has only about 20–60 IU/L vitamin D, which is insufficient to maintain normal vitamin D concentrations in the infant and $25(OH)D$ concentrations in breastfed infants primarily reflect their exposure to sunlight. Thus, infants at highest risk of nutritional rickets are dark skinned, breastfed infants who do not receive vitamin D supplementation and who are not exposed to adequate sunlight. It has been estimated that, during the summer months, breastfed infants in the northern USA need 30 min/week exposure to the sun in a diaper only and no sunscreen or 2 h/week if fully clothed but not wearing a hat. Infant formulas contain 400 IU/L vitamin D and 500 mL/day thus provides 200 IU/day vitamin D, which is considered adequate.

Diets low in calcium may exacerbate the effects of vitamin D deficiency. Poor calcium intake leads to increased catabolism of $25(OH)D$ by increasing PTH, which increases $1,25(OH)_2D$ production. $1,25(OH)_2D$ may increase the clearance of $25(OH)D$ by the liver, thus worsening $25(OH)D$ deficiency. This mechanism of the development of rickets may be a common cause of rickets in adolescents in whom calcium intake is low while calcium requirements are increasing as the skeleton is growing.

Calcium deficiency alone is an uncommon cause of rickets and is found primarily in developing countries.

Stages of vitamin D-deficient rickets

The progression of vitamin D-deficient rickets can be broken down into three stages (Table 7.3), each with characteristic biochemical findings. Stage 1, which is usually transient and can be mild, is characterized by hypocalcemia. The decreased amount of $25(OH)D$ results in decreased $1,25(OH)_2D$, which impairs intestinal calcium absorption. The hypocalcemia leads

Table 7.3 25(OH)D, calcium, PTH, phosphorus, and alkaline phosphatase in the three stages of rickets.

	Stage 1	Stage 2	Stage 3
25(OH)D	Decreased	Further decreased	Further decreased
Calcium	Decreases	Increases to low-normal range	Decreases
PTH	Starts to rise	Elevated	Increases further
Phosphorus	Normal	Decreases	Low
Alkaline phosphatase	Increases	Increases	Increases

to increased alkaline phosphatase and secondary hyperparathyroidism. Clinical manifestations in infants include apnea, seizures, tetany, or stridor. Bone changes have not had time to be manifest.

In stage 2, the hypocalcemia leads to secondary hyperparathyroidism, which results in normalization of the calcium concentrations. Calcium is mobilized from bone and reabsorbed from kidney, leading to further increases in alkaline phosphatase. In addition, the elevated PTH concentrations stimulate increased conversion of 25(OH)D to $1,25(OH)_2D$, increasing intestinal absorption of calcium. These effects together normalize serum calcium concentrations. Secondary hyperparathyroidism also results in hypophosphatemia due to the action of PTH on the kidney. During stage 2, radiographic and clinical manifestations of rickets emerge.

In stage 3, rickets becomes severe. The homeostatic mechanisms in place to normalize calcium fail and hypocalcemia recurs as the secondary hyperparathyroidism progresses but with diminishing effect. Depletion of calcium results in decreased PTH-stimulated calcium release from bone, despite high PTH concentrations. Further depletion of 25(OH)D results in relative deficiency of $1,25(OH)_2D$. The hypocalcemia combined with hypophosphatemia leads to the severe clinical and radiological manifestations of rickets.

Laboratory changes in nutritional rickets

Low concentrations of 25(OH)D define vitamin D-deficient rickets, although there is some debate as to what is normal. Despite the normal range in many laboratories being quoted at 9–74 ng/mL, many consider a level of <15 ng/mL to represent vitamin D deficiency and a level of 15–20 ng/mL to represent vitamin D insufficiency. Once the clinical diagnosis of rickets is made, finding a low 25(OH)D level confirms the diagnosis of vitamin D deficiency.

$1,25(OH)_2D$ concentrations are more problematic and variable. They can be elevated because of increased conversion of 25(OH)D to $1,25(OH)_2D$ by PTH. Since $1,25(OH)_2D$ is the active form of vitamin D, it is puzzling that rickets occurs when $1,25(OH)_2D$ concentrations are elevated. It may be that, in stage 1 with low 25(OH)D concentrations, concentrations of $1,25(OH)_2D$ decrease, leading to hypocalcemia. Secondary hyperparathyroidism then occurs in stage 2, increasing the conversion of 25(OH)D to $1,25(OH)_2D$ and thus correcting the hypocalcemia by increasing intestinal absorption of calcium and increasing bone resorption. By stage 3, there is insufficient 25(OH)D to maintain normal $1,25(OH)_2D$ concentrations and the concentrations may be inappropriately low given the degree of elevation of PTH.

Calcium concentrations in nutritional rickets are often normal. Although hypocalcemia does occur in stages 1 and 3, hypocalcemia is not evident in many children with rickets. However, even the mild, transient hypocalcemia in stage 1 leads to secondary hyperparathyroidism, which characterizes nutritional rickets. Hypophosphatemia occurs because of the effect of PTH on the kidney to decrease TRP and increase phosphate loss. However, phosphate concentrations are often normal or elevated, which may be a result of PTH resistance. Urinary calcium excretion is decreased and there can be aminoaciduria and increased loss of bicarbonate in the urine.

Alkaline phosphatase concentrations are increased, even though osteoblastic activity is decreased. Caution must be taken in interpreting alkaline phosphatase concentrations, since the liver isoenzyme represents a large portion of the total alkaline phosphatase and liver disease can also raise alkaline phosphatase concentrations. In addition, alkaline phosphatase concentrations vary with age, pubertal status, growth rate, and nutritional status, further confounding interpretation but alkaline phosphatase is the best marker to follow the progression of rickets with therapy.

Treatment and prevention

Vitamin D deficiency is treated with oral vitamin D2 or D3. Treatment regimens include 5–15 000 IU/day for 4–8 weeks or a single oral or intramuscular dose of 2–600 000 IU. The improvement in biochemical parameters is faster (4–7 days) when a large oral dose of 600 000 IU of vitamin D is given, compared with the smaller daily dose (2–3 weeks). There is no evidence that the large oral dose leads to vitamin D intoxication and one advantage is that compliance is not an issue.

Whatever the regimen used, 25(OH)D concentrations should be measured after several months and, if the response has been inadequate, the treatment should be repeated.

Calcium supplementation should also be given, especially if the intake of calcium is less than 600–1000 mg/day (depending on the size of the child). Symptomatic hypocalcemia should be treated with a slow intravenous infusion of calcium gluconate, 1–2 mg/kg of a 10% solution.

Sun exposure will prevent vitamin D deficiency but there may be barriers to adequate exposure to UV irradiation, such as latitude, religious customs, use of sunscreens and hats, increased melanin pigmentation, overcrowding, and living in an urban environment. Thus oral intake of vitamin D is the best method to assure adequate vitamin D and prevent rickets. To address the issue of vitamin D deficiency in infants due to inadequate vitamin D concentrations, all infants should have a minimum intake of 200 IU of vitamin D per day beginning during the first 2 months of life. In addition, it is recommended that an intake of 200 IU of vitamin D per day be continued throughout childhood and adolescence, because adequate sunlight exposure is not easily determined for a given individual. It is likely that 200 IU/day is the minimum; doses of 400–600 IU/day are safe and will not cause vitamin D intoxication.

Genetic forms of calciopenic rickets

Vitamin D 1α-hydroxylase deficiency

Deficiency of 1α-hydroxylase occurs when loss-of-function mutations in the gene render it inactive and 25(OH)D is not converted to the active form, 1,25(OH)$_2$D. The resulting rickets has been called pseudo-vitamin D-deficient rickets or vitamin D-dependent rickets type I but, now that the cause is known, the term vitamin D 1α-hydroxylase deficiency is most appropriate.

Children usually present in the first 2 years of life with symptoms and signs of severe rickets. Laboratory findings are similar to those seen in vitamin D-deficient rickets, including hypocalcemia, hypophosphatemia, elevated alkaline phosphatase, and elevated PTH. However, the distinguishing feature is a very low 1,25(OH)$_2$D level and normal 25(OH)D.

Calcitriol 0.25–2.0 µg/day cures the disease, although treatment must be lifelong. An adequate intake of calcium must be maintained, especially during the healing phase. Calcium concentrations should be maintained in the low-normal range and PTH concentrations should be allowed to remain in the high-normal range to avoid hypercalciuria and nephrocalcinosis.

Hereditary 1,25(OH)$_2$D-resistant rickets

Hereditary 1,25(OH)$_2$D-resistant rickets (HVDRR) (aka pseudo-vitamin D-deficient rickets type II, vitamin D-dependent rickets type II, and calcitriol-resistant rickets) is due to mutations in the VDR that lead to resistance of target tissues to vitamin D. Patients present with symptoms and signs similar to those with nutritional rickets and vitamin D 1α-hydroxylase deficiency but many have alopecia, which is a distinguishing feature.

Biochemical features are similar to those with the other forms of calciopenic rickets but, unlike other forms of calciopenic rickets, 1,25(OH)$_2$D concentrations are vastly elevated and the 25(OH)D concentrations are normal.

Treatment is more difficult than for the other forms of calciopenic rickets because of the resistance to vitamin D. High doses of 25(OH)D or 1,25(OH)$_2$D are moderately effective. Patients with alopecia are the least responsive to therapy, probably because the presence of alopecia is a marker for a more severe defect. Infusions of large doses of calcium have been effective in some patients with refractory rickets but are complicated by cardiac arrhythmias and nephrolithiasis.

Phosphopenic rickets

Phosphopenic rickets can be due to a defect that leads to renal phosphate wasting, dietary phosphorus deficiency or impaired absorption of phosphate by the intestine, either as a result of disorders of the gastrointestinal system that affect phosphate absorption or of phosphate binders, such as aluminum salts or calcium carbonate.

Genetic causes of renal phosphate loss include familial hypophosphatemic rickets (FHR), which may be X-linked due to abnormalities in the PHEX gene or autosomal dominant due to mutations in FGF23. FHR is the second most common cause of rickets after nutritional rickets. Hereditary hypophosphatemic rickets with hypercalciuria (HHRH) is a genetic cause which is much rarer than FHR; the underlying etiology is unknown. Tumor-induced osteomalacia (TIO) is a condition that has all the features of FHR.

Other disorders of the kidney can lead to phosphopenic rickets. Fanconi syndrome, which involves multiple defects of the proximal renal tubule and renal tubular acidosis, causes phosphate wasting. Inborn errors of metabolism, such as glycogen storage disease, galactosemia, cystinosis, tyrosinemia, and hereditary fructose intolerance, lead to phosphopenic rickets. Hypophosphatemia can also be seen in polyostotic fibrous dysplasia.

Familial hypophosphatemic rickets

X-linked hypophosphatemic rickets (XLH)

XLH is relatively common in children. The clinical manifestations are similar to those of nutritional rickets but persist through childhood. Unlike other forms of rickets, dental abscesses are common. The primary defect is undermineralized dentin, leading to expansion of the pulp chambers and weakening of the enamel barrier. This results in penetration by microorganisms and abscesses, often in the absence of dental caries. Treatment, which has a positive impact on most features of XLH, does not affect the dental manifestations.

Short stature is common. Individuals with XLH continue to have bone and joint problems, including decreased joint mobility, degeneration of knee joints, bone and joint pain, and pseudofractures as adults.

Hypophosphatemia is the hallmark of XLH. Phosphate concentrations are normally higher in children than in adults so it is important to know the normal range for age, in order not to miss the diagnosis. Hypophosphatemia results from decreased TRP, the fraction of phosphate that is reabsorbed by the kidney.

Another hallmark is normal or mildly decreased $1,25(OH)_2D$ concentrations. Hypophosphatemia normally stimulates 1α-hydroxylase activity, leading to increased concentrations of $1,25(OH)_2D$. The lack of elevation of $1,25(OH)_2D$ distinguishes XLH from renal tubular disorders that lead to hypophosphatemia, where the $1,25(OH)_2D$ concentrations are elevated.

Alkaline phosphatase concentrations are high but not as high as in other forms of rickets. They go down with treatment and are a good way of assessing healing. Calcium and $25(OH)D$ concentrations are normal and PTH is normal or slightly increased, which distinguishes XLH from calciopenic rickets.

Treatment is palliative. Phosphorus and calcitriol are the mainstays. The treatment regimen is difficult, since phosphorus must be taken frequently and compliance is almost never complete. Treatment usually improves the radiographic findings and the alkaline phosphatase decreases. Complications of therapy with calcitriol include hypercalcemia and hypercalciuria and excessive phosphate can result in hyperpara-thyroidism. Nephrocalcinosis is a common complication, the pathogenesis of which is not clear. Frequent monitoring of PTH and urinary calcium excretion and monitoring for nephrocalcinosis by renal ultrasound is crucial. Serum phosphate concentrations should never be used to make changes in phosphorus dosing, since they virtually never normalize. If phosphate concentrations are normal, the dose of phosphorus is probably too high.

Autosomal-dominant hypophosphatemic rickets (ADHR)

ADHR is a rare disorder with clinical manifestations similar to XLH. However, unlike XLH, the penetrance is variable. Within the same family, some members with the disorder present in childhood, some in adulthood and some obligate carriers never manifest the disease. In addition, some individuals lose the phosphate-wasting defect.

ADHR results from mutations in FGF23, a novel member of the fibroblast growth factor family. Mutations that lead to ADHR are in a region of the protein that is a recognition sequence for proteolytic enzymes and thus may protect FGF23 from degradation. It is hypothesized that FGF23 is a 'phosphotonin' and lowers phosphate concentrations by increasing renal phosphate excretion. Mutations in FGF23 lead to an increase in circulating concentrations of FGF23 in patients with ADHR and thus higher concentrations of a protein that causes phosphate wasting. One proposal is that PHEX, an endopeptidase, acts normally to cleave FGF23. Mutations in PHEX also lead to elevated concentrations of FGF23 and phosphate wasting by inhibiting this activity.

Tumor-induced osteomalacia (TIO)

TIO is an acquired condition that mimics XLH. Symptoms and signs are usually more severe than in XLH, with lower phosphate concentrations and lower $1,25(OH)_2D$ concentrations and more bone pain and muscle weakness. TIO results most frequently from benign mesenchymal tumors but other tumors have been described and not all are benign. The disease is cured by removal of the tumor. The cause is not clear.

Hereditary hypophosphatemic rickets with hypercalciuria (HHRH)

HHRH is similar to XLH in that there is hypophosphatemia, renal phosphate wasting and an elevated alkaline phosphatase but, unlike XLH, there is hypercalciuria, suppressed PTH and an elevated $1,25(OH)_2D$ (an appropriate response to the hypophosphatemia). The high $1,25(OH)_2D$ leads to hyperabsorption of calcium from the intestinal epithelium. Renal stones occur, probably secondary to the hypercalciuria. The skeletal phenotype consists of osteopenia and osteomalacia. Treatment is with oral phosphorus. By increasing the serum phosphate concentrations, $1,25(OH)_2D$ concentrations go down, the hyperabsorption of calcium and hypercalciuria improve. The osteopenia also improves.

McCune–Albright syndrome

McCune–Albright syndrome (MAS) is due to gain-of-function mutations in GNAS, the gene that encodes for the $Gs\alpha$ subunit of the GTP protein that couples hormone receptors for the activation of adenlyate cyclase. The mutation results in constitutive activation of cAMP–PKA. Fibrous dysplasia of bone is common and osteomalacia has been noted due to hypophosphatemia secondary to renal phosphate wasting in a number of patients. The underlying etiology of the phosphate wasting in MAS is unclear.

Renal tubular disorders: Fanconi syndrome

Fanconi syndrome is a renal tubular disorder characterized by defects in the reabsorption of ions, organic solutes, and proteins, including magnesium, phosphate, and calcium, as well as sodium, potassium, bicarbonate, glucose, and amino acids. Causes of Fanconi syndrome include hereditary disorders, such as cystinosis, Lowe syndrome, type I tyrosinemia, galactosemia, and mitochondrial disorders. Acquired causes include nephrotic syndrome, amyloidosis, paroxysmal nocturnal hemoglobinuria, and a variety of drugs, heavy metals, or other toxin exposures. Osteomalacia with or without rickets is universal. The primary cause of the bone disease is hypophosphatemia secondary to renal phosphate wasting. Abnormalities in vitamin D metabolism are common in Fanconi syndrome and may contribute to the bone disease. In particular, 1α-hydroxylation of 25-(OH)D may be impaired on account of the renal tubular disease. Treatment includes oral phosphate and usually calcitriol.

Hypophosphatasia

Hypophosphatasia can present with rickets in children and with osteomalacia. There is absence of dental cementum leading to premature loss of teeth. Hypophosphatasia is caused by a genetic defect in the TNAP (liver/bone/kidney), termed TNSALP. Osteoid volume is decreased and correlates with the decrease in the alkaline phosphatase. Biochemically, hypophosphatasia is characterized by low alkaline phosphatase activity in the blood, although alkaline phosphatase activity can be low in other conditions.

Hypophosphatasia is classified into perinatal, infantile, childhood, or adult onset forms. In the perinatal form, the lack of mineralization *in utero* is severe, long bones are deformed and the cranium is severely undermineralized. Children are often stillborn or live only a few days because of pulmonary and/or neurological compromise.

In the infantile form, infants often appear normal at birth but rickets and failure to thrive are present by 6 months of age. Hypocalcemia occurs and may be symptomatic. Radiographs show demineralization and metaphyseal changes characteristic of rickets. The chest is often deformed, which may lead to respiratory difficulties and pneumonia. The sclerae can be blue. Craniosynostosis may occur because of premature closure of the sutures. If children survive, the long-term prognosis is reasonably good.

The childhood form of hypophosphatasia usually presents in the second or third year of life with signs of rickets on physical examination and radiographically. The clinical features that distinguish hypophosphatasia from rickets include exfoliation of the teeth, craniosynostosis involving all sutures leading to shallow orbits and ocular prominence. The bone disease may remit in adolescence but may recur in adulthood.

The adult form of hypophosphatasia is mild but can be debilitating. Osteomalacia can be associated with pseudofractures, bone pain, and traumatic fractures. Dental disease is also common.

In odontohypophosphatasia, only the dental disease is present and there is no bone disease. Loss of teeth occurs, including early loss of deciduous teeth and unexplained loss of permanent teeth. Excessive bone resorption leads to a reduction in the alveolar ridge. The pulp chambers enlarge and there is hypomineralization of the dentin.

There is no good treatment for hypophosphatasia. Because hypercalcemia and hyperphosphatemia occur in the more severe forms, treatment with vitamin D and calcium should be avoided.

Systemic conditions associated with hypocalcemia

Tumor lysis syndrome occurs in about 30% of children during the initial phases of treatment of some hematological tumors. The release of large quantities of phosphate, potassium, and uric acid results in hyperphosphatemia, hyperuricemia, hyperkalemia, uremia, and hypocalcemia. The hypocalcemia is largely consequent upon the hyperphosphatemia, which itself occurs secondarily to the acute renal failure of hyper-uricemia. The condition can be prevented by a combination of forced alkaline diuresis and the use of the recombinant urate oxidase inhibitor, rasburicase.

Chronic renal failure (CRF) has a serious impact on calcium metabolism. Reduced GFR results in retention of phosphate, plasma levels of which begin to rise once GFR falls below $30\,mL/min/1.73\,m^2$. Since the kidney is the only site of 1α-hydroxylase activity, levels of $1\alpha,25(OH)_2D$ fall. Metabolic acidosis, either directly as a result of the CRF or caused by renal tubular disorders that may have led to the CRF, is often a factor. Hypocalcemia results, which induces secondary hyperparathyroidism. Renal osteodystrophy therefore consists of a spectrum of both high turnover resulting from the hyperparathyroidism and low turnover secondary to the osteomalacia. Additional factors influencing renal osteodystrophy include calcium, phosphorus, vitamin D analogs, and aluminum.

The principles of minimizing renal osteodystrophy depend upon preventing hyperphosphatemia and reversing the effects of the reduced 1α-hydroxylase activity. Oral phosphate-binding agents are used for the former and calcium carbonate is the most commonly used agent. Alfacalcidol or calcitriol is used to maintain $1\alpha,25(OH)_2D$ levels but must be monitored carefully to prevent hypercalciuria or hypercalcemia, which might worsen the renal failure.

Childhood hypercalcemia

Mild hypercalcemia may be asymptomatic but, as the calcium concentration rises above 3.0 mmol/L (12 mg/dL), symptoms become more common. Infants present with failure to thrive, vomiting, and constipation. Muscle hypotonia, lethargy, anorexia, abdominal pain, and constipation may be present in older children. Polyuria and polydipsia result from a concentrating defect in the renal tubule and longstanding hypercalciuria can lead to nephrocalcinosis, kidney stones, and renal failure. Occasionally, psychiatric disturbance accompanies hypercalcemia and reverses when calcium returns to normal.

Disorders of the calcium-sensing receptor (CaSR)

Although not as common as the disorders causing hypocalcemia, many of these are also genetic in origin.

Familial benign hypercalcemia (FBH) or familial hypocalciuric hypercalcemia (FHH) is an autosomal-dominant condition and most of the patients are heterozygous. It is often identified incidentally or as a result of investigation of FBH kindreds. In some families, there is a history of parathyroidectomy for presumed hyperparathyroidism. Plasma calcium usually remains elevated throughout life. There is a high degree of penetrance and hypercalcemia has usually developed before 10 years of age but often much earlier. Most patients remain asymptomatic, although some infants may develop mild symptoms during the first year. Pancreatitis has been described as a rare complication in FBH. It is not clear whether or not this is a true association or whether the hypercalcemia itself may be the cause. Some mutations may confer susceptibility to pancreatitis in a subgroup of patients.

FBH must be distinguished from primary hyperparathyroidism. Although plasma calcium is elevated, sometimes above 3.0 mmol/L (12 mg/dL), PTH remains normal unless attempts have been made to reduce the plasma calcium with low-calcium diets, etc. The PTH has normal biological activity. However, in contrast to hyperparathyroidism, plasma magnesium is usually slightly elevated, urinary calcium excretion is inappropriately low for the degree of hypercalcemia and nephrocalcinosis does not develop. Treatment of FBH is usually unnecessary and, when the condition is diagnosed in a child of a kindred known to carry the gene, reassurance is all that is required.

Another phenotype similar to FBH is associated with the presence of CaSR blocking antibodies that lead to secondary hyperparathyroidism. The principal difference between this and primary hyperparathyroidism is absence of hypercalciuria, of raised plasma magnesium and normal PTH levels. The natural history is not known but it may remit spontaneously as antibody levels decline.

Disorders of the parathyroid glands

Primary hyperparathyroidism can result from generalized PT gland hyperplasia or single adenomas, which may be isolated and sporadic or form part of one of the inherited multiple tumor syndromes. In many instances, in both the sporadic and the inherited forms of tumor, mutations in one of the oncogenes, tumor suppressor genes, or the PTH gene have been demonstrated.

Multiple endocrine neoplasia type 1 (MEN1) is characterized by a combination of PT (90% of patients), pancreatic endocrine (40%), and anterior pituitary (30%) tumors. Adrenocortical and carcinoid tumors as well as lipomas, angiofibromas, and collagenomas may also occur. The etiology is probably an inactivating mutation of the MEN1 gene, located on chromosome 11q13, which normally codes for a tumor suppressor protein MENIN. PT tumors are usually the first to present, generally in late adolescence or the twenties or thirties.

Three different variants of multiple endocrine neoplasia type 2 (MEN2) are described. Different mutations have been found in all three variants. Identification of them is useful in the diagnosis and management of family members at risk of developing these tumors.

In MEN2a, PT tumors (20%) are associated with medullary carcinoma of the thyroid (MCT) and pheochromocytomas. MEN2b is an association of pheochromocytomas, mucosal neurofibromas, and intestinal autonomic ganglion dysfunction.

In the third variant, MCT only, no tumors other than MCT occur.

Hyperparathyroid-jaw tumor syndrome (HYP-JT) is an autosomal-dominant syndrome. PT adenomas and carcinomas are associated with mandibular and maxillary jaw tumors that are fibro-osseous in nature.

Familial isolated primary hyperparathyroidism (FIHP) has also been described in several families. It appears to be a variant of MEN1, FBH, or occasionally HYP-JT in some. In others, no genetic abnormalities have been detected and it is not clear if this is a separate entity.

PT carcinoma can be difficult to distinguish histologically from PT adenoma, unless metastases are present. All cases have been associated with allelic deletions of the retinoblastoma (Rb) gene, which has three polymorphic markers, located on chromosome 13q14. Loss of heterozygosity (LOH) of at least one of the markers at the Rb locus of the gene occurs in all cases of carcinoma but also occurs in some cases of PT adenoma. However, all PT adenomas show some positivity for the Rb protein (pRb), whereas this is lacking in carcinomas. Lack of translation of the pRb seems to be the distinguishing feature. Treatment is surgical.

Diagnosis and treatment of hyperparathyroidism

Hypercalcemia and hypophosphatemia are associated with raised PTH. Urinary calcium excretion is raised and a partial Fanconi syndrome (generalized aminoaciduria and mild metabolic acidosis) is usually present. Plasma magnesium is often slightly low, in contrast to FBH. Radiological examination may reveal the presence of subperiosteal microcysts and severe hyperparathyroidism can be confused with rickets.

Localization of PT tumors is best undertaken with the aid of radionuclide scanning with ^{99m}Tc-MIBI (methoxyisobutyl isonitrile) or ^{99m}Tc-tetrofosmin. These methods are more sensitive than either ultrasonography or magnetic resonance imaging (MRI) scanning and have proved invaluable in locating persistent tumors, especially after primary surgery has failed to eradicate the problem. They are sometimes combined with thyroid subtraction scintigraphy and, if performed shortly before surgery, can be combined with the use of a handheld gamma camera to pinpoint the tumor at operation.

Treatment consists of surgical removal of the tumors. It may be necessary to control the hypercalcemia before surgery by the use of forced diuresis and frusemide/furosamide. Failing this, bisphosphonates (e.g. pamidronate given in a dose of 0.5 mg/kg daily for 2–3 days) is usually sufficient to restore plasma calcium to normal. Plasma calcium usually declines post-operatively within a few hours and the patient may become hypocalcemic and remain so for some while if hyperparathyroidism has been longstanding. In this case, a 'hungry bone' syndrome develops that requires infusion of calcium in large quantities.

Disorders of the PTH1R

Jansen's disease is an autosomal-dominant condition that presents in the neonatal period with apparent hyperparathyroidism but without detectable PTH or PTHrP. It is characterized by short-limbed short stature caused by abnormal regulation of chondrocyte proliferation and differentiation in the metaphyseal growth plate. It is caused by mutations of the PTH/PTHrP receptor, which autoactivate in the absence of either hormone. Treatment is difficult but the condition is said to respond to calcitonin and, theoretically, bisphosphonates should be of value.

Hypercalcemia associated with abnormal vitamin D metabolism

Subcutaneous fat necrosis usually occurs in term infants who have suffered a mild degree of birth asphyxia. Firm lumps appear in the subcutaneous tissues and may be multiple in number. Hypercalcemia develops within the first few weeks after birth and is accompanied by hypercalciuria and nephrocalcinosis. The skin lesions are invaded by macrophages and

the etiology of the hypercalcemia is thought to be inappropriate activation of 1α-hydroxylase within the macrophages, which results in high concentrations of circulating $1\alpha,25(OH)_2D$. The condition is self-limiting within a few weeks but steps may need to be taken in the meantime to reduce the plasma calcium level. Calcium and vitamin D restriction, steroids, and bisphosphonates may be of value.

A similar process is thought to occur in sarcoidosis and other granulomatous diseases, including tuberculosis and cat-scratch disease. The hypercalcemia usually resolves with treatment of the underlying condition.

Vitamin D in very large doses may cause hypercalcemia because of the high concentrations of $25(OH)D$. Although $25(OH)D$ has limited activity, high concentrations cause increased bone resorption. A more common cause of hypercalcemia as a result of vitamin D excess is seen in patients treated with excess doses of alfacalcidol or calcitriol. The symptoms are those typical of hypercalcemia from other causes. Complications of prolonged hypercalcemia are ectopic calcification, nephrocalcinosis, and impaired renal function. Hypercalcemia following excess vitamin D is usually more prolonged than that caused by the vitamin D metabolites because vitamin D itself is stored in fat, whereas the metabolites have a shorter half-life. Treatment is directed toward restricting the source of vitamin D. If acute symptoms are present, steroids or bisphosphonates may be of value.

Idiopathic infantile hypercalcemia (IIH) was originally described in infants born to mothers who had been ingesting large quantities of vitamin D and the incidence declined with a general reduction in vitamin D supplementation. However, some cases continued to occur with no evidence of excess vitamin D intake. Familial cases have been described. Some of the features of this condition show similarities to Williams syndrome and can include hypertension, strasbismus, and radio-ulnar synostosis with failure to thrive, poor feeding, etc. The dysmorphic features are usually absent and correction of the hypercalcemia allows normal development, although the tendency to hypercalcemia may last beyond the first year. Lack of mutations in the elastin gene allows this condition to be distinguished from Williams syndrome.

The etiology of this condition is uncertain. Treatment consists of lowering the plasma calcium with a calcium- and vitamin D-restricted diet, steroids, and bisphosphonates if necessary. Cellulose phosphate has been used to limit calcium absorption.

Other causes of hypercalcemia in childhood

Williams syndrome is autosomal dominant but usually sporadic. Infants have a characteristic phenotype consisting of 'elfin facies' caused by periorbital fullness, a long philtrum, malar hypoplasia, and an open-mouthed appearance caused by an arched upper lip and full lower lip. As they get older, features change, become coarsened and some skeletal abnormalities such as radio-ulnar synostosis may develop. Many patients develop hypercalcemia during infancy, which rarely lasts beyond the first year. Subsequently, cardiac anomalies are often present, particularly sub-valvar aortic stenosis or peripheral pulmonary stenosis. Developmental delay is a feature and patients develop a tendency to 'cocktail party' conversation as children and young adults, in which it appears that they are conducting an intelligent conversation which, on reflection, is largely meaningless.

Most patients have a microdeletion of chromosome 7q11.23, which encompasses the elastin gene. Infant patients present with failure to thrive, poor feeding, and irritability. Treatment of the hypercalcemia consists of giving a low-calcium diet. A low-calcium milk (Locasol) is useful in this respect if available. It should be noted that, where patients live in hard water areas, there may be sufficient calcium in the water to negate the effect of Locasol. If symptoms are severe, a short course of prednisolone, 1 mg/kg/day, is useful and can usually be stopped after a few weeks. Correcting the hypercalcemia has no effect on the progress of the other features of the disease, which may evolve without hypercalcemia ever having been present.

Immobilization

Hypercalcemia occurs in a small proportion of patients who are immobilized following quadriplegia or other neurological insults. It is more common in adolescents whose bone turnover is naturally more rapid than in adults. The symptoms are non-specific and consist of lethargy, mood changes, nausea, vomiting, and ano-rexia but may be overlooked in the context of the other problems. They usually arise within a few days or weeks of the original insult. Hypercalcemia and hypercalciuria are present and nephrocalcinosis can result. Bone biopsy shows loss of trabecular volume, increased osteoclast and decreased osteoblast activity with an overall increase in bone turnover as demonstrated by raised bone turnover markers. The etiology is uncertain and is probably multifactorial, including lack of mechanical stress, poor vascularity, metabolic changes in bone and denervation. If remobilization is not possible and conventional treatment with intravenous fluids and loop diuretics (which may increase urinary calcium excretion) are ineffective in controlling the hypercalcemia, infusion of pamidronate, 0.5 mg/kg daily for 2–3 days is usually effective in correcting the hypercalcemia. This effect may last for several weeks. Calcitonin has been used but the effect is not so rapid and it has to be given in divided daily doses for more prolonged periods.

Hypercalcemia of malignancy

Hypercalcemia is a rare complication of malignancy in childhood and has been reported to occur in about 0.4% of cases. It may be a presenting feature of leukemia but also occurs in Hodgkin disease, non-Hodgkin lymphoma, and a variety of solid tumors, such as rhabdomyosarcoma, hepatoblastoma, neuro-blastoma, and angiosarcoma.

As with other conditions complicated by hypercalcemia, the symptoms may be overlooked. The cause is usually related to excess secretion of PTHrP and PTH levels are low. Bone turnover is increased and, if the hypercalcemia does not remit on treatment of the underlying malignancy, it usually responds well to bisphosphonate therapy as for immobilization.

Tertiary hyperparathyroidism

This occasionally occurs in children after chronic hyperstimulation of the PT glands, particularly in CRF. PTH levels are usually very elevated and the hyper-plastic glands become susceptible to developing auton-omous nodules. It is not clear whether or not this adenomatous formation is polyclonal or monoclonal in origin but recent studies have suggested, somewhat surprisingly, that the latter may be present in a major-ity of cases. Treatment consists of parathyroidectomy.

Osteoporosis

Osteoporosis and osteopenia are due to a decrease in bone formation or an increase in bone resorption.

Osteomalacia, which is also associated with a low bone mass, is due to a mineralization defect of bone so that unmineralized bone matrix (osteoid) accumulates. Thus, osteoporosis and osteomalacia are both associated with a low bone mass but the mechanisms that lead to the low bone mass are different.

The diagnosis of osteoporosis and osteopenia is difficult in children because measurements of bone mineral density (BMD), by which they are defined in adults, are unreliable. In adults, the definitions are based on bone densitometry (as measured by a dual-energy X-ray absorptiometry or DEXA scan). A decrease in BMD as measured by a DEXA scan in an adult of 1.0 SD is associated with a two- to threefold increase in the risk of fracture. There are no comparable data in children. In addition, DEXA scans measure areal BMD in g/cm^2, which is not a true volumetric measurement. The areal BMD is highly dependent on bone size and thus increases with age as the size of the bones increases. Thus, instead of comparing BMD with peak bone mass (T-score), bone density in children should be compared only with that of age-matched control subjects (Z-score).

Primary osteoporosis

Primary osteoporosis results from intrinsic skeletal defects. Most of these are heritable disorders of connective tissue, with the exception of idiopathic juvenile osteoporosis.

Osteogenesis imperfecta (OI) is the most common cause of primary osteoporosis in children and is divided into up to seven types (types I–VII). Types I–IV are due to mutations in the COL1A1 and COL1A2 genes that encode the type Ia collagen chains. The defects in the more recently described (and much rarer) types V and VI are unknown. Type II is the lethal neonatal form and type III is the classic severe OI, with multiple fractures, blue sclerae, and skeletal deformities. Type IV and especially the mildest form, type I, may be difficult to diagnosis clinically, as blue sclerae (particularly in type IV) and skeletal deformities (particularly type I) may be absent. In all forms of OI, fractures tend to decrease in frequency in puberty. A mild form of OI (type I or IV) should be suspected in anyone with a low BMD, low-trauma fractures, and no secondary causes of osteoporosis. In order to make the diagnosis, the mobility of collagen from a fibroblast culture from a skin biopsy can be studied.

A genetic diagnosis can also be made by mutational analysis of the COL1A1 or COL1A2 genes. Treatment is generally palliative, although cyclic pamidronate has been shown to increase BMD, decrease fractures, and improve bone pain and mobility in children with OI.

Other connective tissue disorders that lead to primary osteoporosis include Marfan and Ehlers–Danlos syndromes.

Idiopathic juvenile osteoporosis is a rare cause of primary osteoporosis in children that presents in previously healthy prepubertal children (usually 2–3 years before puberty) and resolves spontaneously over 2–5 years. The disorder is not inherited and the cause is unknown. Pain and fractures, including vertebral compression factures, are common. The bone density is markedly decreased. There is no treatment, other than optimizing vitamin D and calcium intake. Bisphosphonates may be considered under certain circumstances.

Secondary osteoporosis

Secondary osteoporosis is due to an underlying disorder or its treatment. Any disorder resulting in decreased mobilization leads to secondary osteoporosis. Under these conditions, osteoporosis results from chronic disuse and lack of mechanical stress on bone. In children, the result is lack of adequate accrual of bone.

Causes include cerebral palsy, primary disorders of muscle, such as muscular dystrophy and a number of chronic illnesses, such as hematological (leukemia), gastrointestinal (anorexia nervosa, inflammatory bowel disease), pulmonary (cystic fibrosis), neuromuscular, rheumatological, and endocrine diseases and organ transplantation. Lack of normal activity, poor nutrition, and treatment with medications such as glucocorticoids may all contribute to the low BMD. Individuals with seizures are often on anticonvulsants that interfere with vitamin D metabolism. Endocrine disorders, such as growth hormone deficiency, Turner syndrome, delayed puberty, hyperthyroidism, and diabetes mellitus, are all associated with decreases in BMD, although the clinical significance of the changes in bone mass are not clear.

Some causes of secondary osteoporosis can be treated, such as growth hormone deficiency and hypogonadism associated with Turner syndrome.

However, many of the causes cannot be reversed and prevention of secondary osteoporosis often involves the recognition and treatment of contributing factors, such as inadequate nutritional intake, especially of calcium and vitamin D and lack of exercise. Vitamin D deficiency should be excluded. Drugs that interfere with bone mass accumulation, such as glucocorticoids, should be avoided whenever possible and individuals on anticonvulsants should be on twice the recommended daily intake of vitamin D. Bisphosphonates increase the BMD of children with secondary osteoporosis.

8   Water Balance

Learning Points

- Maintenance of plasma osmolality is by thirst and urine output, which is controlled by arginine vasopressin/antidiuretic hormone (AVP/ADH)
- Extracellular volume is regulated by the renin–angiotensin–aldosterone system
- Vasopressin deficiency causes diabetes insipidus (DI)

- Symptoms of DI are polydipsia and polyuria and distinction must be made between DI and primary polydipsia
- Resistance to vasopressin action causes nephrogenic DI (NDI)
- The syndrome of inappropriate ADH secretion must be distinguished from cerebral salt wasting when hyponatremia follows central nervous system injury

---

Water intake and excretion varies widely in normal persons but plasma osmolality is maintained strictly within the range of 275–295 mOsm/kg. Plasma osmolality above or below the range results in alterations in intracellular solute concentrations, patterns of cellular depolarization, cell morphology and critical aspects of cell function that can become life threatening.

To limit excursions in osmolality, thirst controls water intake and arginine vasopressin (AVP) controls urine concentration. Intact function of either thirst or vasopressin secretion can maintain normal plasma osmolality independently with adequate access to water.

The regulation of extracellular fluid volume is primarily under the control of the renin–angiotensin–aldosterone system (see Chapter 6) and occurs by modulation of sodium intake and excretion, in contrast to the regulation of osmolality by water intake and excretion.

Handbook of Clinical Pediatric Endocrinology, 1st edition. By Charles G. D. Brook and Rosalind S. Brown. Published 2008 by Blackwell Publishing, ISBN: 978-1- 4501-6109-1.

Body water and electrolytes

In term neonates and young infants, 75–80% of body weight is water, with 45–50% of body weight extracellular water and 30% of body weight intracellular water. During the first few days of life, there is a rapid diuresis of 7% of total body water from the extracellular compartment. This trend slows but continues over the first year of life so that the adult distribution of intracellular, extracellular and total body water of 40%, 20% and 60%, respectively, is achieved during childhood.

Daily water intake and loss can vary 10-fold between individuals and within a given individual due to changes in diet, environmental conditions and state of health (for example, increased losses with febrile illness or gastroenteritis). Water losses occur through the respiratory tract and skin (insensible losses), the gastrointestinal (GI) tract and urine. Urine volume, and thus water losses, depends upon the amount of solute required to be excreted and the concentration of the urine in which it is excreted. These parameters can vary over a wide range as a result of changes in the solute composition of infant formula, milk, juice and other dietary components introduced over the first year of life, together with improved renal concentrating capacity over the first months.

Normal daily obligate solute excretion is approximately $500\,mOsm/m^2/day$. To excrete this solute in urine in the middle of the concentration range (osmolality $500–600\,mOsm/kg$) would require approximately $900\,mL/m^2/day$ urine. Combined with respiratory and skin losses of $750\,mL/m^2/day$, GI losses of $100\,mL/m^2/day$ and gain of total body weight due to water of oxidation generated during metabolism of energy sources of $250\,mL/m^2/day$, this yields an average net loss of approximately $1500\,mL/m^2/day$. This volume is the amount of maintenance fluid needed to maintain homeostasis. Under conditions in which urine cannot be diluted or concentrated to the mid-range, this maintenance volume can lead to overhydration or dehydration with resultant abnormalities in plasma osmolality.

Physiology of osmotic regulation

To maintain plasma osmolality in the range that allows optimal cellular function requires sensitive mechanisms for detecting deviation from a normal set point and neural and biochemical pathways that implement a means of restoring the system to that set point. Osmosensors within the central nervous system (CNS) modulate two pathways to maintain homeostasis, thirst to change water intake and posterior pituitary vasopressin secretion to alter renal water excretion.

Vasopressin and water excretion

Biochemistry
AVP (aka antidiuretic hormone, ADH) regulates plasma osmolality by controlling renal free water excretion. AVP is a cyclic nonapeptide that, like its evolutionarily related counterpart oxytocin, consists of a six-member disulfide ring and a three-member tail on which the carboxy-terminal group is amidated (Fig. 8.1a). AVP differs from oxytocin only in replacement of phenyl-alanine for isoleucine at position 3 and of arginine for leucine at position 8 of the molecule. These structural differences allow activation of receptors relatively

specific for either AVP or oxytocin and thereby separation of biological effects. While AVP has potency in activating renal V_2-type vasopressin receptors, the affinity of oxytocin is two orders of magnitude lower, so that it cannot compensate for loss of vasopressin in promoting free water reabsorption.

The AVP and oxytocin genes are located on chromosome 20. AVP is synthesized as a preprohormone (Fig. 8.1b) which is processed to the mature peptide by cleavage of the signal peptide and then self-association leading to neurosecretory granules, initially as dimers.

As the granules traffic toward the axon terminal, the prohormone is cleaved by endo- and exopeptidases, releasing AVP, neurophysin II and copeptin. The hormone is amidated at its C-terminus by a monooxygenase and lyase present as insoluble complexes with neurophysin II within granules. The vasopressin-containing granules are stored in the nerve terminals until neuronal activation occurs causing calcium entry into the nerve terminal and subsequent exocytosis.

Once in plasma, the AVP–neurophysin complex dissociates and the hormone circulates in a free form. Increases in secretion of AVP are coupled to increases in synthesis but this compensatory response may not always balance the increased rate of release. A chronic severe stimulus, such as prolonged water deprivation or nephrogenic diabetes insipidus (NDI), may thus severely deplete the posterior pituitary stores of vasopressin, as can be seen by an absence of the pituitary bright spot on magnetic resonance imaging (MRI).

Detailed structure–function analyses of specific amino acids within the vasopressin and oxytocin peptides has generated new molecules that are advantageous in the management of states of vasopressin deficiency. For example, replacement of L-arginine with D-arginine at position 8 of vasopressin together with its amino-terminal deamidation resulted in a vasopressin analog with more potent and pro-longed antidiuretic activity, which is now widely used clinically (desamino-D-arginine vasopressin (dDAVP), Fig. 8.1).

Anatomy
AVP is synthesized by neurons in the bilateral hypothalamic supraoptic and paraventricular nuclei. The large magnocellular neurons within these nuclei send axons toward the midline to terminate at various concentrations within the pituitary stalk or in the

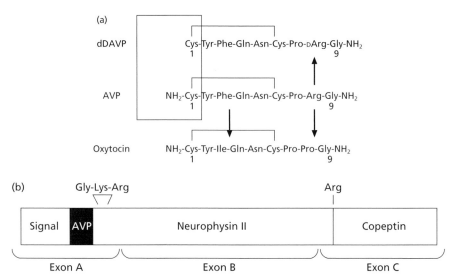

Figure 8.1 AVP protein and gene structure. (a) Amino acid comparison of AVP and the structurally related molecules oxytocin and dDAVP. Amino acids are numbered from the amino-terminus of each molecule, and differences in amino acids between these molecules are shown by the arrows. The box indicates the deamidation of the amino-terminus in dDAVP compared with AVP. (b) Relationship of AVP to its preproAVP precursor. Intron–exon boundaries of the gene relative to the coding sequences are shown, as are the di- and monobasic cleavage sites essential for protein processing.

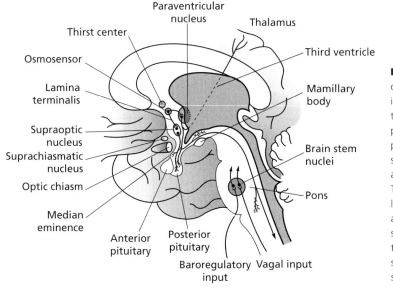

Figure 8.2 Anatomy of AVP-producing cells in the hypothalamus and their projections to the posterior pituitary. AVP is produced by neurons in the supraoptic, paraventricular and suprachiasmatic nuclei. The magnocellular neurons located in the supraoptic and paraventricular nuclei send axonal projections to the posterior pituitary for secretion of AVP into the systemic circulation.

posterior pituitary (neurohypophysis) itself (Fig. 8.2). AVP is released from these neurosecretory granule-rich terminals in the posterior pituitary and stalk into the systemic circulation. The superior and inferior hypophyseal arteries, distal branches of the internal carotid artery, provide the blood supply to the posterior pituitary.

There is a second group of smaller parvocellular neurons that also synthesize AVP in the paraventricular nucleus of the hypothalamus. In contrast to the magnocellular neurons, the parvocellular neurons give rise to axons that terminate at the median eminence and secrete AVP into the portal-hypophyseal vascular plexus to augment adrenocorticotrophic hormone

(ACTH) synthesis and release from anterior pituitary corticotrophs.

Regulation of AVP secretion

Osmotic regulation

The set point for initiation of AVP secretion occurs at a plasma osmolality of 280 mOsm/kg, although this can vary between 275 and 290 mOsm/kg based upon interindividual genetic differences, other hormonal signals and volume status.

When serum osmolality falls below the osmotic threshold for AVP release, plasma AVP concentration falls below 1 pg/mL, the sensitivity limit of most radioimmunoassays. This reduction in AVP promotes excretion of maximally dilute urine. The resultant loss of free water increases serum osmolality and limits further dilution of intracellular and extracellular fluids.

Once serum osmolality exceeds the threshold for AVP release, increasing plasma osmolality 1% increases plasma vasopressin by approximately 1 pg/mL (1 pmol/L), an amount sufficient to alter urine concentration and flow (Fig. 8.3). Peak antidiuresis and production of a maximally concentrated urine occurs at a plasma AVP concentration of 5 pg/mL. Osmotic stimulation linearly increases plasma AVP to as high as 20 pg/mL at a plasma osmolality of 320 mosm/kg

or above but this causes no further change in urine concentrating ability.

Many solutes contribute to plasma osmolality but sodium and its anions constitute the majority and they modulate vasopressin release. Increases in osmolality by sugars such as mannitol augment vasopressin release through the osmosensors but not all solutes that contribute to plasma osmolality have the capacity to stimulate AVP release. Non-stimulatory solutes include glucose and urea in healthy individuals but hyperglycemia does stimulate AVP release in the context of insulin deficiency, which may possibly exacerbate progression of hyponatremia during treatment of diabetic ketoacidosis.

Non-osmotic regulation

Other homeostatic and environmental factors influence AVP secretion. Of these, acute changes in intravascular volume and pressure are particularly important. Baroreceptors in the cardiac atria and aortic arch are activated by blood vessel wall stretching due to increased intravascular volume and activate neurons within the brainstem. These neurons synapse upon neurons within the supraoptic and paraventricular nuclei and inhibit vasopressin release. Conversely, when intravascular volume falls or blood pressure decreases, inhibition of vasopressinergic neurons

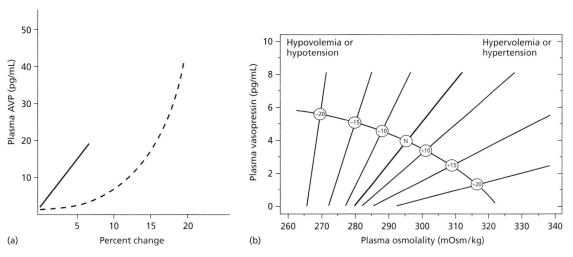

Figure 8.3 Interactions of osmolality and hemodynamic stimuli in the regulation of AVP secretion. (a) Plasma AVP concentration in relation to percentage increase in blood osmolality (solid line) or percentage decrease in blood volume (dashed line). (b) Changes in hemodynamic status alter the sensitivity of AVP secretion into the plasma.

within the hypothalamus is diminished, resulting in augmented AVP release.

In contrast to the subtle changes in plasma osmolality that modulate AVP secretion, larger changes in intravascular volume are needed to initiate AVP release. Vasopressin concentration does not increase until intravascular volume deficits exceed 8% (Fig. 8.3). When intravascular volume depletion exceeds this threshold, plasma AVP concentrations increase exponentially so that decreases in intravascular volume of 20–30% increase plasma vasopressin to concentrations far greater than those required for maximum antidiuresis and maximal concentrations seen with osmotic stimulation.

Osmotic and hemodynamic stimuli interact to enhance the AVP response generated by each independent stimulus (Fig. 8.3). For example, hypovolemia or hypotension lowers the threshold and increases the gain for AVP release imparted by the osmoregulatory system, increasing the stimulatory effect of a given level of plasma osmolality. Conversely, increased intravascular volume or hypervolemia dampens the AVP response to increases in plasma osmolality. This interaction suggests that the osmo- and baroregulatory systems, although anatomically distinct, converge upon the same population of neurosecretory neurons.

Nausea strongly promotes vasopressin secretion and circulating concentrations of AVP may exceed those associated with maximal osmotic stimulation. This is probably mediated by afferents from the area postrema in the brainstem, a key emetic center. Nicotine, acute hypoglycemia, hypoxia and hypercapnia, as well as many drugs and hormones are strong stimuli of AVP release. AVP secretion is inhibited by glucocorticoids.

Many drug effects on AVP secretion are thought to occur indirectly by providing hemodynamic or emetic stimuli. Psychological or physiological stress caused by pain, emotion, physical exercise or other deviations from homeostasis has long been thought to cause the release of vasopressin but this may be due indirectly to other factors, such as the hypotension or nausea that often accompany vasovagal reactions.

Vasopressin metabolism

AVP has a half-life of 5–10 min in the circulation, being quickly degraded by vasopressinase. Because of its resistance to amino-terminal degradation, the synthetic AVP analog dDAVP has a much longer half-life, 8–24 h.

Biological action of AVP

The crucial action of AVP is to limit the excretion of water by increasing the permeability of the distal nephron to luminal water, thereby increasing reabsorption of free water and reducing urine output. To achieve this, AVP acts upon specific vasopressin receptors on the serosal surface of the distal and collecting renal tubules (Fig. 8.4). Three subtypes of vasopressin receptors (V_{1a}, V_{1b} (V_3) and V_2) each arise from a different genes coding for a member of the seven-transmembrane G-protein-coupled receptor family.

The V_2 receptor accounts for the antidiuretic effects of AVP in the kidney. Mutations in the gene (at Xq28) result in X-linked NDI. V_2 receptors are located in the distal nephron and in the thick ascending limb of Henle's loop and periglomerular tubules. V_2 receptors are also found on vascular endothelial cells promoting vasodilation and the actions of von Willebrand factor, factor VIIIa and tissue plasminogen activator. The prothrombotic actions of AVP, and

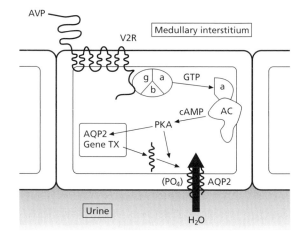

Figure 8.4 Renal actions of AVP. In the collecting duct epithelium, AVP binding to the V_2 receptor results in Ga-mediated activation of cAMP production from adenylyl cyclases. The elevation in intracellular cAMP causes activation of protein kinase A (PKA), which then phosphorylates aquaporin 2 (AQP-2) at serine 256. This phosphorylation event promotes aggregation of AQP-2 homotetramers in subapical membrane vesicles and their fusion with the apical plasma membrane. The insertion of the water channels into the luminal membrane allows the flow of water from the urine within the duct lumen into the hypertonic medullary interstitium, decreasing free water clearance.

specifically of dDAVP, have been used to treat bleeding disorders associated with von Willebrand disease and hemophilia.

V_{1a} receptors mediate extrarenal effects including contraction of vascular smooth muscle, stimulation of hepatic glycogenolysis and aggregation of platelets. V_{1b} receptors are primarily located on ACTH-producing corticotrophs in the anterior pituitary, where activation increases ACTH release during acute and chronic stress.

In the absence of vasopressin, the distal nephron is largely impermeable to water and solutes. Dilute tubular fluid passes without additional concentration. Urine is maximally dilute (osmolality <100 mOsmol/kg) and a high rate of urine flow ensues at or above 3 L/m^2/day, depending on the amount of solute requiring excretion.

In the presence of vasopressin, V_2 receptors are activated and insert preformed, subapical vesicular water channels, aquaporin-2 (AQP-2), into the apical membrane, which results in a large increase in water permeability, allowing diffusion of water into the hypertonic inner medullary interstitium.

The water channels themselves belong to a family of related proteins, the AQP, which differ in their sites of expression and pattern of regulation. AQP-2 comprises the specifically vasopressin-regulated water channel in the kidney, its predominant site of expression. AQP-1, -3 and -4 are also expressed in the kidney but play a less prominent and AVP independent, role in water balance.

An increase in plasma vasopressin of 0.5 pg/mL raises urine osmolality by approximately 150–250 mOsm/kg. Maximum antidiuresis occurs when plasma vasopressin concentration reaches 2–5 pg/mL. Vasopressin may also play a role in limiting insensible water loss but this effect is small and easily overcome by changes in environmental conditions such as temperature and humidity, as well as exercise.

Thirst

Restoration of deficits in body water due to urinary and insensible losses occurs normally by ingestion of water. Thirst is regulated by many of the same physiological factors that regulate vasopressin release, of which plasma osmolality is the most potent. Anatomically, osmotic regulation of thirst occurs by osmosensors in the anterior hypothalamus and includes modulatory

activity by neurons in the ventromedial nucleus of the hypothalamus.

Hypovolemia and hypotension also increase thirst. The magnitude of intravascular depletion or hypotension needed to stimulate thirst has not been defined but is probably larger than that associated with AVP release.

Fluid intake often occurs for reasons other than thirst, such as social cues of others drinking, pleasurable taste or other effects of an ingested beverage, hunger or dry mouth resulting from factors independent of hydration such as anxiety or medication. When water intake exceeds requirements, plasma vasopressin decreases to undetectable concentrations, allowing excretion of the extra water. With defects in either thirst or urine concentrating ability on their own, plasma tonicity can still be maintained within the normal range so, in AVP deficiency, random plasma osmolality is usually normal if the patient has access to water since an intact thirst mechanism stimulates water ingestion up to 10 L/m^2/day. Similarly, normal vasopressin regulation can mask impairment of thirst by avidly retaining water. When thirst and vasopressin secretion are both disrupted, life-threatening dysregulation of plasma osmolality and intravascular volume may occur.

Volume sensor and effector pathways

Renin–angiotensin–aldosterone system
The primary regulator of vasopressin and thirst is osmolality and, although vasopressin and thirst do respond to large changes in intravascular volume, the renin–angiotensin system is the primary regulatory network for maintaining euvolemia. This system acts in a classical endocrine manner (see Chapter 6).

The natriuretic peptide system
The natriuretic peptides (atrial natriuretic peptide (ANP), brain natriuretic peptide (BNP) and C-type natriuretic peptide (CNP)) contribute to salt and water balance by promoting renal salt excretion and altering vasopressin secretion from the hypothalamus, respectively.

ANP synthesis occurs in both the left and the right atria in response to increasing wall pressure and increased heart rate. Ventricular production of ANP increases with ventricular hypertrophy. ANP produced within the brain is also modulated in a volume-dependent manner. ANP released into the peripheral circulation has a number of renal effects, inhibiting sodium reabsorption in the medullary collecting duct, impairing the salt-retaining actions of angiotensin II on the proximal tubule and the renal effects of vasopressin in water retention. In addition, ANP inhibits aldosterone synthesis in adrenal zona glomerulosa cells by inhibiting actions of aldosterone secretagogues, particularly the action of angiotensin II. ANP reduces plasma renin activity, which reduces the generation of angiotensin II, further diminishing aldosterone secretion and renal salt reabsorption.

BNP is synthesized in the ventricle with production augmented in congestive heart failure and hypertension; it causes renal and adrenal effects similar to ANP. The brain is the primary site of CNP production and CNP expression overlaps with ANP expression in the hypothalamus.

Disorders of water balance

Vasopressin deficiency

Deficiencies in AVP secretion or action result in polyuria and polydipsia. The signs and symptoms of DI are urinary frequency, nocturia and persistent enuresis or delayed toilet training in younger children. These symptoms are accompanied by thirst and increased fluid intake throughout the day and night.

Diagnostic approach

Patients presenting with polyuria and polydipsia should have diabetes mellitus (DM) excluded promptly, the possibility of DI then being considered. Fluid intake and output should be measured to see whether either exceeds $2 L/m^2/day$.

If pathological polyuria or polydipsia is present, serum osmolality and concentrations of sodium, potassium, glucose, calcium and urea should be measured as an outpatient; urinalysis, including measurement of osmolality, specific gravity and glucose, should be performed. A urine osmolality >600 mOsm/kg excludes DI and DI is also unlikely if the serum osmolality and sodium are low or low normal, results most consistent with primary polydipsia. Serum sodium above 145 mmol/L or serum osmolality >300 mOsm/kg with urine osmolality <600 mOsm/kg confirms the diagnosis of DI and a water deprivation test is superfluous.

The water deprivation test should be done in a controlled setting, either at an outpatient site appropriate for 8–10 h of observation and assessment or as an inpatient. Because patients with DI can become dehydrated in a few hours, it is not appropriate to restrict fluid before the patient arrives for the test. During the test, the environment must be controlled to avoid surreptitious water intake, since the intense drive to drink can lead to fluid intake from unusual sources. Physical signs and biochemical parameters are measured hourly (Fig. 8.5) and the laboratory should be aware of the need for prompt assessment of the specimens.

A common recommendation is to stop a test based on a 5% loss of body weight but this may result in the test being stopped before a diagnosis can be made. Unless vital signs or other symptoms suggest significant

Water deprivation phase

- Obtain initial weight, vitals, and document duration of pretest water restriction (if any)
- Place intravenous line to assist with repeated blood drawing, and place foley catheter in children too young to provide hourly voided urine specimens
- Obtain baseline serum Na, vasopressin, urine osmolality, and urine specific gravity
- Begin (or continue) water deprivation
- Measure and record hourly on a flow sheet:
  – Weight, HR, BP, urine output, and urine specific gravity
  – Stat laboratory testing: serum sodium and urine osmolality
- If Na < 145, urine osmolality < 600, and there is no clinical evidence of significant, symptomatic hypovolemia, continue water deprivation
- If urine osmolality is above 1000, or above 600 and stable over two measures, stop test. Patient does not have diabetes insipidus
- If serum osmolality is above 300 and urine osmolality is below 600, the patient has diabetes insipidus. Proceed to vasopressin response phase

Vasopressin response phase

- Collect blood for vasopressin level
- Administer Pitressin, 1 unit/m^2, SQ
- Allow the patient to eat and drink, limiting fluid intake to the volume of urine produced during the entire testing period (water deprivation and vasopressin response)
- 30 and 60 min after Pitressin, measure vital signs, urine output, and urine specific gravity, and send urine to laboratory for osmolality
- A twofold increase in urine osmolality indicates central diabetes insipidus
- An increase of less than twofold in urine osmolality is consistent with nephrogenic diabetes insipidus

Figure 8.5 Protocol for water deprivation testing for diagnosis of DI.

clinical hypovolemia, the test should proceed until diagnostic results are obtained.

If a diagnosis of DI is made, subcutaneous aqueous vasopressin (Pitressin) can differentiate central and nephrogenic forms. This is frequently done immediately following the water deprivation test but can be done independently of it. Following administration of vasopressin, fluid restriction should be stopped, since continued restriction in a child with NDI will result in progressive dehydration. Intake should be limited to protect against excessive water consumption with resultant hyponatremia. Owing to its longer duration of action, dDAVP is not recommended for this test, since it can cause water intoxication. Patients with long-standing primary polydipsia may have mild NDI because of dilution of their renal medullary interstitium.

Central diabetes insipidus

Central (neurogenic, pituitary, hypothalamic, cranial or vasopressin-responsive) diabetes insipidus (CDI) results when pituitary AVP production is reduced. Losses of up to 90% of normal AVP secretion can occur without overt clinical manifestations in otherwise well individuals. Further loss of AVP secretion results in onset of clinically apparent polyuria and polydipsia. Therefore, onset of symptoms is generally perceived as abrupt and patients or their families often identify a discrete time of onset. Once symptoms develop, the degree of polyuria and polydipsia depends both on the degree of AVP deficiency and other factors, such as the integrity of thirst, renal function, dietary salt load and normality of other endocrine systems. Urinary losses as high as $400\,\mathrm{mL/m^2/h}$ have been documented. CDI responds well to AVP replacement therapy with vasopressin or its more stable analog, dDAVP.

Causes of CDI

Genetic causes
The inherited forms of CDI account for <10% of cases of DI in most patient populations (Tables 8.1 and 8.2). *Familial autosomal-dominant neurohypophyseal DI* (ADNDI) is caused by mutations in the AVP–NPII gene. Symptoms appear in the first decade of life, usually before 7 years of age but are not apparent at birth.

Table 8.1 Causes of central diabetes insipidus (CDI).

Genetic
AVP
  Neurophysin gene
    Autosomal dominant
    Autosomal recessive
Wolfram syndrome

Congenital
Septo-optic dysplasia
Midline craniofacial defects
Holoprosencephalic syndromes
Agenesis of the pituitary

Acquired
Neoplasms
  Craniopharyngioma
  Germinoma
  Pinealoma
  Leukemia/lymphoma
Inflammatory/infiltrative
  Langerhans cell histiocytosis
  Systemic lupus erythematosus
  Neurosarcoidosis
  Lymphocytic neurohypophysitis
Infectious
  Meningitis
  Encephalitis
  Congenital infection
Traumatic injury
  CNS surgery
  Head trauma
  Hypoxic injury
Idiopathic

Vasopressin secretion declines gradually until DI of variable severity supervenes.

Autosomal-recessive familial neurohypophyseal DI is due to a single mutation in the AVP–NPII gene. Affected children are asymptomatic for the first year or more of life.

Wolfram syndrome is a rare, progressive, neurodegenerative condition also known as DIDMOAD (DI, DM, optic atrophy and deafness). The minimal features required for diagnosis are juvenile-onset insulin-dependent diabetes and optic atrophy. DI, sensorineural deafness, urinary tract atony, ataxia, peripheral neuropathy, mental retardation and psychiatric illness develop in the majority of patients. Onset of DI is usually in the second decade.

Congenital intracranial anatomic defects

Midline brain defects are associated with CDI and account for 5–10% of pediatric cases. DI may become apparent in the first weeks of life but diagnosis may be delayed. The most frequent defect associated with congenital CDI is septo-optic dysplasia (SOD, De Morsier syndrome) characterized by hypoplasia of the optic nerves with other midline cerebral anomalies and pituitary hormone deficiencies. Mutations in the homeobox gene HESX1 have been associated with some cases of SOD but most cases do not have a gene defect identified.

Other anomalies associated with CDI include nasal encephalocele, porencephaly, holoprosencephaly, hydrocephalus and hydranencephaly. MRI evaluation generally reveals an absent posterior pituitary bright spot, in addition to the accompanying CNS lesions. Visible midline craniofacial defects associated with congenital CDI include single central incisor, cleft lip or palate, high arch palate, micrognathia, synophrys, hypotelorism, flat nasal bridge or other midface hypoplasia but many children with congenital CDI have no external evidence of midline abnormalities. Deficiencies of anterior pituitary hormones and defects in thirst perception are not uncommon. In patients who have cortisol deficiency, symptoms of DI may be masked because cortisol deficiency impairs renal free water clearance. In such cases, glucocorticoid therapy may unmask AVP deficiency and precipitate polyuria.

Acquired CDI

Non-familial, acquired forms of DI account for the majority of CDI cases.

Brain tumors are the most common cause (10–15% in children) and include germinoma, astrocytoma, pinealoma, CNS lymphoma, glioma and craniopharyngioma. Although craniopharyngioma infrequently causes DI before surgery, the majority of children develop DI following resection and craniopharyngiomas ultimately account for the majority of tumor-associated CDI in children. Including those who develop DI following surgery, brain tumors account for up to 50% of acquired DI.

Because hypothalamic AVP neurons are distributed over a large area within the hypothalamus, tumors that cause DI must be large, infiltrative or located at the point of convergence of the hypothalamo-neurohypophyseal axonal tract in the infundibulum. Because germinomas and pinealomas typically arise near the base of the hypothalamus, where AVP axons converge as they enter the posterior pituitary, they are the tumors most commonly associated with DI at diagnosis. Germinomas causing DI can be small and undetectable by MRI for several years following the onset of DI. The β-subunit of human chorionic gonadotropin and α-fetoprotein are often secreted by germinomas and pinealomas and repeated measurements and MRI scans should be performed in children with idiopathic or unexplained DI. Tumor-associated DI is rare before 5 years of age.

Neurosurgical intervention is one of the most common causes of CDI. In the post-operative period, it is important to distinguish polyuria associated with DI from polyuria due to the normal diuresis of fluids given during surgery and polyuria associated with cerebral salt wasting (CSW). In both DI and normal diuresis, the urine may be very dilute and of high volume but, with post-surgical diuresis, serum sodium and osmolality will be normal, whereas they will be high in DI if the patient does not have free access to water.

In CSW, urine volumes are also high but urinary sodium concentrations are high and serum osmolality and sodium are low. Post-surgical DI is characterized by an abrupt onset of polyuria, usually within the first 12–24 h. This phase is often transient, resolving spontaneously in 1–2 days and thought to be due either to acute injury to the neurohypophysis with inhibition of AVP secretion or to release of biologically inactive AVP-like peptide hormones from the damaged hypothalamo-neurohypophyseal system that interfere with the binding of AVP to the V_2 receptor.

Not infrequently, a 'triple-phase' response is seen. Following the initial DI, the syndrome of inappropriate ADH secretion (SIADH) is seen, typically after 4–5 days, which can last for 10 days and is due to the unregulated release of vasopressin from dying neurons. A third phase of permanent DI follows if sufficient numbers of vasopressin-producing cells were destroyed. Although cranial irradiation is associated with the development of anterior pituitary hormone deficiencies, it is never associated with DI.

Infections involving the base of the brain, such as meningococcus, group B streptococci, *Haemophilus influenzae, Streptococcus pneumoniae*, cryptococcal and listeria meningitides, congenital cytomegalovirus, tuberculoma or toxoplasmosis can cause CDI, which may be transient or permanent. When permanent, DI is often combined with anterior pituitary endocrinopathies.

Langerhans cell histiocytosis (LCH) is the most common infiltrative disorder causing CDI (10% of acquired cases). It is characterized by a clonal proliferation of abnormal dendritic histiocytes (Langerhans cells) with an accompanying infiltration of lymphocytes, eosinophils and neutrophils. It can involve many body organ systems or tissues and the disease often targets the posterior hypothalamo-pituitary region.

About 50% of patients with LCH have DI. A minority has concurrent anterior hormone deficiencies, which can develop many years after the onset of DI but rarely without it. DI associated with LCH is almost always a multisystem disease, with lesions in bone (68%), skin (57%), lung (39%) and lymph nodes (18%). X-ray evaluation for skeletal lesions and clinical symptoms of multisystem disease should be sought when LCH is considered in a differential diagnosis. Thickening of the pituitary stalk may be seen on cranial MRI but the pituitary stalk can also appear normal.

Trauma to the base of the brain can cause swelling around or severance of the magnocellular neurons, resulting in DI, even after seemingly minor trauma. As in CNS surgery, the DI associated with trauma may develop rapidly after the injury and can be transient or permanent. Occasionally, onset can be delayed as the magnocellular neurons degenerate.

Autoimmune DI is associated with autoantibodies to AVP-secreting cells; these are present in more than half of adults < 30 years of age presenting with idiopathic DI and are much more common in individuals with a history of prior autoimmune disease or pituitary stalk thickening. Based on the presence of these antibodies, it has been suggested that auto-immune lymphocytic neurohypophysitis may account for a significant proportion of patients with idiopathic DI but 16% of patients with non-idiopathic CDI also have the antibodies. It is possible that anti-bodies directed against vasopressin-containing cells are not pathogenic but are markers of previous neuronal cell destruction. In addition, patients with other autoimmune diseases may have AVP-secreting cell antibodies without evidence of DI.

Hypoxic injury caused by carbon monoxide poisoning, smoke inhalation, respiratory failure, cardiopulmonary arrest, septic shock and sudden infant death syndrome may cause CDI. The interval between the insult and development of DI ranges from a few hours to many days. Because the neurohypophyseal system has a bilateral blood supply and is relatively resistant to hypoxic injury, the appearance of DI following hypoxic injury is ominous and generally indicative of widespread neurological damage. Thus, DI is present in approximately 40% of children with brain death and CDI should be considered in the differential diagnosis of polyuria occurring in any patient who has suffered hypoxic injury.

Idiopathic DI occurs in 12–20% of cases. MRI may be normal or the pituitary stalk may be thickened. Thickening is observed in approximately one-third of children with CDI. Some of these have a cause for their DI at presentation, most often LCH, but most have idiopathic DI. Patients with idiopathic DI and thickening of the pituitary stalk appear to be more likely to have or to develop anterior pituitary hormone deficiencies but all patients should have anterior pituitary function tests at presentation and during follow-up. Patients with or without thickening of the pituitary stalk should be followed with repeated MRI since DI is the most common initial presentation of germinoma and may occur before radiographic evidence of the tumor is present. Evidence of a tumor is usually within 2.5 years after diagnosis and 1.3 years after thickening of the pituitary stalk is noted on MRI. Gonadotropin deficiency is a marker for organic disease.

Treatment of CDI

Treatment of CDI is usually lifelong because recovery from a deficiency lasting more than a week is uncommon, even if an underlying cause is eliminated. With intact thirst and free access to water, an individual with DI will drink sufficiently to maintain normal serum osmolality and high-normal serum sodium. To relieve the symptoms of polyuria and polydipsia, the treatment of choice is administration of dDAVP (desmopressin) by subcutaneous injection, nasal solution or orally. Oral dDAVP is highly effective and safe in children in doses of 50–600 mg (0.05–0.6 mg) every 8–12 h.

Treatment should begin with the lowest amount that gives the desired antidiuretic effect. Dosing can be once or twice per day and patients with intact thirst should be allowed to escape from the antidiuretic effect briefly at least once a day to allow excessive water to be excreted and reduce the risk of water intoxication.

dDAVP cannot reduce fluid output below the level of water intake in a standard diet, so hyponatremia should not occur in the absence of excess fluid intake. Patients and parents should be educated about the risk of excessive fluid intake and the signs and symptoms of water intoxication. Patients and families should be counseled that intake should be guided solely by thirst and children should be taught to avoid incidental or social drinking.

Treatment of CDI in the setting of hypodipsia or adipsia

Thirst is normal in more than 90% of patients with pituitary DI but a few, mostly those with a history of congenital midline CNS malformations, head trauma, hypothalamic surgery, ruptured anterior communicating artery aneurysms or suprasellar malignancy, have hypodipsia or adipsia. This greatly complicates the management, since changing urine output is no longer compensated by spontaneous adjustment in fluid intake. Many such patients also have significant defects in cognitive function.

Management of DI in this situation requires a fixed dose of dDAVP and a daily water intake to meet fluid needs under usual conditions of treatment, diet, temperature and activity. This is usually close to $1 \, L/m^2/day$ in the absence of significant diuresis. Frequent monitoring of serum sodium is essential. Daily weight can be helpful in determining the need to make interval adjustments in the daily fluid intake but target weights need to be recalibrated periodically to compensate for growth.

Treatment of post-operative CDI

In the acute post-operative management of DI, vasopressin therapy can be used but hyponatremia can occur if the child is receiving an excessive amount of fluid. Vasopressin will mask the emergence of the SIADH phase of the triple-phase response to neurosurgical injury or resolution of the DI. For these reasons, it is often best to manage post-operative DI in children with fluids alone. When intravenous therapy is used, input is matched with output hourly, with an initial limit imposed on total fluid administration at 3–$5 \, L/m^2/day$.

A basal infusion rate of $1 \, L/m^2/day$ ($40 \, mL/m^2/h$) should be given as 5% dextrose in 0.22% saline. No additional fluid should be administered for hourly urine volumes under $40 \, mL/m^2/h$. For hourly urine volumes above $40 \, mL/m^2/h$, the additional volume should be replaced with 5% dextrose water to a maximum of 120–$200 \, mL/m^2/h$ (3–$5 \, L/m^2/day$). For urine outputs above $120 \, mL/m^2/h$, the initial total infusion rate should be $120 \, mL/m^2/h$ and may be adjusted up to $200 \, mL/m^2/h$ if needed. In the presence of DI, this will result in serum sodium in the $150 \, mmol/L$ range. This mildly volume-contracted state should produce a prerenal reduction in urine output, generally avoiding the need to give larger volumes of fluid and will also allow the assessment of thirst and the return of normal vasopressin function or the emergence of SIADH.

Patients may become mildly hyperglycemic with this regimen, particularly if they are also receiving post-operative glucocorticoids. Frequent assessment of fluid balance, urine-specific gravity and serum electrolytes to determine appropriate adjustments in therapy are essential to avoid fluctuations in volume status, particularly in cases where the triple-phase response develops. If the child is awake and able to drink, free access to water based on thirst should be allowed with advice to avoid non-thirst-mediated fluid intake. If there is concern about impaired thirst oral intake should be matched to urine output using the same parameters given for intravenous fluid administration.

If therapy with AVP or dDAVP is used, fluid intake should be limited to $1 \, L/m^2/day$, unless unusual non-renal fluid losses are anticipated. Therapy with aqueous vasopressin (Pitressin) is preferred, since its effect is more rapidly reversed and the dose can be titrated to achieve the desired urine output. Occasionally, following hypothalamic surgery, higher concentrations of vasopressin are required initially to treat acute DI, which may be attributable to the release of biologically inactive vasopressin-like peptides acting as antagonists to normal vasopressin activity. If dDAVP is used, the need for additional doses should be determined by whether or not polyuria and hypernatremia recur following each dose. Patients treated with vasopressin for post-neurosurgical DI should be switched from intravenous to oral fluid intake at the earliest opportunity, because thirst sensation, if intact, will help to regulate blood osmolality and minimize the risk of significant hypernatremia or hyponatremia.

Nephrogenic diabetes insipidus

NDI (vasopressin resistant), which is characterized by impaired urinary concentrating ability despite normal or elevated plasma concentrations of AVP, can be genetic or acquired. Genetic etiologies are diagnosed during childhood and are generally more severe than acquired causes. Acquired NDI can occur as a component of acquired kidney disease, in the setting of a number of metabolic abnormalities or in response to drugs.

Causes of NDI

Genetic NDI

There are three genetic causes of NDI, all of which are rare (Table 8.2) . The symptoms are the same but they can be differentiated by their pattern of inheritance. Polyuria and polydipsia are present from birth with NDI and pregnancies involving affected infants can be complicated by hydramnios. Unless the disease is recognized early, affected children have repeated episodes of dehydration, sometimes complicated by convulsions and death. Affected infants are irritable

Table 8.2 Causes of nephrogenic diabetes insipidus (NDI).

Genetic
X-linked recessive (AVP-V_2 receptor)
Autosomal recessive (AQP-2)
Autosomal dominant (AQP-2)

Acquired
Drugs
  Lithium
  Foscarnet
  Demeclocycline
  Many others
Metabolic
  Hyperglycemia
  Hypercalcemia
  Hypokalemia
  Protein malnutrition
Renal
  Chronic renal failure
  Ischemic injury
  Impaired medullary function
  Outflow obstruction

and present with symptoms such as vomiting, anorexia, failure-to-thrive, fever and constipation. Serum sodium is generally elevated at presentation.

Growth failure in the untreated child may be secondary to the ingestion of large amounts of water, which the child may prefer over other higher calorie substances and/or due to general poor health resulting from dehydration and hypernatremia. Mental retardation of variable severity has historically been the norm but it is probable that this results from frequent episodes of dehydration and can be prevented by early recognition and appropriate management. Even with early institution of therapy, short stature remains common in children with congenital NDI. Some patients develop severe dilation of the urinary tract, which may predispose to rupture after minor trauma. Intracranial calcification has been described in NDI.

Congenital X linked NDI accounts for more than 90% of cases. It is caused by loss-of-function mutations in the AVP V_2 receptor, which is located in the chromosome region Xq28. Although it is X-linked, heterozygous females may rarely be affected, presumably as a result of X-chromosome inactivation of the wild-type locus.

Autosomal NDI constitutes <10% of cases of NDI and is caused by mutations in the AQP-2 gene, located in the 12q13 chromosome region.

Acquired NDI

Approximately 50% of patients receiving lithium have impaired urinary concentrating ability and 10–20% of them develop symptomatic NDI on long-term therapy. Lithium appears to act by decreasing AQP-2 targeting to the apical membrane. The risk of symptomatic DI increases with duration of lithium therapy and NDI may be very slow to recover or may persist following discontinuation of lithium therapy.

Other drugs that have been reported more rarely to be associated with NDI include foscarnet, cidofovir, clozapine, fluvoxamine, amphotericin, gentamicin, demeclocycline, cyclophosphamide, isophosphamide, methotrexate, cimetidine, verapamil, methoxyflurane, colchicine and glyburide.

Metabolic causes of NDI (hyperglycemia, hypokalemia and hypercalcemia) are associated with AVP-resistant polyuria and polydipsia. Hyperglycemia causes an osmotic diuresis; in hypokalemia, the DI is not as severe as that seen with familial or lithium-induced NDI but does appear to result from a true reduction in

AVP responsiveness, probably by a reduction in total AQP-2. Hypercalcemia-associated polyuria and polydipsia is associated with AQP-2 downregulation and diminished trafficking of AQP-2 to the collecting duct apical membrane.

Impaired urinary concentrating capacity and unresponsiveness to AVP occurs in acute and chronic renal failure. Protein malnutrition or low-sodium intake can also lead to diminished tonicity of the renal medullary interstitium and diminish the driving force for water reabsorption. Urinary tract obstruction produces polyuria, which appears to be multifactorial but includes decreased AQP-2.

Management

Treatment focuses on elimination of the underlying disorder or drug, if possible. In congenital NDI, the main goals are to ensure an adequate intake of calories for growth and to avoid severe dehydration. Therapies for congenital NDI do not completely eliminate polyuria but reduction of polyuria to $3–4\,L/m^2/day$ is often achievable.

Foods with the highest ratio of calorie content to osmotic load should be used to maximize growth and minimize the urine volume required to excrete solute. Thiazide diuretics in combination with amiloride or indomethacin are the most useful pharmacological agents. Thiazides inhibit the NaCl co-transporter in the distal convoluted tubule.

Indomethacin potentiates the thiazide effect but can be associated with significant side-effects, most notably GI bleeding. The combination of thiazide and amiloride diuretics is the most commonly used combination regimen for the treatment of congenital NDI. When thiazides are used alone, potassium depletion can occur and hypokalemia itself can cause vasopressin-resistant polyuria. Amiloride, used at a dose of $0.3\,mg/kg/day$ divided three times per day, counteracts thiazide-induced hypokalemia, avoids the toxicity associated with indomethacin therapy and is well tolerated, even with prolonged treatment.

Polydipsia

Polyuria and polydipsia with low vasopressin concentrations can result from excessive intake of water and may be mistaken for DI. However, in contrast to DI, hypernatremia is never seen. Excessive intake of water slightly reduces the effective osmotic pressure of body fluids. Inhibition of the secretion of vasopressin allows water diuresis to compensate for the increased intake. This condition, primary polydipsia, must be distinguished from DI because dDAVP, which may cause water intoxication, is contraindicated in most cases.

Psychogenic polydipsia

Primary polydipsia can occur as part of a general cognitive defect associated with schizophrenia or other psychiatric disorders, which is usually called psychogenic polydipsia or compulsive water drinking. With rare exception, patients do not complain of thirst and usually attribute their polydipsia to disordered beliefs. Treatment focuses on the underlying psychiatric disorder. If water intake has been sufficient to cause hyponatremia in the absence of dDAVP, the patient may need supervised care to control access to water.

Dipsogenic polydipsia

In dipsogenic polydipsia, an increase in thirst may be seen due to diseases involving the hypothalamus, although it is most often idiopathic. Management should include a search for the cause and for the presence of associated defects in hypothalamic and anterior pituitary function. Some cases result from resetting the osmotic threshold for thirst below the threshold for vasopressin release. Because vasopressin secretion is suppressed at the thirst osmotic threshold, ingested water is rapidly excreted and thirst persists. dDAVP therapy may be beneficial in cases where thirst and AVP osmotic threshold are reversed, because it allows the serum osmolality to fall below the threshold for thirst, thereby suppressing water ingestion.

Iatrogenic polydipsia

Primary polydipsia can also be prompted by incorrect advice or incorrect understanding of advice offered by physicians, nurses, folk practitioners or the lay media. It is usually mild and rarely results in urine outputs of more than $5\,L/day$. It can be corrected if those involved are amenable to adopting more appropriate fluid intake practices.

Hypernatremia

Hypernatremia (serum sodium concentration >145 mmol/L) is caused by loss of water or gain of sodium. Because the increased serum osmolality associated with hypernatremia induces intense thirst, even a modest rise in serum sodium stimulates water ingestion, preventing progression of hypernatremia. Therefore, in a normal ambulatory individual with intact thirst, hypernatremia rarely occurs, even in the setting of DI. A prerequisite for hypernatremia is impaired water intake relative to water requirement.

Adipsic hypernatremia

Primary adipsia is usually caused by lesions in the anterior hypothalamus and is often accompanied by DI with impaired AVP release in response to increasing serum osmolality but adipsia can occur without DI, as can adipsic hypernatremia. The absence of thirst in a conscious hypernatremic child can be assessed by offering water and observing the response. The water intake associated with a normal diet is insufficient to match insensible water losses and absent thirst can lead to hypernatremic dehydration. Hypernatremia can develop slowly and even moderate to severe elevations in plasma sodium may be well tolerated and cause no obvious clinical abnormalities. If hypernatremic dehydration develops rapidly or is particularly severe, it usually results in overt clinical signs of hypovolemia and damage to the brain and other organs can occur.

As with DI, adipsia requires an evaluation of the cause, including cranial MRI to evaluate the hypothalamus. The long-term management of patients with adipsic hypernatremia should prevent or minimize recurrences of hypertonic dehydration by minimizing urinary water losses using dDAVP if DI is present and ensuring that fluid intake is sufficient to replace total water output. Even in the absence of dDAVP, caution should be taken to avoid excessive fluid intake as some of these individuals will have an impaired ability to downregulate AVP secretion and, in the setting of increased fluid intake, may be at risk of water intoxication.

Adipsic hypernatremia should be distinguished from the presence of physical obstacles to drinking, such as occur in patients who are debilitated by acute or chronic illness, have neurological impairment or are at the extremes of age.

Excessive free water losses (other than DI)

When an acute illness results in inadequate fluid intake or excessive free water losses, hypernatremia can result. Gastroenteritis, burns and high fever are the most common examples.

Excessive sodium intake

Increased sodium intake can be due to accidental ingestion or deliberate administration of large quantities of salt or intravenous administration of hypertonic solutions. Increased water intake corrects the hyperosmolality and excess sodium is rapidly excreted as long as thirst and renal function are intact and there are no physical limitations preventing access to water. In infants, severely ill or debilitated patients, excessive sodium administration can result in persistent hypernatremia until adequate free water is provided to allow salt diuresis.

Treatment

The initial treatment of hypernatremia should replace the water deficiency and minimize further losses. Free water should be given orally if possible but it can also be infused intravenously either as 5% dextrose in 0.225% saline or as 5% dextrose water (if hyperglycemia is not present). The net increase in body water that must be achieved to correct the deficit can be estimated by the formula:

$$\Delta H_2O = [(P_{Na}-140)/140] \times 0.6 \times BW$$

where ΔH_2O is the estimated water deficit in liters, P_{Na} is the plasma sodium concentration expressed in mmol/L and BW is the body weight in kilograms.

Non-acute hypernatremic dehydration or hypernatremic dehydration of uncertain duration should be corrected gradually because intracellular dehydration will lead to cellular swelling if hypernatremia is corrected too rapidly. The target should be to replace the free water deficit over a minimum of 24–48 h and to avoid changes in sodium concentration exceeding 0.5–1 mmol/L/h. During the correction of hypernatremia, fluid intake, output and plasma sodium (and glucose if hyperglycemia is present) should be monitored frequently and the treatment plan adjusted as necessary to achieve the desired rate of correction.

Hyponatremia

Vasopressin excess

The primary defense against developing hyponatremia is the ability to generate dilute urine and excrete free water, a process inhibited by vasopressin. Clinical manifestations include anorexia, headache, nausea, vomiting, muscle cramps and weakness. As hyponatremia advances, symptoms include impaired responsiveness, bizarre behavior, hallucinations, obtundation, incontinence, seizures and respiratory insufficiency. In its most severe form, hyponatremia may progress to cerebral edema and impending herniation, including decorticate or decerebrate posturing, bradycardia, hyper- or hypotension, altered temperature regulation, dilated pupils and respiratory arrest. The severity of the neurological effects depends on the degree of hyponatremia, the rate of decline and the age of the patient. Children appear to be more susceptible to symptomatic hyponatremia

after closure of the fontanelles, which leaves less room for brain expansion.

Determining the etiology of the hyponatremia is critical, since management depends on the diagnosis.

Diagnostic approach

The first step in the evaluation of hyponatremia is confirmation that it is associated with hypotonicity by measuring serum osmolality (Fig. 8.6). The most common cause of hypertonic hyponatremia is hyperglycemia.

Inappropriate AVP secretion

Osmotically inappropriate AVP secretion that cannot be accounted for by a non-osmotic stimulus implies a primary abnormality in the regulation of vasopressin secretion, the SIADH. Patients with SIADH fail to suppress AVP secretion even when plasma osmolality falls below the normal osmotic threshold for stimulated AVP release. This results in impaired renal free water clearance, total body free water excess and hypo-natremia. SIADH is the most common etiology of severe hyponatremia but the mechanism is not fully understood.

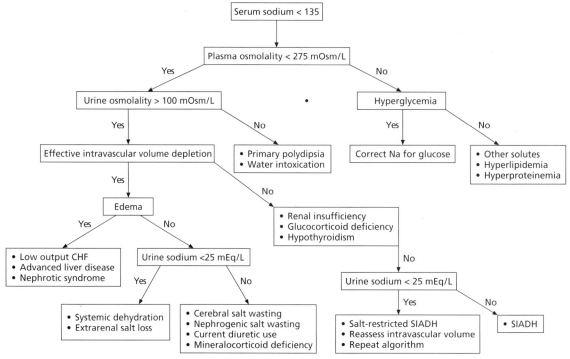

Figure 8.6 Diagnostic approach to hyponatremia.

Table 8.3 Drugs associated with impaired water clearance.

Class	Common drugs
Angiotensin-converting enzyme inhibitors	Lisinopril
Anticonvulsants	Carbamazepine
	Oxacarbazepine
	Valproic acid
Antineoplastics	Cis-platinum
	Cyclophosphamide
	Vinblastine
	Vincristine
Antiparkinsonian	Amantadine
	Trihexyphenidyl
Antipsychotics	Haloperidol
	Thioridazine
Antipyretics	Acetaminophen
Hypolipidemics	Clofibrate
Oral hypoglycemics	Chlorpropamide
	Tolbutamide
Selective serotonin uptake inhibitors	Fluoxetine
	Sertraline
Tricyclic antidepressants	Imipramine
	Amitriptyline
Other	Ecstasy

SIADH was first described with bronchogenic carcinoma and has since been recognized in patients with several other types of tumors, particularly of neuroendocrine origin.

Drugs associated with impaired free water clearance are listed in Table 8.3.

CNS disorders include systemic lupus, sarcoid, Guillain–Barré syndrome and infectious causes, such as meningitis and encephalitis. Tuberculous meningitis has an unusually high association with SIADH, with 70% of tuberculous meningitis cases in children affected. SIADH has also been seen in association with CNS mass lesions, such as tumors or brain abscesses, following cerebrovascular accident and following CNS surgery or traumatic injury. In CNS injury, care must be taken to distinguish SIADH from CSW, which also causes hyponatremia but requires markedly different management.

Non-malignant pulmonary disorders such as hypoxia and hypercapnia elevate plasma AVP concentrations. SIADH generally occurs with acute respiratory failure and is also seen in advanced chronic obstructive pulmonary disease and several other pulmonary disorders, including tuberculosis, severe asthma, respiratory syncytial virus (RSV) bronchiolitis, cystic fibrosis (CF) exacerbation and pneumonia.

The use of hypotonic saline for hydration during acute post-surgical management puts patients at risk of hyponatremia and, for this reason, isotonic saline solutions are widely used for fluid support following surgery. However, despite these practices, more than 50% of children sustaining neurological morbidity and mortality associated with hospital-acquired hyponatremia became hyponatremic following minor surgical procedures while receiving hypotonic fluids.

An SIADH-like syndrome occurs in patients with adrenal insufficiency, which impairs free water excretion. Severe hypothyroidism can also produce an SIADH-like hyponatremia, the etiology of which is unknown. SIADH should not be diagnosed until hypothyroidism and adrenal insufficiency have been excluded.

Management

The underlying cause should be identified and treated and the excess in body water should be corrected but much of the time the abnormal vasopressin secretion cannot be corrected and must be allowed to run its course until spontaneous recovery occurs. Fortunately, SIADH is generally temporary and therapy with fluid restriction will be necessary only until it remits.

Body water can also be reduced by inhibiting the antidiuretic effects of vasopressin using demeclocycline, a tetracycline derivative that causes a reversible form of NDI in almost all patients with SIADH in a week or more.

Brain edema associated with hyponatremia can result in decreased cerebral blood flow, hypoxic brain injury, herniation and cardiopulmonary arrest. Symptomatic hyponatremia is a medical emergency, requiring prompt treatment to prevent permanent brain damage or death. Fluid restriction should be instituted but hypertonic saline should be used in addition in symptomatic or severe hyponatremia to raise serum sodium more rapidly. Urine output as well as plasma sodium should be monitored at least every 2 h during hypertonic saline infusion and every 2–4 h during subsequent fluid restriction.

Once symptoms associated with hyponatremia have remitted, hypertonic saline infusion should be stopped and further correction should be achieved with fluid restriction alone.

During treatment of severe chronic hyponatremia, overtreatment leading to an increase in sodium above 10–12 mmol/L/24 h may occur despite careful monitoring. If overcorrecting is associated with a change in mental state, suggesting possible brain injury or is >15 mmol/L/24 h, it may be appropriate to lower the sodium again to concentrations at which the patient's symptoms improve or the daily increase in sodium remains below 10 mmol/L/24 h. This can be accomplished with infusion of 5% dextrose or 5% dextrose following administration of dDAVP if the SIADH has resolved. Once the patient has stabilized at the lower sodium, the process of correction can be restarted at a slower rate.

Appropriately increased secretion of vasopressin

Hypovolemic hyponatremia

Osmotically inappropriate but physiologically appropriate thirst and vasopressin secretion occur during large reductions in extracellular volume. The syndrome of hypovolemic hyponatremia can result from a number of salt- and water-depleting diseases, such as severe gastroenteritis, renal tubular acidosis, medullary cystic disease of the kidney, pyelonephritis, deficiency of aldosterone or aldosterone action and during diuretic therapy.

During systemic dehydration, there is a fall in the renal glomerular filtration rate (GFR) that results in an increase in proximal tubular sodium and water reabsorption, with a concomitant decrease in distal tubular water excretion. This, along with the associated stimulation of the renin–angiotensin–aldosterone system and suppression of ANP secretion by decreased vascular volume, results in the excretion of a concentrated urine that is very low in sodium. As dehydration progresses, hypovolemia and/or hypotension become major stimuli for AVP release, even in the presence of hypotonicity. These physiological responses, although they preserve volume, can cause hyponatremia, especially if water replacement in excess of salt replacement is given. Hyponatremia may be evident from physical signs, such as increased heart rate and decreased skin turgor; laboratory studies will show hemoconcentration and elevated blood urea nitrogen.

In contrast to the hyponatremia associated with SIADH, patients with systemic dehydration should be rehydrated with isotonic salt-containing fluids, such as normal saline or lactated Ringer's solution. Because of activation of the renin–angiotensin–aldosterone system, the administered sodium will be avidly conserved and a water diuresis will ensue as volume is restored and vasopressin concentrations fall. Hypernatremic fluid administration should not be needed and care must be taken to prevent too rapid correction of hyponatremia to avoid central pontine myelinolysis by controlling the rate of fluid administration if the hyponatremia has been prolonged.

When salt loss exceeds intake, sodium deficiency can result in hyponatremia. Causes include primary renal diseases, such as congenital polycystic kidney disease, acute interstitial nephritis and chronic renal failure, deficient mineralocorticoid secretion or action, diuretic use, burns and CF. Hyponatremia is countered by suppression of vasopressin release, which results in increased watetr excretion. With continuing salt loss, hypovolemia develops, resulting in non-osmotic stimulation of vasopressin. Hypovolemia leads to increased thirst and the ingestion of fluids with low solute content contributes to the hyponatremia.

Patients with hyponatremia due to salt loss require isotonic saline replacement but also ongoing supplementation with sodium chloride and fluids.

Hypervolemic hyponatremia

Severe low-output congestive heart failure, advanced liver cirrhosis with ascites and nephrotic syndrome are all characterized by increased total body sodium and water, resulting in peripheral edema. They also have a decrease in 'effective' intravascular volume due to decreased cardiac output and/or reduction in blood volume caused by a shift of salt and water from plasma to the interstitial space. As with systemic dehydration, the renin–angiotensin–aldosterone system is stimulated and water and salt excretion by the kidney is reduced. As the disease progresses, decreases in baroreceptor stimulation result in a compensatory increase in vasopressin secretion, leading to a further reduction in water clearance. If water intake is not restricted, hyponatremia can develop and hyponatremia in these clinical situations is common, although severe hyponatremia is rare.

When possible, the underlying disease should be treated but often this is not possible. Fluid and salt restriction and diuretics are commonly used but can worsen hyponatremia.

As with SIADH, acute treatment of symptomatic hyponatremia can be accomplished with hypertonic saline but the underlying disorder makes it difficult to maintain the administered fluid within the intravascular space. Frequent monitoring of sodium and fluid balance is critical and, once symptoms have been controlled, therapy should be adjusted so that the hyponatremia is corrected slowly to avoid the risk of neurological injury associated with overly rapid correction.

Other causes of hyponatremia

Water intoxication

Water intoxication as a cause of hyponatremia in the absence of any of the disease processes described above is seen primarily in pyschogenic polydipsia but infants fed overly dilute formula or water in place of formula are at risk of water intoxication.

Cerebral salt wasting

Following CNS injury, a syndrome of hyponatremia associated with increased urine sodium concentration, increased urine volume and volume depletion known as CSW can develop. This is associated with primary renal salt losses in the absence of primary renal disease. It is critical to distinguish CSW from DI and SIADH. Each of these syndromes shares some clinical features (Table 8.4), yet the distinction between the disorders is of considerable clinical importance, given the wholly divergent nature of the treatments. Fluid restriction is the treatment of choice for SIADH, whereas the treatment of CSW involves vigorous sodium and volume replacement and DI requires volume replacement with fluids of low salt content. DI and CSW can be distinguished easily by measuring serum sodium. Determination of volume status is the key to distinguishing SIADH from CSW.

CSW is transient but appropriate management while it persists involves vigorous administration of intravenous isotonic saline solutions. Since this therapy would be expected to worsen hyponatremia in SIADH and worsen hypernatremia in DI, the diagnosis and clinical and laboratory markers of volume status and serum osmolality should be reassessed frequently during therapy. As might be expected with the inappropriately low aldosterone, the efficacy of hypervolemic therapy appears to be improved by administration of fludrocortisone to help inhibit the natriuresis.

Table 8.4 Comparison of findings in syndrome of inappropriate ADH secretion, cerebral salt wasting and central diabetes insipidus.

	SIADH	CSW	CDI
Plasma volume	↑	↓	↓
Clinical evidence of volume depletion	−	+	+
Serum sodium/osmolality	↓	↓	↑
Urine sodium/osmolality	↑	↑↑	↓
Urine flow rate	↓	↑↑	↑
Plasma renin activity	↓	↓	↑
Plasma aldosterone concentration	↓ or →	↓	↑
Plasma AVP concentration	↑	↑ or →	↓
BUN/creatinine	↓/↓	↑/↑	↓/↑
Hematocrit	↓	↑	↑
Albumin concentration	↓	↑	↑
Serum uric acid concentration	↓	↓ or →	↑
Plasma ANP or BNP concentration	↑	↑	↓
Treatment	Fluid restriction	Salt and fluid replacement	Salt-poor fluid replacement

9 Polyglandular Syndromes

Learning Points

- Autoimmune polyglandular syndrome (APS) type 1 requires the presence of two of chronic mucocutaneous candidiasis, autoimmune hypoparathyroidism and autoimmune adrenal failure
- When any of these is diagnosed, the others should be sought
- APS2 is defined by the presence of primary adrenocortical insufficiency with either autoimmune thyroid disease or type 1 diabetes

- APS3 is the association between autoimmune thyroid disease and an autoimmune disease other than Addison disease. There are many variants
- Other associations are important because of the necessity not to miss the treatment of their evolving manifestations, which can be life threatening
- APS1 usually presents in children and APS2 and APS3 later in life

A high index of suspicion needs to be maintained whenever one organ-specific autoimmune disorder is diagnosed in order to prevent morbidity and mortality from the index disease as well as associated diseases.

Autoimmune polyglandular syndrome type 1 (APS 1)

The clinical presentation of APS1 is very variable. Diagnosis can be difficult initially when only one manifestation is present and it often takes years for others to appear. Increased awareness of the condition, combined with analysis of specific autoantibodies and mutational analysis of the *autoimmune regulator* (*AIRE*) gene, should help to diagnose this condition earlier and prevent serious and fatal complications.

Handbook of Clinical Pediatric Endocrinology, 1st edition. By Charles G. D. Brook and Rosalind S. Brown. Published 2008 by Blackwell Publishing, ISBN: 978-1- 4501-6109-1.

APS1, known as the autoimmune polyendocrinopathycandidiasis-ectodermal dystrophy syndrome (APECED), is a debilitating disorder of childhood. It is inherited as an autosomal-recessive condition; heterozygotes have no manifestations. The female–male ratio is close to 1. The clinical diagnosis requires the presence of two of the three cardinal components: chronic mucocutaneous candidiasis (CMC), autoimmune hypoparathyroidism and autoimmune adrenal failure. Only one of these is required if a sibling has the syndrome. There is a spectrum of associated minor components, which include endocrine and non-endocrine manifestations.

The gene defect is located on chromosome 21q22.3. It is named the *AIRE* gene. *AIRE* encodes a putative nuclear protein expressed in a variety of tissues of the immune system but particularly in the epithelial antigen-presenting cells in the thymus, where it is thought to play an important role in the central induction of self-tolerance, being involved in the negative selective of potentially autoreactive thymocytes.

Over 45 disease-causing mutations have been described in the *AIRE* gene which include point mutations, insertions and deletions, and are spread through the whole coding region of the gene. Mutations affecting splice sites have also been reported.

It is possible that the specific manifestations that develop in a particular APS1 patient may depend on alleles at other loci such as human leukocyte antigens (*HLA*), because the same *AIRE* mutations are associated with varying phenotypes. No consistent associations between APS1 manifestations and *HLA* alleles have been found but *HLA* polymorphisms may explain some of the variability in phenotype seen in APS1.

The pathogenesis of many of the manifestations of APS1 is unclear but autoimmunity is involved in the development of the endocrinopathies and patients have circulating autoantibodies to a variety of antigens from other affected tissues.

Measurement of autoantibodies is of limited use in patients with APS1 in determining their risk of developing new components because the sensitivity of the antibody test may frequently be less than the patient's pre-existing risk of the complication.

Clinical features

The first manifestation is typically mucocutaneous candidiasis, which develops in infancy or early childhood. Hypoparathyroidism characteristically develops around the age of 7 years and adrenal failure by 13 years. The complete evolution of the three cardinal features usually occurs in the first 20 years, with additional minor manifestations continuing to appear at least until the fifth decade. Although this sequence of appearance of the major manifestations is frequently observed in childhood, APS1 subjects not uncommonly present in other ways, either with one cardinal feature and several minor manifestations or with several minor manifestations and ectodermal dystrophy.

The median number of disease components is four, with up to 10 manifestations in some subjects. The cardinal triad occurs in around 60% of subjects and there may be a delay in diagnosis in the early years when rarer components may dominate the clinical picture. Patients who present initially with adrenal insufficiency rather than candidiasis tend to develop fewer components than others. It has also been reported that the earlier the first component presents, the more likely is it that multiple components will develop.

Table 9.1 Frequencies of the major and main minor components of APS1.

Disease	Frequency (%)
Main manifestations	
CMC	72–100
Autoimmune hypoparathyroidism	76–93
Autoimmune adrenal failure	73–100
Common minor manifestations	
Autoimmune endocrinopathies	
Hypergonadotrophic hypogonadism	17–61
Autoimmune thyroid disease	4–18
Type 1 diabetes mellitus	0–23
Pituitary defects	7
Gastrointestinal components	
Pernicious anemia	13–31
Malabsorption	10–22
Cholelithiasis	44
Chronic active hepatitis	5–31
Skin autoimmune diseases	
Vitiligo	8–26
Alopecia	29–40
Urticarial-like erythema with fever	9
Ectodermal dysplasia	
Nail dystrophy	10–52
Dental enamel hypoplasia	40–77
Tympanic membrane calcification	33
Other manifestations	
Keratoconjunctivitis	2–35
Asplenia	15

Data from European and North American patients. Iranian Jews have distinctly different frequencies from the other populations and have been excluded.

Table 9.1 lists the cardinal and more common minor manifestations together with their frequency.

Cardinal manifestations

Chronic or periodic mucocutaneous candidiasis (CMC) may occur as early as 1 month of age but more typically in the first 2 years of life. It is frequently mild or intermittent and responds well to periodic systemic anti-candidal treatment. In some subjects, CMC does not develop until adulthood but it is the most frequently occurring cardinal manifestation, present in 73–100% of patients. Oral candidiasis is the commonest presentation but esophagitis is also found, causing substernal pain, especially on swallowing. Infection of the intestinal mucosa leads to abdominal discomfort and diarrhea. Candidal infection can also affect the vagina, nails and skin.

Hypoparathyroidism has a peak incidence between 2 and 11 years of age in around 75–95% of patients with a slightly reduced penetrance in males. It may be asymptomatic or present with tetany and grand mal seizures. Presentation may be precipitated by factors such as fasting, low calcium or high phosphate intake. The diagnosis is confirmed by a low or undetectable plasma parathyroid hormone (PTH) concentration in the presence of hypocalcemia. Hyperphosphatemia and hypomagnesemia are common, with low urinary calcium excretion. Autopsy studies of parathyroid glands show atrophy and an infiltration of the parathyroids with mononuclear cells.

Autoimmune adrenal failure (Addison disease) is typically the third of the cardinal manifestations to present in APS1, with a peak incidence around 13 years. In most populations of APS1 patients, it occurs less frequently than the other major components. Destruction of the adrenal cortex may develop gradually and deficiencies of cortisol and aldosterone can appear in either order up to 20 years apart. At autopsy, the adrenals of these patients are atrophic, with the adrenal cortex being almost completely destroyed and having an extensive inflammatory cell infiltrate. Diagnosis of adrenal insufficiency is confirmed by a normal or low cortisol concentration with increased adrenocorticotrophic hormone (ACTH) and a subnormal cortisol response to ACTH stimulation. Deficiency of aldosterone is confirmed by a raised plasma renin activity even before the development of overt electrolyte disturbance.

Minor manifestations

Primary hypogonadism is the commonest minor manifestation. It is almost invariably accompanied by adrenal failure. Females present with primary or secondary amenorrhea. Male hypogonadism has been reported from puberty onwards.

Type 1 diabetes mellitus is relatively infrequent with a peak presentation in the teenage years.

Hashimoto thyroiditis or primary atrophic thyroiditis are uncommon. The age of presentation varies from around 10 years for Hashimoto thyroiditis to 17 years for primary atrophic thyroiditis. Hyperthyroidism is very rare.

Pituitary defects have occasionally been described and can induce single or multiple hormonal defects.

Chronic atrophic gastritis affects up to a third of patients with APS1, with a peak incidence at 10–20 years. It can lead to a megaloblastic anemia due to vitamin B12 deficiency or to a microcytic anemia because of iron deficiency.

Malabsorption presents with periodic or chronic diarrhea, usually with steatorrhea but may be associated with constipation. It can be a characteristic feature of an early atypical presentation of APS1 in the first year of life. It can be due to villous atrophy, exocrine pancreatic insufficiency, intestinal infections (*Giardia lamblia* or *Candida*), defective bile acid reabsorption and intestinal lymphangiectasia. There is a strong association with the hypocalcemia of hypoparathyroidism, since hypocalcemia impairs the secretion of cholecystokinin leading to a failure of normal gall bladder contraction and pancreatic enzyme secretion.

Cholelithiasis is present in up to 40% by ultrasonography, is frequently asymptomatic and is thought to be secondary to disruption of the enterohepatic circulation.

Chronic active hepatitis develops in 5–30% of cases. The clinical course varies from chronic but asymptomatic in the majority of cases to the development of cirrhosis or fulminant hepatic failure with a potentially fatal outcome in some. It may present in early childhood and can be the first manifestation of APS1.

Vitiligo can appear at any age, but most commonly in childhood, affecting up to a quarter of APS1 patients. It is highly variable in extent and often worsens with time.

Alopecia affects about a third of patients and can involve all body sites in varying degrees. It can develop rapidly at any age.

Recurrent urticaria with fever has been reported in about 10% of patients during childhood. It may persist for many years and is strongly associated with uveitis. High concentrations of immunoglobulin G (IgG) and circulating immune complexes are found and skin biopsy reveals a lymphoplasmacytic vasculitis.

Ectodermal dystrophy affects the nails and tooth enamel (Fig. 9.1). The pitted nails are unrelated to candidal infection and can be an important clue to the diagnosis. Dental enamel hypoplasia is common but deciduous teeth are never affected. Enamel hypoplasia

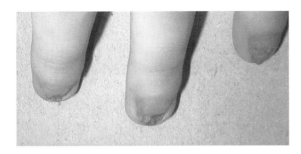

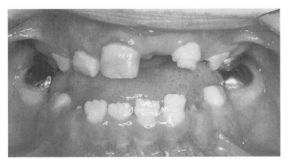

Figure 9.1 Ectodermal features of APS1 illustrating the nail dystrophy and the dental enamel hypoplasia.

can precede hypoparathyroidism and is unrelated to serum calcium concentrations. Even in the absence of ear infection, a third of patients have calcified plaques on the tympanic membranes.

Keratoconjunctivitis is the first manifestation in some cases. The initial symptoms are intense photophobia, blepharospasm and lacrimation; permanent visual impairment and even blindness are not infrequent. Some patients enter a quiescent phase around 10 years after onset.

Asplenia or hyposplenism has been documented by ultrasonography or suggested by hematological parameters in up to 15% of APS1 cases. It may be congenital or acquired, secondary to progressive autoimmune-mediated destruction or vascular insult to the spleen. It is suspected by a typical blood smear including Howell–Jolly bodies and thrombocytosis. It causes secondary immunodeficiency, rendering subjects susceptible to pneumococcal sepsis.

Several cases of selective *IgA deficiency and hypergammaglobulinemia* have been reported. Many patients have tuberculin anergy but whether this indicates an abnormal susceptibility to tuberculosis is unclear.

Impairment of renal function, due to interstitial nephritis or iatrogenic nephrocalcinosis necessitates, transplantation in some cases.

Neoplasia, most commonly squamous carcinoma of the oral mucosa in subjects with chronic oral *Candida* who smoke and adenocarcinoma of the stomach, is also seen.

Follow-up

The aim is the recognition of new disease components because some manifestations are life threatening. Each visit requires a thorough history and examination, particularly for oral mucocutaneous candidiasis and signs of evolving adrenal insufficiency, such as postural change in blood pressure. Blood should be taken for basal hormone, hematological and biochemical markers and an occasional antibody screen performed (Table 9.2). This, together with a high index of clinical suspicion, allows earlier diagnosis and treatment of additional components as they develop.

The early diagnosis of Addison disease is of particular importance and an annual measurement of ACTH is needed until adrenocortical failure develops. Plasma renin activity should be measured at the same time. Adrenal failure can evolve rapidly and annual assessment may not be sufficient to prevent acute presentations. The patient, immediate family and primary health care team must be made aware of the signs and symptoms of adrenal failure. Postural blood pressure and serum electrolytes should be determined at each clinic visit, together with periodic screening for 21-hydroxylase autoantibodies.

Treatment

Treatment of the individual disorders is no different from treating patients with the isolated disorders, except that polypharmacy is the rule and malabsorption may complicate therapy.

Live vaccines must be avoided in view of the underlying immunodeficiency but, since splenic atrophy is a common component, all APS1 patients should receive polyvalent pneumococcal vaccine with measurement of antibody response 6–8 weeks later. Non-responders or those who are asplenic should receive prophylactic daily antibiotics.

Prognosis

Many patients feel chronically unwell and the physical and psychological impacts of the multiple problems should not be underestimated. Despite improved survival, mortality rates are still high at 10–20% from

Table 9.2 Investigations recommended in the routine follow-up of APS1 patients to attempt to identify early development of new complications.

Disease component	Blood screening investigation
Major manifestation	
Addison disease	U&E, ACTH, plasma renin activity, annual synacthen test
Hypoparathyroidism	Serum calcium, phosphate, and magnesium
Minor manifestation	
Hypogonadism	Gonadotropin levels
Type 1 diabetes	Glycosylated hemoglobin
Autoimmune thyroid disease	fT3, fT4 and TSH
Autoimmune hepatitis	Liver function tests
Atrophic gastritis/pernicious anemia	FBC[a]
Hypo/asplenism	FBC,[a] blood smear[b]

[a]The presence of anemia on full blood count (FBC) results needs further investigation with ferritin, transferrin, and serum iron levels if the anemia is microcytic, and vitamin B12 levels if macrocytic.
[b]A blood smear indicating hypo/asplenism (Howell–Jolly bodies, anisocytes, poikilocytes, target cells and burr cells) and/or the presence of thrombocytosis needs follow-up with an abdominal ultrasound to assess spleen presence and size.

adrenal crisis, diabetic ketoacidosis, fulminant hepatic failure oral carcinoma, septicemia, hypocalcemia, generalized candidal infection during immunosuppressive treatment, complications of kidney failure and alcoholism. Around 3% die before the diagnosis of APS1 has been made, with adrenal failure the likely cause. Suicide is high among this patient group. Working capacity may be maintained in subjects with a limited number of manifestations but many are significantly incapacitated.

Autoimmune polyglandular syndrome type 2 (APS2)

APS2 is defined by the presence of primary adrenocortical insufficiency with either autoimmune thyroid disease or type 1 diabetes in the same individual. An autoimmune origin of all the major components should be demonstrated for a correct diagnosis. The association of autoimmune Addison disease with autoimmune thyroid disease is known as Schmidt syndrome and of Addison disease with type 1 diabetes as Carpenter syndrome. Other endocrine and nonendocrine autoimmune disorders occur with increased frequency in these individuals and their families.

Clinical features

Clinical presentation of APS2 can be at any age but is most frequently in early adulthood, with a peak onset in the fourth decade. It is less common in children and adolescents. It affects both sexes, with a female–male ratio of 3:1.

APS2 is a genetically complex disease aggregating in families and appearing to show an autosomal-dominant pattern of inheritance with incomplete penetrance in some. Susceptibility is determined by multiple genetic loci that interact with environmental factors. Only two genes have shown consistent association with *APS2*, *HLA* and *CTLA4*. Of these, *HLA* appears to have the strongest gene effect.

Addison disease is always present in APS2; autoimmune thyroid disease (Hashimoto thyroiditis, atrophic hypothyroidism, Graves' disease and postpartum thyroiditis) occurs in 70–80% and type 1 diabetes in 30–50%. Only about 10% have the complete triad. Adrenal failure is the first endocrine abnormality in around 50% but several minor APS2 components are often present at the diagnosis of adrenal failure, raising the possibility of APS2. On presentation with Addison disease, type 1 diabetes already exists in around 20% and autoimmune thyroid disease in around 30% but they can present more than 20 years before the diagnosis of adrenal failure.

Delayed diagnosis and preventable deaths still occur in patients with undiagnosed adrenal failure because signs and symptoms are non-specific until an adrenal crisis ensues. Adrenal insufficiency often presents as hypoglycemic seizures in children. Hyperpigmentation may be observed but may be absent in fair or red-headed subjects.

In those who already have type 1 diabetes, deterioration of glycemic control with recurrent hypoglycemia can be the presenting sign. The onset of autoimmune hyperthyroidism or thyroxine replacement for newly diagnosed hypothyroidism leads to enhanced cortisol clearance and can precipitate adrenal crisis in subjects with subclinical adrenocortical failure. Clinicians should maintain a high degree of alertness for underlying adrenal failure before initiating thyroid hormone replacement. Conversely, cortisol inhibits thyrotrophin release, so thyroid-stimulating hormone (TSH) concentrations are often high at the initial diagnosis of adrenal insufficiency (typically 5–10 mU/L) but return to normal after initiation of glucocorticoid replacement in the absence of co-existent thyroid disease. Adrenal insufficiency can mask the hyperglycemia of type 1 diabetes.

Incomplete APS2

Patients with autoimmune thyroid disease or type 1 diabetes with adrenal autoantibodies in the serum or patients with Addison disease and either thyroid and/or islet cell autoantibodies are sometimes classified as incomplete APS2. Self-evidently, these patients may develop APS2 in the future, particularly those with evidence of subclinical disease such as an elevated TSH or impaired glucose tolerance. Annual screening

by ACTH and renin measurement, together with education about the likely presentation of adrenal failure, is recommended for such individuals. About 30% of subjects with positive adrenal antibodies progress to adrenal failure over a 6-year period. Patients with either autoimmune thyroid disease or type 1 diabetes alone who have a sibling with APS2 are also classified by some as having incomplete APS2.

Autoimmune polyglandular syndrome type 3 (APS3)

APS3 is defined as the association between autoimmune thyroid disease and an additional autoimmune disease other than Addison disease. Many clinical combinations can be found in APS3 and it can therefore be subdivided into 3A to D, depending on the associated conditions (Table 9.3).

Hashimoto thyroiditis is the commonest form of autoimmune thyroid disease, although Graves' disease and post-partum thyroiditis are also seen. Autoimmune thyroid diseases tend to increase in incidence in the teenage years, with a peak in the fourth decade for Graves' disease and in the fifth and sixth decades for autoimmune hypothyroidism. Autoimmune thyroid disease is most commonly isolated and polyglandular involvement in the form of APS3 or APS2 is rare. Only 1% of patients with autoimmune thyroid disease have adrenal autoantibodies (with risk of APS2), whereas 3–5% have either pancreatic islet autoimmunity and/or clinical type 1 diabetes.

Autoimmune thyroid disease is more commonly associated with pernicious anemia, vitiligo, alopecia, myasthenia gravis and Sjögren syndrome and autoimmune thyroid disease should be sought prospectively

Table 9.3 Classification of APS3.

Autoimmune thyroid disease plus	Autoimmune endocrinopathy excluding Addison disease (e.g. type 1 diabetes, premature ovarian failure, lymphocytic hypophysitis)	3A
	Autoimmune gastrointestinal disease (e.g. pernicious anemia, celiac disease, autoimmune hepatitis)	3B
	Skin or neurological manifestations (e.g. alopecia, vitiligo, myasthenia gravis)	3C
	Connective tissue disease (e.g. SLE, rheumatoid arthritis, Sjögren syndrome)	3D

SLE, systemic lupus erythematosus.

in patients with these conditions. Around 30% of subjects with vitiligo have another autoimmune disorder, with autoimmune thyroid disease and pernicious anemia being the most common. Many patients with vitiligo are asymptomatic and other autoimmune diseases are diagnosed only by prospective screening, including evaluation of autoantibody status. Up to 15% of patients with alopecia and nearly 30% of those with myasthenia gravis have autoimmune thyroid disease.

Management

Hormone replacement or other therapies for the component diseases of APS2 are similar whether the disease occurs in isolation or in association with other conditions and disorders should be treated as they are diagnosed. However, certain combinations of diseases require specific attention. Most importantly, thyroxine therapy for hypothyroidism can precipitate a life-threatening adrenal crisis in a patient with untreated and unsuspected adrenal insufficiency. Thus, to avoid adrenal crisis, clinicians should maintain a high degree of suspicion for co-existing adrenal failure in subjects who are hypothyroid. Hyperthyroidism increases cortisol clearance so, in patients with adrenal insufficiency who have unresolved hyperthyroidism, glucocorticoid replacement should be at least doubled until the patient is euthyroid. Decreasing insulin requirements or increasing occurrence of hypoglycemia in type 1 diabetes can be one of the earliest indications of adrenocortical failure. One of the most important aspects of managing these patients is to be continually alert to the possibility of the development of further endocrinopathies to insure early diagnosis and treatment.

Follow-up

Once APS2/3 is suspected, a full assessment of endocrine function is needed. The number of disorders that will develop and the age at which they will present is unpredictable, so long-term follow-up is needed. A high clinical index of suspicion needs to be maintained, particularly in those subjects who have yet to develop adrenal failure or diabetes. Presymptomatic recognition of autoimmune disease minimizes associated morbidity and mortality. There is a clear link between the presence of organ-specific autoantibodies and the progression to disease, although there

is often an asymptomatic latent period of months or years. The absence of autoantibodies does not exclude the risk of a disease component.

In all patients with Addison disease, there is a need to screen for other endocrine disorders, particularly autoimmune thyroid disease and type 1 diabetes. At diagnosis, screening for thyroid peroxidase (TPO) and GAD65 autoantibodies is worthwhile. If negative, this should be repeated occasionally, perhaps every 2–3 years.

The determination of thyroid function should be carried out at least annually for early recognition of thyroid disease in all subjects with type 1 diabetes and Addison disease. The determination of P450c17 and P450scc antibodies in females with Addison disease and APS2 may identify subjects at high risk from primary hypogonadism before gonadotropins become elevated. Such subjects may be suitable for cryopreservation of embryos, ovarian material or sperm.

Screening for APS2-associated disorders should also be performed in women with primary or secondary amenorrhea or premature ovarian failure and young patients with vitiligo. As APS2 shows strong familial tendencies, family members should also be checked for features of associated endocrine conditions.

Miscellaneous disorders

Immune dysregulation, polyendocrinopathy and enteropathy (X-linked) syndrome (IPEX) is a rare and devastating X-linked condition of male infants, affecting immune regulation and resulting in multiple autoimmune disorders. The first feature is commonly intractable diarrhea and failure to thrive due to autoimmune enteropathy occurring around 3–4 months of age. Type 1 diabetes and autoimmune hypothyroidism develop in the first year of life in around 90% and 50% of males, respectively. Additional clinical features include eczema, autoimmune hemolytic anemia, autoimmune thrombocytopenia, recurrent infections, lymphadenopathy, membranous nephropathy and striking growth retardation. Other autoimmune features are less frequent. Sepsis may result from a primary defect in immune regulation but is exacerbated by autoimmune neutropenia, immunosuppressive drugs, malnutrition, enteropathy and eczema.

The onset of *autoimmune lymphoproliferative syndrome (ALPS)* is usually in the first 2 years of life and the characteristic feature in all cases is massive generalized lymphadenopathy. Hepatosplenomegaly and hematological autoimmunity (hemolytic anemia and thrombocytopenia) are also frequent manifestations. Other autoimmune conditions, including thyroid autoimmunity and type 1 diabetes, have occasionally been reported as part of this syndrome. ALPS follows a chronic course, with the response to immunosuppressive drugs varying. Splenectomy is usually performed to reduce the lymphadenopathy and improve the thrombocytopenia and hemolytic anemia, although this leads to an increased risk of infections in patients who are often neutropenic. Long-term outcome is variable, although survival into adulthood has been reported, when an increase in malignancy is seen. Allogenic bone marrow transplantation has been successful in a few children.

Kabuki make-up syndrome (KMS) is a probably genetic syndrome consisting of five characteristic manifestations: (1) dysmorphic face with eversion of the lower lateral eyelid, arched eyebrows with sparseness of their lateral one-third, long palpebral fissures with long eyelashes, depressed nasal tip and prominent large ears (100%); (2) unusual dermatoglyphic patterns (96%); (3) skeletal abnormalities and hypermobile joints (88%); (4) mild to moderate mental retardation (84%); and (5) postnatal growth retardation with short stature (55%). Other features include dental abnormalities, susceptibility to infections, particularly recurrent otitis media, cardiovascular anomalies, renal and urinary tract anomalies, biliary atresia, diaphragmatic hernia and anorectal anomalies. Less common associations include growth hormone deficiency, primary ovarian dysfunction, Hashimoto thyroiditis and vitiligo. Patients often survive with a good prognosis unless they have severe complications such as cardiovascular, hepatic or renal disease. Males and females are affected equally and most cases are sporadic, although a few familial cases have been reported. KMS may be inherited as an autosomal-recessive disorder. As yet, there is no evidence or clues to the underlying cause of the syndrome. The endocrinopathies should be treated along standard lines.

10 Hypoglycemia

Learning Points

- Maintenance of a normal blood glucose concentration is critical to brain development and function so hypoglycemia is a medical emergency
- The risk of harm is greater in infants and children because brain size is relatively greater to body size than later in life
- Glucose is the prime source of energy for the brain but ketones can provide an alternate source in chronic hypoglycemia
- Control of blood glucose is by an equilibrium being maintained between glucose production and glucose utilization

- Obtaining specimens of blood and urine in appropriate containers for laboratory analysis at the time of hypoglycemia assists diagnosis of the cause and obviates the need for a fasting study
- Absence of ketonuria at the time of hypoglycemia suggests hyperinsulinemia or a defect of fatty acid oxidation
- Hepatomegaly suggests a defect of glycogen storage or release

Maintenance of a normal blood glucose concentration involves interaction between plasma glucose, insulin, glucagon, epinephrine, cortisol and growth hormone (GH). Glucose metabolism accounts for approximately half of daily energy needs.

Glucose can be stored as glycogen or fat and can be used for the synthesis of proteins and structural components such as cell membranes via the recycling of its carbon atom. Normal blood glucose concentration is maintained by a balance between glucose production and glucose utilization and anything that alters this equilibrium leads to hypoglycemia. Insulin decreases glucose production and increases glucose utilization, whereas glucagon, epinephrine, cortisol and GH increase glucose production and decrease glucose utilization.

The definition of hypoglycemia is confusing and controversial because there is poor correlation between plasma glucose concentrations, the onset of clinical symptoms, the duration of hypoglycemia and long-term neurological sequelae. If hypoglycemia is defined by a concentration <2.5 mmol/L (45 mg/dL), ~20% of normal full-term infants have blood glucose concentrations lower than this in the first 48 h. It is assumed that these infants, who have concurrent hyperketonemia, are protected against neural dysfunction by the availability of alternative fuels for brain metabolism.

Hypoglycemia is a potent cause of neurological damage when persistent or recurrent. Even mild hypoglycemia, at concentrations that were previously thought to be innocuous, may be associated with serious long-term effects in preterm infants, so prompt diagnosis of the cause (Table 10.1) and early treatment are critical.

When confronted with a child with hypoglycemia, a blood sample for detailed investigations should be

Handbook of Clinical Pediatric Endocrinology, 1st edition. By Charles G. D. Brook and Rosalind S. Brown. Published 2008 by Blackwell Publishing, ISBN: 978-1-4501-6109-1.

Table 10.1 Summarizing the different causes of hypoglycemia in the neonatal, infancy and childhood period.

Hyperinsulinism
Transient: Infant of diabetic mother/perinatal asphyxia/rhesus disease/intrauterine growth retardation/Beckwith–Weidemann syndrome/'idiopathic'
Congenital: SUR1/KIR6.2/glucokinase/glutamate dehydrogenase mutations
    Defects in the metabolism of fatty acids (SCHAD)
    Carbohydrate-deficient glycoprotein syndrome (CDG)
    Insulinomas

Hormonal deficiency
Cortisol/growth hormone/ACTH/glucagon/epinephrine

Defects in hepatic glycogen release/storage
Glycogen storage diseases: glucose-6-phosphatase, amylo 1,6 glucosidase deficiency, liver phosphorylase deficiency, hepatic glycogen synthase deficiency

Defects in gluconeogenesis
Fructose-1,6-bisphosphatase deficiency, phosphoenolpyruvate carboxykinase (PEPCK) deficiency, pyruvate carboxylase deficiency

Defects of fatty acid oxidation and carnitine metabolism
Very-long-chain acyl-CoA dehydrogenase (VLCAD) deficiency
Medium-chain acyl-CoA dehydrogenase (MCAD) deficiency
Short-chain acyl-CoA dehydrogenase (SCAD) deficiency
Long-/short-chain-L-3-hydroxy-acyl CoA (L/SCHAD) deficiency
Carnitine deficiency (primary and secondary)
Carnitine palmitoyltransferase deficiency (CPT 1 and 2)

Defects in ketone body synthesis/utilization
HMG CoA-synthase deficiency/HMG CoA-lyase deficiency
Succinyl-CoA: 3-oxoacid CoA-transferase (SCOT) deficiency

Metabolic conditions (relatively common ones)
Organic acidemias (propionic/methylmalonic)
Maple syrup urine disease, galactosemia, fructosemia, tyrosinemia
Hereditary fructose intolerance
Glutaric aciduria type 2
Mitochondrial respiratory chain complex deficiencies

Drug induced
Sulfonylurea/insulin/beta-blocker/salicylates/alcohol

Miscellaneous causes (mechanism may not be so clear)
Idiopathic ketotic hypoglycemia (diagnosis of exclusion)
Infections (sepsis, malaria), congenital heart disease

Table 10.2 The intermediary metabolites and hormones to be measured in the initial investigations of hypoglycemia.

Blood	Urine
Glucose	Ketones
Insulin	Reducing substances
Cortisol	Organic acids
Growth hormone	
Non-esterified fatty acids	
Acetoacetate	
3β-hydroxybutyrate	
Carnitine (free and total)	
Blood spot acyl-carnitine	
Ammonia	
Lactate	

taken before giving enteral feeds or intravenous glucose, because this sample enables the defect in the many metabolic and endocrine pathways involved in the etiology of the hypoglycemia to be identified. A urine sample should be saved at the same time. The substances to be measured are shown in Table 10.2; Table 10.3 lists the more detailed investigations required if there is a clue from the preliminary investigations of the cause of the hypoglycemia.

Glucose production

In addition to ingestion, glucose can be produced from fat, from protein by gluconeogenesis and from glycogen stored in the liver. Glycogen breakdown by glycogenolysis accounts for about 30–40% of overall hepatic output of glucose. This results in a readily available source of glucose for the brain and other neural tissues which are obligate glucose users.

The liver also provides glucose by gluconeogenesis, which involves the synthesis of glucose from lactate and alanine. Gluconeogenesis contributes 50% of glucose production in children.

Glucose utilization

The factors that determine glucose utilization include plasma glucose concentration, the tissue requirement for glucose, the availability of alternative substrates and, in certain tissues, their sensitivity to insulin.

Table 10.3 More detailed investigations will depend on the possible etiology of the hypoglycemia.

Hyperinsulinism (or insulin-like action)
C-peptide
Proinsulin, preproinsulin
IGFBP-I (inverse relation to insulin)
Transferrin isoelectric focusing (especially if hyperinsulinism associated with syndrome)
'Abnormal' IGF-II forms
Insulin autoantibodies

Hormonal
Growth hormone provocation testing
Glucagon (extremely rare)
Epinephrine/norepinephrine (extremely rare)

Fatty acid oxidation disorder
Fatty acid flux studies (skin biopsy for fibroblast culture)

Glycogen storage disease
Cholesterol, triglycerides
Urate, LFTs

Gluconeogenesis
Leukocyte fructose 1,6 bisphosphatase activity
Liver phosphorylase

Hepatic glycogen synthesis disease
Pre- and post-prandial blood glucose and lactate profiles

Ketone body synthesis/utilization disorder
HMG Co-A/succinyl-CoA: 3-oxoacid CoA-transferase (SCOT) mutational analysis
Liver biopsy

'Metabolic'
Red cell galactose-1-phosphateuridyltransferase activity (galactosemia)
Plasma amino acids (maple syrup urine disease)
Urinary succinylacetone (tyrosinemia)
Transferrin isoelectric focusing (CDG syndromes)
Pyruvate
Acetoacetate
Mitochondrial respiratory chain complex activity

Unexplained
Urine toxicology (specifically request for the possible offending agent)

The transport of glucose into tissues depends on specific glucose transporters, GLUT 1–5.

GLUT 1, which is responsible for glucose transport across the blood–brain barrier is an insulin-independent transporter found in all cells. GLUT 2, which is insulin independent, is a low-affinity transporter not easily saturated even at high plasma glucose concentrations. It is the main GLUT in liver and pancreatic β cells. GLUT 3 is the insulin-independent GLUT in the central nervous system with the highest affinity for glucose. GLUT 4 is an insulin-dependent transporter in muscle and adipose tissue. GLUT 5, primarily expressed in the jejunal brush border, is mainly a fructose transporter.

Insulin regulates the steady-state concentration of the insulin-dependent transporters by promoting their synthesis but also causes mobilization of these transporters to the cell membrane when the plasma glucose concentration increases.

Glucose may be stored in cells as glycogen or fat, be oxidized to carbon dioxide or converted to lactate. The proportions of glucose directed to these fates depend upon the degree of fasting, the hormonal milieu and the presence of alternative energy substrates.

Changes associated with feeding and fasting

Insulin regulates glucose production and utilization in both the fed and the fasted states. After a meal, plasma glucose concentration starts to increase within 15 min, which stimulates insulin secretion. Plasma glucose concentrations peak at 30–60 min and decline until absorption is complete, usually about 4–5 h later. Plasma insulin concentrations follow a similar time course.

After a meal, there is marked suppression (50–60%) of hepatic glucose production. Post-prandial plasma glucose concentrations are determined by the balance between the rates of glucose removal from and delivery to the systemic circulation. Lipolysis, ketogenesis, glycogenolysis and gluconeogenesis are all suppressed post-prandially. The liver, small intestine, brain, muscle and adipose tissue are mainly responsible for the removal of glucose from the circulation, the magnitude of glucose uptake by the tissues, being determined largely by the plasma insulin concentration, although glucose uptake by the brain is independent of insulin and determined by the plasma glucose concentration.

A steady state is reached 4–6 h after a meal when glucose production equals glucose consumption and plasma glucose concentrations are maintained within a narrow range. Glucose turnover (glucose production and utilization) is then approximately 10 mmol/kg/min. Non-insulin-dependent utilization of glucose in this state accounts for 80%, mainly by the brain (which accounts for 50% of the total), red blood cells, kidneys and the gastrointestinal system. The glucose concentrations are maintained by the usual hormonal interactions:

• Glucagon allows the controlled release of stored glycogen from the liver.
• Insulin restrains the effects of glucagon by preventing accelerated lipolysis and proteolysis.
• Cortisol and GH play permissive roles in setting the sensitivity of the peripheral tissues to glucagon and insulin.
• Epinephrine promotes hepatic glycogenolysis.
• Norepinephrine is less potent than epinephrine in promoting glycogenolysis but more potent in mobilizing free fatty acids.

As the period of fast lengthens, tissue glucose utilization decreases while utilization of free fatty acids and ketone bodies increases. Hepatic glucose output is reduced by a decrease in glycogenolysis, with an increase in the rate of gluconeogenesis. Glucagon secretion with reduced insulin allows stored fats to be converted to glycerol and fatty acids and proteins to be converted to amino acids for gluconeogenesis. The liberated free fatty acids are transported to the liver bound to albumin, where they can either undergo β-oxidation in the mitochondria to yield ketone bodies or be re-esterified to triacylglycerols and phospholipids.

Muscle and other tissues become progressively more dependent on free fatty acids and ketone bodies for their continued energy requirements as fasting persists. Ketone bodies produced in the liver from the oxidation of fatty acids are exported to peripheral tissues as an energy source. They are particularly important for the brain, which has no other substantial non-glucose-derived energy source. Ketone bodies replace glucose as the predominant fuel for nervous tissue, thereby reducing the obligatory requirement of the brain.

Glucose and the brain

Some parts of the brain, for example the cortex, are more susceptible to hypoglycemic damage than others, such as the cerebellum, probably because of regional differences in cerebral metabolic capacity. During moderate acute hypoglycemia, there are no changes in cerebral functional activity but when hypoglycemia is severe (lower than 2 mmol/L, 36 mg/dL), cerebral glucose utilization decreases and blood flow increases.

During chronic hypoglycemia, the brain increases the number of GLUT sites and decreases glucose utilization. Cerebral blood flow is increased more than during acute hypoglycemia. Neuronal damage due to severe and prolonged hypoglycemia occurs as a result of active release of excitatory amino acids mainly in the cerebral cortex, hippocampus and caudate putamen.

The utilization of alternative substrates may provide another mechanism of protection against hypoglycemia. In adults infused with β-hydroxybutyrate during insulin-induced hypoglycemia, the counter-regulatory hormonal response to hypoglycemia is lowered, as is the delay in cognitive dysfunction. The fetus and neonate can take up and oxidize ketone bodies. The uptake of ketone bodies by the brain is proportional to the circulating concentration and the uptake is higher in neonates than in adults.

Young children have glycogen stores adequate for a period of starvation of only about 12 h, after which the maintenance of normal blood glucose is dependent on gluconeogenesis. During a brief period of fasting, they convert more rapidly to a fat-based fuel economy.

Children have higher glucose production rates in comparison with adults in order to meet the increased metabolic demands of the brain because the brain relative to body size is much larger than in adults. Brain size is the principal determinant of factors that regulate hepatic glucose output throughout life. Fasting newborn and young children demonstrate a high glucose utilization rate per kg body weight relative to adult requirements, which is why they are more susceptible to hypoglycemia than adults.

Diagnostic approach

Hypoglycemia occurs more frequently during the first days than at any other time of life. This is transient in the majority of cases but symptoms may be very non-specific (Table 10.4), so any child with symptoms must have a blood glucose concentration measured and documented.

Table 10.4 The symptoms of hypoglycemia may be very non-specific.

Any non-specific symptom may indicate hypoglycemia
Feeding poorly
Irritability
Lethargy
Stupor
Apnea, cyanotic spells
Hypothermia
Hypotonia, limpness
Tremor
Seizures
Coma

In many conditions, hypoglycemia occurs only in relation to periods of starvation. Starvation tests are potentially very dangerous and must be conducted only under strictly controlled conditions by staff experienced in their administration, with a secure intravenous infusion available for immediate correction of hypoglycemia. The hazards are greatest in defects of fatty acid oxidation, since the induced hyperfatty acidemia carries a risk of inducing a cardiac arrhythmia. Sequential measurements of intermediary metabolites and glucose are taken throughout the fast, with the crucial blood sample being drawn when hypoglycemia occurs. The urine sample passed then or after restoration of normoglycemia should be deep frozen for measurement of organic acids and other abnormal metabolites.

Other measurements from this specimen obtained at the time of hypoglycemia can help in diagnosis. Cortisol deficiency may be revealed and further tests to define the integrity of the hypothalamo-pituitary–adrenal axis then become mandatory. Low GH concentrations at the time of fasting hypoglycemia do not exclude or confirm deficiency.

The documentation of abnormal urinary organic acids is particularly helpful when hypoglycemia is due to methylmalonic acidemia, maple syrup urine disease (MSUD) or mitochondrial β-oxidation defects.

Causes of hypoglycemia

Hypoglycemia in childhood can be broadly divided into those resulting from hormonal abnormalities (hyperinsulinism, cortisol or GH deficiency), defects of hepatic glycogen release/storage, gluconeogenesis, carnitine metabolism, fatty acid oxidation or unknown causes, such as idiopathic ketotic hypoglycemia (Table 10.1).

Hormonal abnormalities

Insulin

Hyperinsulinism of infancy (HI), characterized by excessive and inappropriate secretion of insulin in relation to the prevailing blood glucose concentration, is the commonest cause of recurrent and severe hypoglycemia. It can be transient or persistent.

The transient form, which may be idiopathic, is associated with maternal diabetes mellitus, intra-uterine growth retardation, perinatal asphyxia, erythroblastosis fetalis, Beckwith–Wiedemann syndrome, administration of some drugs (e.g. sulfonylureas) to the mother and after intravenous maternal glucose infusions during labor.

Congenital hyperinsulinism, which presents in the newborn period or during the first 2–6 months after birth, is by far the most difficult to manage. It has a high (and unchanging) incidence (up to 25%) of neurological handicap. Inappropriate secretion of insulin has been called a variety of names, including idiopathic hypoglycemia of infancy, leucine-sensitive hypoglycemia, neonatal insulinoma, microadenomatosis, focal hyperplasia, nesidioblastosis and persistent hyperinsulinemic hypoglycemia of infancy (PHHI). Sporadic and familial variants are recognized, with sporadic forms being uncommon (incidence 1 per 40 000 live births) and familial forms being common (as high as 1 in 2500 live births) in communities with high rates of consanguinity.

The characteristic profile of a blood sample drawn at the time of hypoglycemia is hyperinsulinemia, hypoketotis and hypofatty acidemia with inappropriately raised concentrations of insulin and C-peptide. The concentration of insulin in the blood may not be particularly high but what is an appropriate insulin concentration for normoglycemia becomes inappropriate in the presence of hypoglycemia. Any measurable insulin in a hypoglycemic sample is strong evidence of a failure of basal insulin control.

The immediate imperative of management is to give glucose sufficient to maintain blood glucose concentrations above 3 mmol/L (54 mg/dL). Infusion rates in excess of 4–6 mg/kg/min, even >20 mg/kg/min, may be necessary. Having stabilized the blood glucose concentration, diazoxide and a thiazide diuretic should be given concurrently, in order to overcome the tendency of diazoxide to cause fluid retention and to capitalize on the fact that the drugs have synergistic effects in increasing blood glucose concentration. A convenient starting dose of diazoxide is 5–10 mg/kg/day in three 8-hourly aliquots, increasing to a maximum of 20 mg/kg/day.

The use of a calcium channel-blocking agent, such as nifedipine, has been promoted, with some patients showing good response, but some patients have impairments in voltage-gated calcium entry, so nifedipine may not always be effective.

Because of the anabolic effects of insulin, the hypoglycemia occurs despite a liver engorged with glycogen. This can be mobilized by administration of glucagon given by continuous infusion (starting dose 1.0 mg/kg/h). The glycemia can also usually be improved by an infusion of somatostatin that will switch off insulin secretion. Glucagon given concurrently with the somatostatin analog octreotide (initial dose 10 mg/kg/day) may confer substantial benefit.

When managing a child unresponsive to conventional therapy with diazoxide, the options are long-term combined continuous subcutaneous infusion of glucagon and somatostatin or surgical resection of the pancreas. The operation most commonly performed is a 95% pancreatectomy in the first instance but some children still remain hypoglycemic and a further attempt can then be made to control the procedure with diazoxide. In a minority of cases, total pancreatectomy may be necessary to control the severe hyperinsulinism, which may be exacerbated by regeneration of the pancreatic remnant.

The recognition of focal disease has led to preoperative percutaneous transhepatic pancreatic vein catheterization with the withdrawal of multiple blood samples to identify hotspots of insulin secretion. Rapid-frozen sections are used to identify areas of focal hyperplasia at surgery, which are then resected.

Other hormones

Deficiencies of glucagon, epinephrine, GH or cortisol can cause hypoglycemia. Deficiencies of the first two are very rare. GH and cortisol increase rates of gluconeogenesis and glycolysis and antagonize the effects of insulin. Congenital hypopituitarism may present with life-threatening hypoglycemia, abnormal serum sodium concentrations, shock, microphallus and growth failure later. Causes include septo-optic dysplasia, other midline syndromes and mutations of transcription factors involved in pituitary gland development. The incidence of hypoglycemia in acquired hypopituitarism resulting from tumors (most commonly craniopharyngioma), radiation, infection, hydrocephalus, vascular anomalies and trauma can be as high as 20% and may be a cause of sudden death. Appropriate replacement therapy prevents hypoglycemia.

Hypoglycemia due to defects in hepatic glycogen release

Glucose-6-phosphatase deficiency (glycogen storage disease type I, Von Gierke disease) is the commonest of the glycogen storage diseases. Children present with recurrent hypoglycemia associated with lactic acidosis, hyperuricemia and hyperlipidemia. The aim of treatment is to prevent hypoglycemia using a combination of continuous nasogastric drip feeding and cornstarch.

Deficiency of amylo-1,6-glucosidase causes glycogen storage disease type III, which presents with hepatomegaly, hypoglycemia, hyperlipidemia, short stature and, in a number of subjects, cardiomyopathy and myopathy. Deficiency of liver phosphorylase causes glycogen storage disease VI, which presents with hepatomegaly, growth retardation, variable but mild episodes of fasting hypoglycemia and hyperketosis during childhood. Patients may demonstrate elevated serum transaminases, hyperlipidemia, hypotonia and muscle weakness. These clinical features and biochemical abnormalities generally resolve by puberty. Rare variants may have associated proximal renal tubular acidosis, myopathy or fatal cardiomyopathy.

Hypoglycemia due to defects in gluconeogenesis

Gluconeogenesis, the formation of glucose from lactate/pyruvate, glycerol, glutamine and alanine maintains normoglycemia during fasting. Inborn deficiencies of pyruvate carboxylase, phosphoenolpyruvate carboxykinase (PEPCK), fructose-1,6-bisphosphatase and glucose-6-phosphatase present with fasting hypoglycemia and lactic acidosis. Pyruvate carboxylase deficiency may lead to a more widespread clinical presentation with lactic acidosis, severe developmental retardation and proximal renal tubular acidosis.

Hypoglycemia due to disorders of carnitine metabolism and defects of fatty acid oxidation

Primary carnitine deficiency is an autosomal-recessive disorder of fatty acid oxidation that can present at different ages with hypoketotic hypoglycemia and cardiomyopathy and/or skeletal myopathy.

The commonest disorder of fatty acid β-oxidation is deficiency of medium-chain acyl-CoA dehydrogenase (MCAD). This autosomal-recessive condition is characterized by intolerance to prolonged fasting and recurrent episodes of hypoglycemic coma with medium-chain dicarboxylicaciduria, impaired ketogenesis and low plasma and tissue carnitine concentrations. The disorder may be fatal in young patients. Other defects of β-oxidation may present with hypoketotic hypoglycemia associated with neurological (hypotonia) and cardiovascular complications (cardiomyopathy). The pattern of dicarboxylicaciduria accumulation is characteristic for each enzymatic defect of the β-oxidation pathway.

Hypoglycemia due to defects in ketone body synthesis/utilization

Ketone bodies are an alternative fuel to glucose for the brain. Each ketone body is synthesized from the combination of acetyl-CoA and acetoacetyl-CoA to form hydroxymethylglutaryl-CoA (HMG-CoA). This is split by HMG-CoA lyase to yield acetoacetate, which is then converted to β-hydroxybutyrate. Hypoglycemia may occur as a result of defects in either the synthesis or the utilization of ketone bodies.

Idiopathic ketotic hypoglycemia

Idiopathic ketotic hypoglycemia is common between the ages of 18 months and 5 years and remits spontaneously by the age of 9–10 years. The typical history is of a child who may miss a meal and develop hypoglycemia unpredictably but usually following an upper respiratory tract infection. The hypoglycemia is associated with raised ketone bodies and free fatty acids with suppressed insulin concentrations.

Metabolic causes

Hypoglycemia occurs in galactosemia, fructosemia, tyrosinemia organic acidemias, MSUD, glutaric aciduria type II and mitochondrial respiratory chain defects. Hereditary fructose intolerance, caused by catalytic deficiency of aldolase B (fructose-1,6-bisphosphate aldolase), is a recessively inherited condition in which affected homozygotes develop hypoglycemia and severe abdominal symptoms after taking foods containing fructose and cognate sugars. Continued ingestion of noxious sugars leads to hepatic and renal injury and growth retardation.

Factitious hypoglycemia

Hypoglycemia can be induced pharmacologically, intentionally as a diagnostic tool, accidentally as a complication of the treatment of diabetes mellitus or as a consequence of poisoning either with insulin itself or with drugs such as sulfonylureas, which stimulate insulin release. Whenever severe hypoglycemia with documented hyperinsulinism occurs in a previously healthy child, the possibility of malicious administration of insulin or an oral sulfonylurea should always be suspected. The clue in the biochemistry will be a raised insulin concentration with normal C-peptide in the case of insulin administration.

11 Obesity and Type 2 Diabetes Mellitus

Learning Points

- There is a global epidemic of obesity
- A very few obese children have a monogenic cause of their condition
- Consequences of obesity include insulin resistance and type 2 diabetes, dyslipidemia, hepatic steatosis/steatohepatitis (fatty liver), hypertension, focal glomerulosclerosis, accelerated growth and bone maturation, ovarian hyperandrogenism, gynecomastia, cholecystitis, pancreatitis and pseudotumor cerebri

- Non-metabolic complications include sleep apnea, orthopedic disorders and stress incontinence
- Long-standing obesity and insulin resistance increase the risk of cardiovascular disease, stroke, orthopedic complications, sleep apnea, some malignancies and psychosocial disorders in adults
- Treatment is by lifestyle intervention (including behavior therapy), pharmacotherapy and surgery but success is very limited
- Prevention is better than cure

The prevalence of obesity in children is difficult to determine because there is no internationally accepted definition. A range of methods that estimate total body fat is available but none is easily applicable in practice. Body weight is reasonably well correlated with body fat but also highly correlated with height, so children of the same weight but different heights can have widely differing amounts of fat. Body mass index (BMI: weight (kg) divided by height^2 (m^2)) correlates reasonably well with more specific measurements of body fat in adults but the relation between BMI and body fat in children varies considerably with age and pubertal maturation (see Fig. 3.3).

Childhood obesity is a global problem, representing the archetypal complex multifactorial disease with behavioral, environmental and genetic factors that influence individual responses to diet and physical activity. Weight, like height, is a heritable trait, the genetic contribution to the variance of BMI being 40–70%. Different individuals have a genetic propensity to store excessive calories as fat but the rising prevalence of obesity has not been due to a recent change in the genetics of the world. The ability to store fat in times of nutritional abundance is a trait selected over many thousands of years of human evolution.

The immediate adverse effects of obesity include insulin resistance and type 2 diabetes, dyslipidemia, hepatic steatosis/steatohepatitis (fatty liver), hypertension, focal glomerulosclerosis, accelerated growth and bone maturation, ovarian hyperandrogenism, gynecomastia, cholecystitis, pancreatitis and pseudotumor cerebri. Non-metabolic complications include sleep apnea, orthopedic disorders and stress incontinence. Long-standing obesity and insulin resistance in adults increase the risk of cardiovascular disease, stroke, orthopedic complications, sleep apnea, some malignancies and psychosocial disorders. Since obese children are more likely to become obese adults,

Handbook of Clinical Pediatric Endocrinology, 1st edition. By Charles G. D. Brook and Rosalind S. Brown. Published 2008 by Blackwell Publishing, ISBN: 978-1- 4501-6109-1.

profound public health consequences must be anticipated as a result of the emergence in later life of associated co-morbidities, such as type 2 diabetes mellitus, ischemic heart disease and stroke.

Pathogenesis of insulin resistance and type 2 diabetes

Type 2 diabetes is the endpoint of a process of metabolic decompensation that may evolve over a period of months or years. In most cases, the disease begins with peripheral resistance to insulin action accompanied by fasting hyperinsulinemia and, extrapolating from animal studies, an increase in islet size and β-cell mass. Progression from insulin resistance to impaired fasting glucose (IFG) (blood glucose concentration >6.1 mmol/L and <7.0, 110–126 mg/dL) and impaired glucose tolerance (IGT or 'prediabetes') (2 h blood glucose concentration >11.1 mmol/L, 200 mg/dL) is accompanied by dysregulation of basal insulin secretion with aberrations in the slow oscillations of insulin release, loss of first-phase glucose-dependent insulin secretion and altered insulin processing, revealed as an increase in the circulating ratio of proinsulin to insulin. The phenotype of type 2 diabetes is characterized by a decline in total insulin production, relative or absolute hypoinsulinemia, a reduction in β-cell mass and deposition of amyloid in the pancreatic islets.

The risk of developing type 2 diabetes depends on genetic inheritance, developmental and nutritional factors and energy expenditure. Prevalence increases with the onset of puberty because of the anti-insulin effects of growth hormone (GH) and sex steroids but risk is modified by events before birth, the disease occurring more frequently in children of diabetic mothers and in those born small for gestational age, particularly if there is rapid catch-up growth in early childhood. Girls are affected more frequently than boys and teenage girls and young women with ovarian hyperandrogenism or the polycystic ovarian syndrome (PCOS) are at high risk; prepubertal girls with adrenarche also appear to be vulnerable.

The most important modifiable risk factor is obesity. Insulin sensitivity correlates inversely with BMI and percentage body fat. Severe obesity in prepubertal children and adolescents is commonly associated with IGT (21–25%) and, in some cases (4% of teenagers),

with unsuspected type 2 diabetes. BMI in childhood (ages 7–13 years) correlates with obesity, hypertension, hyperinsulinemia and dyslipidemia in young adults.

Insulin resistance does not guarantee progression to frank glucose intolerance; indeed, most obese, insulin-resistant subjects never develop type 2 diabetes. The development of glucose intolerance requires β-cell dysfunction and loss of glucose-dependent insulin secretion, probably due to a familial or genetic trait. Chronic elevations in free fatty acid (FFA) probably contribute to β-cell failure in obese, insulin-resistant subjects predisposed to developing type 2 diabetes.

Consequences of obesity

Cardiovascular disease

The development of insulin resistance and type 2 diabetes has serious implications for long-term cardiovascular health. Microvascular complications, including neuropathy, retinopathy and microalbuminuria, all occur with increased frequency in adults with IGT and diabetes and rates of myocardial infarction and stroke are increased two- to fivefold.

Obesity and insulin resistance in childhood predispose to vascular complications in later life. Severe obesity in 9- to 11-year-old children is associated with increased stiffness of the carotid arteries and obesity in adolescence predisposes to increased carotid intima media thickness (CIMT) in young adulthood, although weight loss after adolescence may reduce adult CIMT. The combination of multiple risk factors increases exponentially the extent of arterial intimal surface involvement: BMI and abdominal fat mass in young men correlate with the number and size of fatty streaks and raised lesions in the right and left anterior descending coronary arteries. In both women and men, the extent of fatty streaks correlate with glycated hemoglobin concentrations. Severe glucose intolerance probably accelerates the progression of vascular disease.

The pathogenesis of vascular disease involves hormones, growth factors, vasoactive agents, cytokines, oxygen radicals and cellular adhesion molecules. Under normal conditions, insulin stimulates vasodilatation through induction of nitric oxide synthase (NOS) and generation of NO in vascular endothelial cells but, in obesity and other states associated with insulin resistance, the production of NO is disrupted, leading to vasoconstriction and tissue ischemia. Hyperglycemia contributes to endothelial dysfunction and vascular insufficiency through production of superoxide radicals. Oxygen radicals promote the formation of polyols, glucosamine and advanced glycation endproducts and the activation of protein kinase C prompting the development of microvascular and macrovascular disease.

Glucose-dependent expression of growth factors (vEGF, EGF and IGF-I) and cytokines (IL-1, IL-6 and TNF-α) and a reduction in plasma adiponectin concentrations aggravate these effects by stimulating migration and proliferation of smooth muscle cells and increasing leukocyte adhesion to endothelial surfaces. Reduction in NO availability enhances platelet aggregation and limits fibrinolysis, promoting the progression of atheromatous clots. Increases in the concentrations of the prothrombotic plasminogen activator-1, which is also overexpressed by adipose tissue in obesity, may contribute to fibrin deposition on luminal walls. Production of endothelin-1 in terminal blood vessels is increased, promoting vasoconstriction. These effects are exacerbated by dyslipidemia and hypertension.

Hepatic steatosis, cholecystitis, pancreatitis and pseudotumor cerebri

FFA diverted from adipose tissue are synthesized in the liver to triglycerides (TG), leading to fatty infiltration (steatosis) and cirrhosis. Cholecystitis, pancreatitis and pseudotumor cerebri occur more frequently in obese than in normal weight children, especially pancreatitis in teenage girls.

The pathogenesis of pseudotumor cerebri remains obscure. Increases in intra-abdominal pressure may increase central venous and intrathoracic pressures and thereby raise intracranial pressure.

Growth and bone maturation, pituitary and adrenal function and ovarian hyperandrogenism

Rates of growth and bone maturation are often increased in obese prepubertal children, despite marked reductions in basal and stimulated plasma GH concentrations and a reduction in circulating GH half-life. This is particularly relevant in children under 2 years of age.

Total IGF-I and IGF binding protein (IGFBP)-III concentrations in obese subjects are normal or mildly elevated but free IGF-I concentrations are increased. The latter may reflect reductions in circulating IGFBP-I and -II, which are suppressed by insulin and correlate inversely with insulin sensitivity. Together with nutrient excess, the increase in free IGF-I concentrations may accelerate linear growth and bone age.

The effects of IGF-I on growth and bone maturation in obese subjects may be potentiated by hyperleptinemia. Circulating leptin concentrations rise in proportion to body (particularly subcutaneous) fat stores and are higher in girls than in boys. Leptin stimulates proliferation of isolated mouse and rat osteoblasts and increases the width of the chondroprogenitor zone of the mouse mandible *in vivo*. In leptin-deficient ob/ob mice, leptin increases femoral length, bone area and bone mineral content. The effects of leptin may be exerted in concert with IGF-I because leptin increases IGF-I receptor expression in mouse chondrocytes.

Renal dysfunction

Increased glomerular filtration rate, renal hypertrophy and proteinuria may occur in obesity with histological findings of focal segmental glomerulosclerosis, mesangial proliferation and glomerulomegaly, which differ from the appearances seen in nephrotic syndrome. Obesity-related glomerulopathy is associated with hypertension, hyperinsulinemia, increased free IGF-I and hyperlipidemia.

Calcium homeostasis and bone mineralization

Morbid obesity in adolescents and adults is accompanied by altered binding of calcium to plasma proteins, low concentrations of 25OH vitamin D, elevated 1,25 diOH vitamin D and osteocalcin and secondary hyperparathyroidism. Bone mineral content is variably decreased; fracture rates among obese children are unknown. Alterations in calcium dynamics are reversed by weight loss.

Malignancy

Chronic increases in the circulating concentrations of free IGF-I and sex steroids may contribute to increased risks of certain malignancies in obese adults, especially endometrial cancer, cervical cancer and renal cell carcinoma in women and liver cancer (and to a lesser extent gastrointestinal malignancies) in men. It is not yet known whether childhood obesity predisposes to childhood or adult malignancy but low birthweight and rapid weight gain in the first year of life do.

Table 11.1 Assessment of the obese child.

History

- Age of onset – use of growth charts and family photographs. Early onset (<5 years of age) suggests a genetic cause
- Duration of obesity – short history suggests endocrine or central cause
- A history of damage to the CNS (e.g. infection, trauma, hemorrhage, radiation therapy, seizures) suggests hypothalamic obesity with or without pituitary GH deficiency or pituitary hypothyroidism. A history of morning headaches, vomiting, visual disturbances and excessive urination or drinking also suggests that the obesity may be caused by a tumor or mass in the hypothalamus
- A history of dry skin, constipation, intolerance to cold or fatigue suggests hypothyroidism. Mood disturbance and central obesity suggest Cushing syndrome. Frequent infections and fatigue may suggest ACTH deficiency due to POMC mutations
- Hyperphagia – often denied but sympathetic approach needed and specific questions, such as waking at night to eat and/or demanding food very soon after a meal, suggest hyperphagia. If severe, especially in children, suggests a genetic cause for obesity
- Developmental delay – milestones, educational history, behavioral disorders. Consider craniopharyngioma or structural causes (often relatively short history) and genetic causes
- Visual impairment and deafness can suggest genetic causes
- Onset and tempo of pubertal development – onset can be early or delayed in children and adolescents. Primary hypogonadotropic hypogonadism or hypogenitalism associated with some genetic disorders
- Family history – consanguineous relationships, other children affected, family photographs useful. Severity may differ due to environmental effects
- Treatment with certain drugs or medications. Glucocorticoids, sulfonylureas, MAOIs oral contraceptives, risperidone, clozapine

Examination

- Document weight and height compared with normal centiles. Calculate BMI and WHR (in adults). In children, obtain parental heights and weights where possible
- Head circumference if clinically suggestive
- Short stature or a reduced rate of linear growth in a child with obesity suggests the possibility of GH deficiency, hypothyroidism, cortisol excess, pseudohypoparathyroidism or a genetic syndrome such as Prader–Willi syndrome
- Obese children and adolescents are often tall (on the upper centiles), however, accelerated linear growth (height SDS >2) is a feature of MC4R deficiency
- Body fat distribution – central distribution with purple striae suggests Cushing syndrome. Selective fat deposition (60%) is a feature of leptin and leptin receptor deficiency
- Dysmorphic features or skeletal dysplasia
- Hair color – red hair (if not familial) may suggest mutations in POMC in white Caucasians
- Pubertal development/secondary sexual characteristics. Most obese adolescents grow at a normal or excessive rate and enter puberty at the appropriate age; many mature more quickly than children with normal weight, and bone age is commonly advanced. In contrast, growth rate and pubertal development are diminished or delayed in GH deficiency, hypothyroidism, cortisol excess and a variety of genetic syndromes. Conversely, growth rate and pubertal development are accelerated in precocious puberty and in some girls with PCOS
- Acanthosis nigricans
- Valgus deformities in severe childhood obesity

Investigations

- Fasting and 2-h post glucose and insulin levels. Proinsulin if PC1 deficiency considered
- Fasting lipid panel for detection of dyslipidemia
- Thyroid function tests
- Serum leptin if indicated
- Karyotype
- DNA for molecular diagnosis
- Bone age
- GH secretion and function tests, when indicated
- Assessment of reproductive hormones, when indicated
- Serum calcium, phosphorus and parathyroid hormone levels to evaluate for suspected pseudohypoparathyroidism
- MRI scan of the brain with focus on the hypothalamus and pituitary, when clinically indicated

ACTH, adrenocorticotrophic hormone; CNS, central nervous system; PC1, prohormone convertase 1; POMC, pro-opiomelanocortin; WHR, waist-hip ratio.

The clinical approach

The assessment of obese patients should be directed at screening for potentially treatable endocrine conditions and identifying genetic conditions so that appropriate genetic counseling and, in some cases, treatment can be instituted (Table 11.1).

Classically, patients affected by obesity syndromes have been identified as a result of their association with mental retardation, dysmorphic features and/or other developmental abnormalities. More recently, several new monogenic disorders have been identified. Obesity is usually the predominant presenting feature, although often accompanied by characteristic patterns of neuroendocrine dysfunction. For the purposes of clinical assessment, it remains useful to categorize the genetic obesity syndromes as those with and without associated developmental delay (Figs 11.1 and 11.2).

Pleiotrophic obesity syndromes

Obesity runs in families, although the majority of cases do not segregate with a clear Mendelian pattern of inheritance. There are about 30 Mendelian disorders with obesity as a clinical feature, frequently associated with mental retardation, dysmorphic features and organ-specific developmental abnormalities (i.e. pleiotrophic syndromes). A number of families with these rare syndromes have been studied by linkage analysis. In a number of cases, mutations in genes have been identified by positional cloning and the mechanism underlying the development of obesity is becoming clear in some instances.

Human monogenic obesity syndromes

Monogenic syndromes are rare but an improved understanding of the precise nature of the inherited component of severe obesity has undoubted medical benefits and helps to dispel the notion that obesity represents an individual defect in behavior with no biological basis. For individuals at highest risk of the complications of severe obesity, such findings provide a starting point for providing more rational mechanism-based therapies as has successfully been achieved for congenital leptin deficiency.

Congenital leptin deficiency

Congenital leptin deficiency, although rare, is unique in being amenable to therapy. Patients treated with once-daily subcutaneous injections of recombinant human leptin have all lost weight (specifically fat), often with dramatic clinical benefit. The major effect of leptin was on appetite, with normalization of hyperphagia. Although congenital leptin deficiency is an autosomal-recessive condition, heterozygotes or carriers

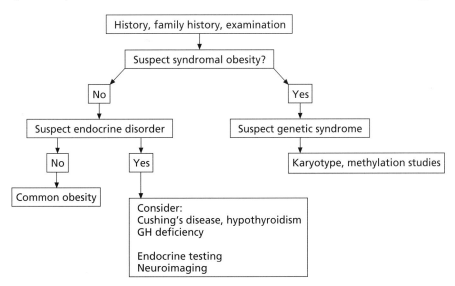

Figure 11.1 Diagnostic algorithm for childhood obesity.

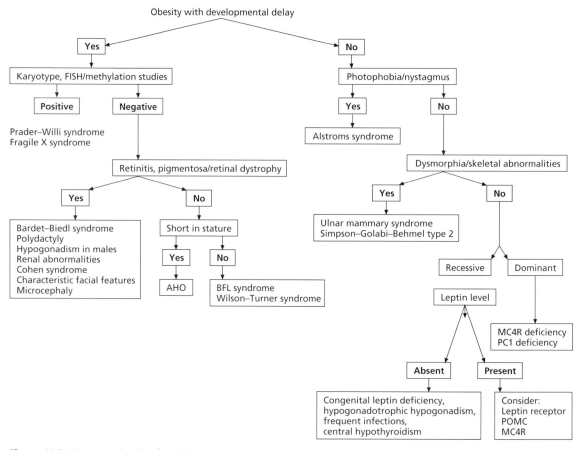

Figure 11.2 Diagnostic algorithm for childhood obesity with developmental delay.

for the ob mutation have partial leptin deficiency that is associated with a 23% increase in body fat.

Leptin receptor deficiency

A mutation in the leptin receptor has been reported. The phenotype has similarities to that of leptin deficiency. Leptin receptor-deficient subjects were also of normal birthweight but exhibited rapid weight gain in the first few months of life, with severe hyperphagia and aggressive behavior when food was denied.

Pro-opiomelanocortin deficiency

Presentation is in neonatal life with adrenal crisis due to adrenocorticotrophic hormone (ACTH) deficiency, because pro-opiomelanocortin (POMC) is the precursor of ACTH. Children require long-term corticosteroid replacement. They have pale skin and red hair due to the lack of melanocyte-stimulating hormone

(MSH) function at melanocortin-1 receptors in the skin, although this may be less obvious in children from different ethnic backgrounds.

POMC deficiency results in hyperphagia and early-onset obesity due to loss of melanocortin signaling at the melanocortin-4 receptor (MC4R) (see below). Although trials of treatment have not been performed, it is plausible that selective MC4R agonists will be available for such patients in the near future.

Prohormone convertase 1 deficiency

Mutations in prohormone convertase 1 (PC1)enzyme, which cleaves prohormones at pairs of basic amino acids leaving C-terminal basic residues that are excised by carboxypeptidase E (CPE) leads to failure to process a number of prohormones, such as pre-progonadotropin-releasing hormone (GnRH), pre-proTRH and POMC. Although the inability to cleave

POMC is a probable mechanism for obesity in these patients, PC1 cleaves a number of other neuropeptides in the hypothalamus, including glucagon-like peptide 1, which may influence feeding behavior.

MC4R deficiency

Heterozygous mutations in MC4R have been reported in obese humans from various ethnic groups with an estimated prevalence of 0.5–1% in obese patients, increasing to 6% in severe, early-onset obesity.

Patients with MC4R deficiency are hyperphagic but this is not as severe as that seen in leptin deficiency, although it often starts in the first year of life. The severity of receptor dysfunction seen in *in vitro* assays predicts the amount of food ingested at a test meal by the subject harboring that particular mutation. As well as the increase in fat mass, MC4R-deficient subjects also have an increase in lean mass not seen in leptin deficiency and an increase in bone mineral density. Thus, they often appear 'big-boned.'

Linear growth is striking, with affected children having a height standard deviation score (SDS) of +2, whereas the mean height SDS of other children with sever early-onset obesity +0.5. MC4R-deficient subjects have higher concentrations of fasting insulin than age, sex and BMI SDS-matched children. The accelerated linear growth does not appear to be due to dysfunction of the GH axis and may be a consequence of the disproportionate early hyperinsulinemia.

One notable feature of this syndrome is that the severity of many of the phenotypic features appears to ameliorate with time. Thus, obese adult mutation carriers report less intense feelings of hunger and are less hyperinsulinemic than children with the same mutation.

MC4R mutations appear to be the commonest monogenic cause of obesity described thus far in humans. The maintenance of this reasonably high disease frequency is likely to be partly due to the fact that obesity is expressed in heterozygotes and that there is no evidence of any apparent effect of the mutations on reproductive function.

Screening of obese children for metabolic complications

Many children and adolescents with insulin resistance, and a subset of those with established type 2

Table 11.2 Screening for glucose intolerance and the metabolic syndrome in children and adolescents.

High-risk populations

Obese (BMI *z*-score >95th percentile) children or adolescent, plus

    High-risk ethnic group and/or

    Family history of type 2 diabetes or GDM and/or

    Acanthosis nigricans and/or

    Prominent abdominal fat deposition

Ovarian hyperandrogenism

Screening procedures

Blood pressure

Fasting glucose and insulin levels

Fasting lipid panel (+FFA if possible)

2-h glucose level (+insulin if possible)

HbA1c (less useful)

GDM, gestational diabetes mellitus; 2-h glucose, plasma glucose 2 h after administration of glucola; HbA1c, hemoglobin A1c.

diabetes, lack classical symptoms of glucose intolerance such as polyuria and polydipsia. Obese children who have one or more of the risk factors listed in Table 11.2 should be screened with a fasting blood sample analysed concomitantly for glucose, insulin and lipid concentrations. Some physicians also measure glucose concentration 2 h after glucose administration (1.75 g/kg up to a maximum of 75 g).

Alternatively, screening can be conducted in children with BMI >85th centile for age and gender with two or more associated risk factors. Particular attention should be focused upon obese children with family histories of type 2 or gestational diabetes and those from high-risk ethnic groups. Progressive abdominal obesity is an ominous finding and the presence of acanthosis nigricans, which suggests insulin resistance, should raise concern.

Management

Treatment of obesity aims to:

1 reduce BMI and visceral fat mass;

2 decrease circulating insulin concentrations;

3 increase insulin sensitivity;

4 decrease hepatic glucose production and fasting and post-prandial glucose concentrations;

5 reduce circulating FFA and TG concentrations;

6 decrease blood pressure;

7 reduce the expression of inflammatory cytokines;

8 normalize vascular and endothelial function.

Lifestyle intervention

Benefits from lifestyle intervention are most likely to be reaped when diet and exercise programs are combined with individual and family counseling and behavior modification. School-based programs, supported by community groups and by state and federal agencies, may assist families and reduce the child's sense of isolation, frustration and guilt.

Long-term success of lifestyle intervention alone has been disappointing. Rates of obesity and insulin resistance in children and adults continue to increase, despite widespread recognition of the dangers of dietary indiscretion and a sedentary existence. This may reflect the resistance of complex feeding and activity behaviors to change as well as the power of social and economic forces that shape lifestyles. The obstacles to success with lifestyle intervention have stimulated interest in pharmacological approaches to the treatment of obesity and the prevention of diabetes and other metabolic complications.

Diet

Mild calorie restriction can be safe and effective when obese children and their families are motivated and willing to change feeding habits but significant reductions in weight are unusual and often transient unless calorie restriction is accompanied by increased energy expenditure. Diets severely restricted in calories produce more dramatic weight loss but cannot be sustained. Very-low-calorie diets are potentially dangerous and may precipitate recurrent and futile cycles of dieting and binge eating.

Obese men and women lose more weight and have more significant reductions in plasma TG concentrations on low-carbohydrate diets than on low-fat diets but the efficacy of low-carbohydrate diets may be related more to decreased calorie intake rather than to reduction in carbohydrate. Elimination of concentrated soft drinks from the diet can reduce calorie intake in some obese adolescents by as much as 500–1000 kcal/day.

Calorie restriction and weight reduction by any means reduce the risk of type 2 diabetes and subsequent cardiovascular disease in obese children. Reduced intake of saturated fats will benefit obese adolescents as well as adults. Reduced consumption of high-glycemic foods is of general health benefit and a balanced diet containing vegetables, fruits, fiber, meat, fish and dairy products is the best prevention against obesity as well as its remedy.

Exercise

A sedentary lifestyle increases the risk of diabetes, while exercise, in combination with calorie and fat restriction, reduces the rate of progression to diabetes in adults with IGT.

The mechanisms by which exercise improves insulin sensitivity and glucose tolerance are complex, involving metabolic adaptations in adipose tissue, liver and skeletal muscle. Exercise has beneficial effects on fat storage and distribution, with losses of visceral fat depots exceeding those of subcutaneous fat stores. Lean body mass increases, thereby augmenting resting energy expenditure. A reduction in visceral fat mass increases adipose tissue sensitivity to insulin, which explains in part the reductions in fasting and post-prandial FFA, LDL and TG concentrations and the increase in plasma HDL concentrations in adults who adhere to a rigorous diet and exercise regimen. Exercise increases hepatic glucose uptake and glycogen synthesis and decreases hepatic glucose production, thereby reducing fasting glucose and insulin concentrations. In skeletal muscle, exercise stimulates insulin-dependent glucose uptake and thereby reduces post-prandial glucose concentrations. Weight loss alone may improve insulin sensitivity but it does not alter fasting rates of lipid oxidation. Weight loss coupled with exercise increases fat oxidation.

Pharmacotherapy

Anorectic agents

Many drugs initially thought to be safe (for example, diethylpropion, fenfluramine, ephedra and phenylpronalolamine) have been withdrawn because they caused life-threatening complications. The only anorectic agent currently approved for use in obese adolescents is *sibutramine*, a non-selective inhibitor of neuronal reuptake of serotonin, norepinephrine and dopamine. It causes hypertension and tachycardia, necessitating reduction in drug dose in a substantial number of patients.

Anorectic agents should complement and never replace a diet and exercise program. They have modest effects on total body weight and responses vary considerably between individuals. Most weight loss from anorectic agents is achieved within the first 4–6 months of treatment; regain of weight is the norm unless drug therapy is maintained.

Drugs that limit nutrient absorption

Orlistat inhibits pancreatic lipase and thereby increases fecal losses of TG. It reduces body weight and total and LDL cholesterol concentrations and reduces the risk of type 2 diabetes in adults with IGT. Side-effects are tolerable as long as subjects reduce fat intake but vitamin A, D and E concentrations may decline, despite multivitamin supplementation. High dropout rates (25% or more) suggest that long-term fat restriction is a problem for teenagers; eating fat while on the drug results in unacceptable flatulence and diarrhea.

Insulin suppressors and sensitizers

The synthesis and storage of TG in adipose tissue is stimulated by insulin. Thus, increases in nutrient-dependent insulin production and/or fasting hyperinsulinemia may contribute to fat storage and limit fat mobilization.

Metformin increases hepatic glucose uptake, decreases gluconeogenesis and reduces hepatic glucose production. It has minor effects on peripheral insulin sensitivity and no effect on skeletal muscle glucose uptake or plasma adiponectin concentrations. Major advantages of the drug include decreased food intake, decreased fat stores (subcutaneous > visceral) and improved lipid profiles and long-term studies suggest that it reduces cardiovascular morbidity and mortality in diabetic adults. It is particularly effective in treating patients with PCOS in whom it reduces plasma insulin, TG and testosterone concentrations and the ratio of LDL to HDL. The addition of flutamide, an androgen antagonist, potentiates these effects and reduces hirsutism scores.

Thiazolidinediones (TZDs) induce the differentiation of small insulin-sensitive adipocytes, increase adipose insulin receptor number, adiponectin expression and adipose tissue glucose uptake and reduce expression of TNF-α. Rates of lipolysis and FFA release are reduced, TG clearance is enhanced and hepatic VLDL synthesis decreases.

TZDs increase insulin sensitivity, improve glucose tolerance and reduce cardiovascular risk in insulin-resistant adults and in women with PCOS. They can, like metformin, reduce the risk of type 2 diabetes and protection from diabetes persists for 3–8 months after the drug was discontinued, suggesting that troglitazone may have altered the natural progression of diabetes and not simply masked progression through a pharmacological action. As with metformin, the duration of this protective action is currently unknown.

Troglitazone was removed from the commercial market because the drug caused fatal hepatic failure in a small number of subjects. Non-lethal hepatotoxicity has also been reported with other currently available TZDs, although at a far lower frequency than with troglitazone. Hepatic dysfunction must be excluded before TZD therapy is initiated and liver function tests should be measured monthly for the first 6 months of treatment, every 2 months for the remainder of the first year and at regular intervals thereafter. Other potential complications of TZD therapy include edema and anemia, so the drug should not be administered to patients with underlying cardiac disease.

Octreotide reduces glucose-dependent insulin secretion. In children with hypothalamic obesity, octreotide reduces insulin secretory responses and rates of weight gain. Unfortunately, the cost of the medication, the need for parenteral administration and the drug's side-effects, which include gastrointestinal distress, edema, gallstones, suppression of GH and thyroid-stimulating hormone (TSH) secretion and cardiac dysfunction, limit its applicability to patients with intractable obesity from hypothalamic injury.

Bariatric surgery

Bariatric surgery may be indicated in selected subjects with extreme obesity and serious co-morbidities. The approaches are most commonly laparoscopic gastric banding and the Roux-en-Y gastric bypass (RYGB).

Laparoscopic adjustable gastric banding (LAGB) utilizes a prosthetic band to encircle the proximal stomach. The ability to adjust band tension as stomach volume changes provides an important theoretical advantage. Results vary widely. Weight regain is common, possibly because high-calorie intake may be maintained through ingestion of concentrated sweet drinks or because the magnitude of decline in plasma concentrations of ghrelin, which stimulates food intake, is less than that in patients subjected to gastric bypass. Gastric banding may cause esophageal dilation and achalasia and may exacerbate gastroesophageal reflux. Other potential complications include port-site malposition or malfunction, balloon rupture and infection. The potential reversibility of the procedure makes gastric banding attractive in children.

RYGB involves the creation of a small stomach pouch into which a distal segment of jejunum is inserted. This procedure combines the restrictive nature of gastrectomy with the consequences of dumping physiology as a negative conditioning response when high-calorie liquid meals are ingested. Food intake may decline as stomach-derived ghrelin concentrations fall.

In adults with morbid obesity, gastric bypass often causes striking weight loss and may reverse type 2 diabetes, hypertension, dyslipidemia, pseudotumor cerebri and degenerative joint disease. Pilot studies report favorable results in morbidly obese adolescents.

Complications of RYGB include iron-deficiency anemia (50%), folate deficiency (30%), cholecystitis (20%), wound infections and dehiscence (10%), small bowel or stomach obstruction (5–10%), atelectasis and pneumonia (12%) and incisional hernia (10%). Prophylactic tracheostomy may be required to maintain airway patency and to correct preoperative hypercapnia. Other possible complications include leaks at the junction of stomach and small intestine requiring reanastomosis, acute gastric dilation, which may arise spontaneously or secondary to intestinal obstruction or narrowing of the stoma, pulmonary emboli and dumping syndrome. Deficiencies of vitamin B12, iron, calcium and thiamine are common. Mortality rates for RYGB range from 1 to 5%

Balancing lifestyle intervention, pharmacotherapy and surgery

All obese children and adolescents require lifestyle intervention. Intensive lifestyle intervention should benefit pediatric patients with IGT or IFG who are at high risk of developing type 2 diabetes and other metabolic complications but lifestyle intervention remains difficult, time-consuming and ineffective in many cases. Treatment failure may prolong or exacerbate insulin resistance, dyslipidemia and glucose intolerance, leading to irreversible β-cell dysfunction, overt type 2 diabetes and progressive cardiovascular disease.

Pharmacological therapy should be considered for severely resistant or glucose-intolerant (IFG or IGT) children or adolescents who fail to respond to a 6–12 month trial of lifestyle intervention despite a 'good faith effort.' This means that the patient has attempted to follow a low saturated fat/low-calorie diet recommended by a dietary counselor and has increased his or her energy expenditure through regular exercise. 'Unsuccessful' means that the elevations of fasting or post-prandial glucose persist or worsen despite lifestyle intervention. The decision to initiate drug therapy relieves neither the child nor the physician of the commitment to long-term lifestyle change; thus, diet and exercise regimens should be maintained, even if they had not proved effective in the absence of medication.

Metformin is the drug of choice for treating the obese child with severe insulin resistance, IFG or IGT. Although lactic acidosis is extraordinarily rare in pediatric patients, metformin should not be administered to children with underlying cardiac, hepatic, renal or gastrointestinal disease. Obese subjects with mild elevations in hepatic enzymes (less than threefold higher than established norms) may receive the drug; indeed, some studies suggest that metformin may be useful in the treatment of hepatic steatosis. Concurrent use of a multivitamin seems reasonable because metformin increases urinary excretion of vitamins B1 and B6.

Given the lack of studies of TZDs in insulin-resistant children or adolescents, their potential, albeit rare, for severe hepatic complications and their tendency to cause weight gain, the use of TZDs should be restricted to adolescents who fail to respond to or cannot tolerate, metformin. Since the danger of hepatic dysfunction with combined therapy in pediatric patients is unknown, TZDs should not be used in conjunction with metformin in non-diabetic children. TZDs are contraindicated in patients with pre-existing hepatic or cardiac disease.

The use of anorectic drugs for treatment of obese children without glucose intolerance cannot be justified.

Bariatric surgery should be reserved for treatment of severely obese (BMI > 40), sexually mature adolescents who have failed other treatment approaches and who have established co-morbidities.

12 Type 1 Diabetes Mellitus

Learning Points

- Type 1 diabetes mellitus is one of the most common chronic diseases of childhood
- Autoantibodies restricted to a single pancreatic antigen have little prognostic value but the presence of antibodies to multiple antigens is highly predictive of disease
- Children with type 1 diabetes mellitus should be treated by a team which includes an endocrinologist, a specialist nurse educator, and a mental health professional
- Therapy must be individualized
- Type 1 diabetes mellitus should be intensively treated to reduce the incidence and progression of long-term complications

- Hypoglycemia is a serious barrier to 'tight' control
- Diabetic ketoacidosis is a preventable, potentially fatal complication of established diabetes which is most commonly due to omission of insulin or the administration of inadequate insulin during infection
- Long-term micro- and macrovascular complications are inevitable but rare before puberty
- Screening for them should start within 5 years of the onset of disease and countermeasures be introduced as early as possible
- Diabetes secondary, for example, to cystic fibrosis is becoming more frequent as prognosis of cystic fibrosis improves

Type 1A diabetes results from chronic progressive T-cell-mediated autoimmune destruction of the β-cells of the pancreas, leading to severe insulin deficiency manifested by low or undetectable plasma concentrations of C-peptide.

Markers of the process include a variety of islet cell autoantibodies present in 85–98% of newly diagnosed children. The disease has strong human leukocyte antigen (HLA) associations, with linkage to the major histocompatibility (MHC) class II genes DQA, DQB, and DRB. Specific HLA-DR/DQ alleles can either predispose to type 1A diabetes or be protective.

The rate of β-cell destruction is variable, being especially rapid infants and young children and slower in adolescents and adults, some of whom may retain the ability to secrete insulin for several years.

The disease occurs throughout life in genetically predisposed individuals but is also related to environmental factors that are poorly understood. Patients with type 1A diabetes are also prone to other autoimmune disorders (see Chapter 9).

Type 1 diabetes with no known etiology, referred to as type 1B diabetes, accounts for a minority of cases. Although strongly inherited, there is no HLA association or evidence of β-cell autoimmunity.

Approximately 85% of new cases of type 1A diabetes occur in persons without an affected first-degree relative. The risk to siblings of an affected child is approximately 6%. The risk to the child of a parent with type 1A diabetes depends on whether the mother or the father has diabetes and is 1.3–4% or 6–9%, respectively. Concordance rates for monozygotic twins

Handbook of Clinical Pediatric Endocrinology, 1st edition. By Charles G. D. Brook and Rosalind S. Brown. Published 2008 by Blackwell Publishing, ISBN: 978-1-4501-6109-1.

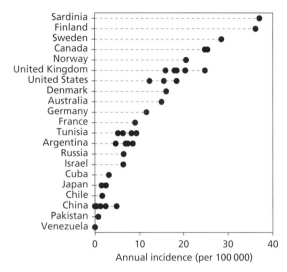

Figure 12.1 Variations in the incidence of type 1 diabetes in children ≤14 years of age among regions of selected countries from six continents. Rates were measured in the early 1990s. Multiple symbols indicate rates measured in different regions within that country.

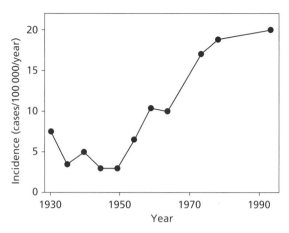

Figure 12.2 Secular increases in the incidence of childhood type 1 diabetes, as measured among Norwegian children <10 years old. Similar trends have been documented in the USA and in many countries in Europe.

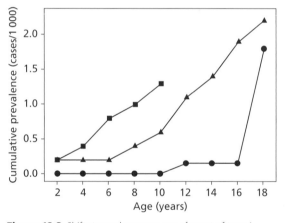

Figure 12.3 Shifts toward younger age of onset of type 1 diabetes in three UK birth cohorts born in 1946 (circles), 1958 (triangles) and 1970 (squares).

are 21–70% and 0–13% for dizygotic twins. These data indicate that both genetic and environmental factors contribute to the pathogenesis of type 1A diabetes.

The environmental factor(s) are not known and there are no interventions that reduce the risk. Possible candidate environmental factors include viral infections, dietary factors, hygiene, and toxins. It is likely that environmental induction of type 1 diabetes relates to the chronology of exposure and interactions with genetic susceptibility.

Epidemiology of type 1 diabetes mellitus

Diabetes mellitus is one of the most common chronic diseases of childhood. The incidence varies widely between geographical regions (Fig. 12.1). A significant portion of this variation is attributable to differences in the prevalence of protective HLA-DQ alleles among populations. Incidence varies among ethnic subgroups within a given geographical area. Some migrant populations retain their original risk of type 1 diabetes, while others show a trend toward acquiring the diabetes risk of their new location.

While the increasing incidence of childhood diabetes may be slowing in western countries (Fig. 12.2),

it is now being detected in other locations, including several eastern European countries. There has also been a trend toward younger age of onset. Diabetes is no longer uncommon in toddlers and preschool-aged children (Fig. 12.3).

Prediction and prevention of type 1 diabetes

The onset of diabetes represents the end of an insidious, progressive, immune-mediated attack on β-cells, and clinical diabetes occurs when approximately

90% of β-cells have been damaged or destroyed. Risk of developing diabetes, both in relatives of a person with type 1 diabetes and in the general population, can be accurately assessed by HLA genotyping and autoantibodies combined with tests of β-cell function. Autoantibodies restricted to a single antigen have little prognostic value but an immune response that has spread to multiple antigens and is stable over time is highly predictive of disease.

The latency period between the detection of antibodies and the clinical onset of disease may extend over several years and offers an opportunity to intervene. Parenteral insulin, oral insulin, and nicotinamide have failed to arrest or retard the diabetes disease process. Since effective preventive intervention does not exist, it is controversial whether screening should be performed outside the context of clinical studies.

At the onset of symptoms, about 10% of β-cells are viable and there is good evidence that residual β-cell function has clinical benefit. Immune intervention at the time of diagnosis is a route to β-cell rescue and trials with continuous cyclosporin A administration have demonstrated this but the benefit disappears when treatment is stopped and the side-effects of cyclosporin A do not justify its long-term use. Other approaches, such as administration of anti-CD3 monoclonal antibody to modulate the T-cell attack on β-cells and possibly to induce immune tolerance, are being investigated.

Atypical diabetes mellitus

Atypical forms of diabetes mellitus have been described in various populations, the hallmark being a propensity to intermittent ketosis or ketoacidosis with no evidence of autoimmunity.

Genetic defects of insulin secretion

Maturity-onset diabetes of the young

Maturity-onset diabetes of the young (MODY) is a form of non-insulin-dependent or 'maturity-onset' type diabetes in children and young adults inherited in an autosomal-dominant pattern. MODY, which may account for 1–5% of all cases of diabetes in industrialized countries, is a heterogeneous group of disorders. MODY is caused by mutations of genes expressed in the β-cell. Mutations in six genes have been described.

Mild asymptomatic hyperglycemia in non-obese children, adolescents, and young adults who have a family history of diabetes in successive generations is the most common clinical presentation. The diagnosis should be considered whenever three or more consecutive generations are affected by diabetes in an autosomal-dominant fashion. Pancreatic auto-antibodies are typically absent. The diagnosis is usually made on clinical grounds. Confirmation of the diagnosis and identification of the specific type of MODY require molecular genetic testing.

Some patients have mild fasting hyperglycemia, whereas others have varying degrees of glucose intolerance for several years before developing persistent fasting hyperglycemia. Because mild hyperglycemia may not cause classic symptoms, diagnosis may be delayed until adulthood. In some cases, progression to overt symptomatic hyperglycemia requiring therapy with an oral hypoglycemic agent or insulin may be rapid.

Most cases of MODY do not require insulin but do require careful monitoring to ensure good glycemic control to avoid complications. Exercise and nutrition to maintain normal weight and insulin sensitivity should be emphasized; pharmacological treatment, when necessary, is tailored to the patient's specific type of diabetes and level of hyperglycemia.

Mitochondrial diabetes

Diabetes may be the presenting manifestation of syndromes caused by mutations in mitochondrial DNA. *Maternally inherited diabetes and deafness syndrome* (MIDD) may present in childhood or adulthood. *Kearns–Sayre syndrome* is characterized by ophthalmoplegia, retinal pigmentary degedneration, and cardiomyopathy, and may include several hormone deficiencies, including diabetes in approximately 13% of cases. Diabetes can be treated initially with diet and sulfonylureas but may require insulin. Patients with impaired mitochondrial function are inherently prone to develop lactic acidosis and, therefore, metformin should not be used.

Genetic defects of insulin signaling

Several rare insulin resistance syndromes are caused by genetic defects in the insulin receptor or its cellular signaling apparatus.

Leprechaunism is the most severe, presenting at birth with low birthweight, characteristic facial features, near total lack of adipose tissue, acanthosis nigricans, and extreme insulin resistance. It is usually fatal in infancy.

Rabson–Mendenhall syndrome is characterized by extreme insulin resistance with acanthosis nigricans, abnormalities of the skeleton, teeth and nails, growth retardation, genitomegaly, and pineal gland hyperplasia.

Type A insulin resistance syndrome presents in thin young women with extreme hyperinsulinism, acanthosis nigricans, glycosuria, hyperandrogenism with virilization and polycystic ovary syndrome (PCOS).

Inherited lipoatrophic diabetes is associated with widespread loss of adipose tissue and severe insulin resistance. Hyperlipidemia, hepatomegaly, acanthosis nigricans, and elevated basal metabolic rate are common findings. Several forms of lipoatrophic diabetes are due to gene defects.

Seip–Berardinelli syndrome is inherited as an autosomal recessive, presenting in the first year of life with lack of subcutaneous (SC) adipose tissue. Insulin resistance, acanthosis nigricans, and diabetes mellitus develop before adolescence.

Familial partial lipodystrophy is autosomal dominant, presenting in adolescence with loss of SC adipose tissue from the trunk and extremities but with excess adipose tissue on the face and neck. Affected women are more likely to develop diabetes.

Acquired insulin resistance

Severe, generalized, acquired lipoatrophy may present during childhood. Diabetes ensues within a few years of the loss of adipose tissue. Some forms of acquired lipoatrophic diabetes are caused by immune-mediated destruction of adipocytes and are frequently associated with other autoimmune diseases. Some patients with HIV disease treated with protease inhibitors develop partial lipodystrophy.

Type B insulin resistance syndrome is a rare cause of diabetes caused by circulating antibodies directed against the insulin receptor.

Diabetes as a component of specific genetic syndromes

Wolfram syndrome is also known as DIDMOAD (diabetes insipidus, diabetes mellitus, optic atrophy, and deafness). Insulin-deficient diabetes mellitus is often the presenting characteristic, with a median age at onset of 6 years. Most cases have a mutation of the Wolframin gene, which is typically inherited in an autosomal-recessive fashion.

Many other syndromes are associated with an increased risk of diabetes. Alstrom, Prader–Willi, and Bardet–Biedl syndromes combine severe obesity with insulin-resistant diabetes mellitus.

Secondary causes of diabetes

Cystic fibrosis-related diabetes (CFRD)

As life expectancy of patients with cystic fibrosis increases, CFRD becomes more common. Insulinopenia is caused by pancreatic destruction and amyloid deposition in the islets. Insulin resistance may be prominent during exacerbations of pulmonary disease and causes deterioration in glycemia. First-phase insulin release is particularly affected but ketoacidosis is rare. Cystic fibrosis-related diabetes can present in the first decade but is usually seen in the second and third decades of life. The development of CFRD is associated with progressive clinical deterioration and increased mortality. Screening for glucose intolerance should begin at the age of 14 years and hyperglycemia should be treated aggressively.

Insulin is the only therapy recommended for CFRD. It prevents protein catabolism, promotes weight gain, and improves pulmonary function. Diet should not be restricted but patients should be taught carbohydrate counting and how to use rapid-acting insulin with meals. Destruction of the pancreatic α-cells results in glucagon deficiency and chronic use of glucocorticoids can cause adrenocortical insufficiency. Patients with CFRD are therefore at increased risk of severe hypoglycemia owing to malabsorption and impaired counter-regulatory responses.

Hemosiderosis

Frequent blood transfusions and chelation therapy have greatly improved the prognosis of β-thalassemia major. Adolescents and young adult patients are, however, at increased risk of developing diabetes mellitus because of the effects of iron overload on β-cell function and insulin sensitivity. Insulin is required for treatment.

Drug-induced diabetes

Various pharmacological agents can cause hyperglycemia, including glucocorticoids, growth hormone (GH), antipsychotic agents, antiretroviral protease inhibitors, beta-adrenergic agents used for treatment of acute asthma, diazoxide, cyclosporin A, and L-asparaginase. Pediatric transplant recipients are especially prone to insulin requiring diabetes when treated with the calcineurin inhibitor tacrolimus.

Neonatal diabetes mellitus

The prevalence of insulin requiring hyperglycemia presenting within the first 4–6 weeks of life is estimated to be 1 in 400 000–500 000 births. Associated findings include intrauterine growth retardation, low birthweight, and decreased adipose tissue. Markers of autoimmunity and insulin resistance are typically absent. Various birth defects may be present in about half the cases.

More than half the cases of neonatal diabetes are transient and resolve within months but mild non-insulin-dependent diabetes may recur in childhood or early adulthood in a substantial proportion of patients. Long-term surveillance is necessary. A number of cases of transient neonatal diabetes have had macroglossia and umbilical hernia. Abnormalities at chromosome 6q24 are found in about 50% of cases.

Presentation of type 1 diabetes mellitus

Children with type 1 diabetes usually present with classic symptoms for a few days to several weeks. The frequency of diabetic ketoacidosis (DKA) at diabetes onset varies widely by geographical location, being more frequent the further from the equator. It is more frequent in infants, toddlers, and preschool-aged children, in children who do not have a first-degree relative with type 1 diabetes and in children whose families are of lower socioeconomic status.

The progression of type 1 diabetes follows a characteristic course with the abrupt onset of symptoms disappearing after starting insulin replacement therapy. This is often followed by a temporary remission ('honeymoon phase') with partial recovery of endogenous insulin secretion, demonstrable by plasma C-peptide concentrations. Recurrence or persistence of the autoimmune attack on β-cells, however, leads to inexorable decline in insulin production until it ceases.

Distinguishing between types 1 and 2 diabetes in children

Both types of diabetes present most frequently during puberty, when a physiological reduction in insulin sensitivity of approximately 30% occurs. With a high prevalence of overweight and obesity in children and adolescents, distinguishing the types of diabetes has become more difficult. About one quarter of patients with type 1 diabetes are obese at the time of diagnosis, irrespective of race, gender, and age. In contrast to type 2 diabetes in adults, in whom ketonuria is unusual, 33% of adolescents with type 2 diabetes have ketosis at presentation and up to 25% present in DKA. Insulin requirements typically decrease after several weeks of treatment of type 2 diabetes, which may resemble the remission or 'honeymoon' period of type 1 diabetes.

Measuring pancreatic autoantibodies and serum insulin and C-peptide concentrations at presentation is recommended to help distinguish types 1 and 2 in obese patients. A plasma C-peptide concentration above or in the upper normal range suggests type 2 diabetes but C-peptide concentrations may initially be temporarily low in type 2 diabetes owing to glucotoxicity and lipotoxicity.

Other causes of glycosuria

Diabetes mellitus is occasionally diagnosed in an asymptomatic individual because glycosuria is discovered incidentally. The diagnosis must always be confirmed by at least two independent measurements of plasma glucose concentration. Glycosuria can occur without hyperglycemia because of renal tubular dysfunction (e.g. Fanconi syndrome) or because of an isolated reduction of the renal tubular threshold for glucose reabsorption (benign glycosuria).

Transient hyperglycemia

The incidence of transient hyperglycemia is estimated to be approximately 1 per 8000 pediatric office visits and 1 per 200 emergency department or hospital visits. A minority of children with transient hyperglycemia develop diabetes mellitus. When transient hyperglycemia is detected in a child who does not have a severe illness, the risk of developing diabetes is much higher than if a severe illness were present. The presence of pancreatic autoantibodies and/or a low first-phase insulin response during an intravenous glucose tolerance test strongly predicts progression to diabetes.

Management

Initial management

Children with signs of severe DKA (long duration of symptoms, compromised circulation, depressed level of consciousness) and those who are at increased risk of cerebral edema (<5 years of age, new-onset diabetes) should be treated in a pediatric intensive care unit or in a children's ward that specializes in diabetes care and can provide comparable resources and supervision of care.

The initial goals of management are:
• to restore fluid and electrolyte balance,
• to stabilize the metabolic state with insulin,
• to provide age- and developmentally appropriate diabetes education and self-care training for the child and other caregivers.

Families require considerable emotional support and time for adjustment and healing and need at least 2–3 days to acquire basic or 'survival' skills while they are coping with the emotional upheaval that typically follows the diagnosis of diabetes in a child. Even if they are not acutely ill, children with newly diagnosed type 1 diabetes are usually admitted to hospital for metabolic stabilization, diabetes education, and self-management training but outpatient or home-based management has been preferred at some centers with the appropriate resources. Outpatient education and stabilization offer several advantages, which include avoiding the stress of a hospital stay. The outpatient setting or patient's home is a more natural learning environment for the child and family and possibly reduces the cost of care.

Psychosocial issues

Issues for families with a diabetic child include parental guilt, resulting in poor adherence to the treatment regimen, difficulty coping with the child's rebellion against treatment, anxiety, depression, fear of hypoglycemia, missed appointments, financial hardship, loss of health insurance affecting the ability

to attend scheduled clinic appointments and/or purchase supplies. Recurrent ketoacidosis is the extreme indicator of psychosocial stress and management of such patients is incomplete without comprehensive psychosocial assessment.

Each phase of childhood has characteristics that complicate treatment, such as the unpredictable eating of toddlers and the unscheduled intense physical play of school-aged children that can hinge on irregular factors such as the weather. Adolescence is characterized by multiple physiological and psychosocial factors that make glycemic control more difficult. Optimal diabetes treatment should thus be tailored to each child and family, based on factors including age, gender, family resources, cognitive faculties, the schedule and activities of the child/family, and the goals and desires of the child and family.

Outpatient diabetes care

The diabetes team

Care of children with type 1 diabetes is complex and time-consuming. Few primary care practitioners or pediatricians have the resources and expertise, nor can they devote the time required to provide all the components of an optimal treatment program for children with diabetes. Children with diabetes should be managed by a multidisciplinary team that should consist of a pediatric endocrinologist (or pediatrician with training in diabetes), a pediatric diabetes nurse educator, a dietitian, and a mental health professional, either a clinical psychologist or a social worker. A member of the diabetes team should always be available by telephone to respond to crises that require immediate intervention and to provide guidance and support to parents and patients.

Initial diabetes education

The diabetes education curriculum should be adapted to the individual child and family. Parents and children are anxious and overwhelmed and cannot assimilate a large amount of information so the education program should be staged. Initial goals should be limited to survival skills so that the child can be safely cared for at home and return to his or her daily routine. Initial education and self-management training should include understanding what causes diabetes, how it is treated, how to administer insulin, basic meal planning, self-monitoring of blood glucose (SMBG) and ketones, recognition and treatment of hypoglycemia and how and when to contact a member of the diabetes team.

Continuing diabetes education and long-term supervision of diabetes care

When the child is medically stable and parents and other care providers have mastered survival skills, the child is discharged from the hospital or ambulatory treatment center. In the first few weeks after diagnosis, frequent telephone contact provides emotional support and helps parents to interpret the results of BG monitoring and adjust insulin doses if necessary. Within a few weeks of diagnosis, many children enter partial remission evidenced by normal or near-normal BG concentrations on a low dose (<0.25 units/kg/day) of insulin. By this time, most patients and parents are less anxious, have mastered basic diabetes management skills through experience and repetition and are more prepared to begin to learn the intricate details of intensive diabetes management. At this stage, the diabetes team should begin to provide patients and parents with the knowledge and skills they need to maintain optimal glycemic control while coping with the challenges imposed by exercise, fickle appetite and varying food intake, intercurrent illnesses and the other variations that normally occur in a child's daily life.

In the first month after diagnosis, the patient is seen frequently by the diabetes team to review and consolidate the education and practical skills and to extend the scope of training. Follow-up with members of the diabetes team should occur at least every 3 months thereafter. Regular visits are to ensure that the child's diabetes is being appropriately managed at home and the goals of therapy are being met. A history should obtain information about self-care behaviors, the child's daily routines, the frequency, severity and circumstances surrounding hypoglycemic events and BG monitoring data should be reviewed.

At each visit, height and weight are measured and plotted on a growth chart. The weight curve is especially helpful in assessing adequacy of therapy. Significant weight loss usually indicates that the prescribed dose is insufficient or the patient is not receiving the prescribed doses of insulin. A physical examination should be performed at least twice each year focusing on blood pressure, stage of puberty,

evidence of thyroid disease, mobility of the joints in the hands, scarring of the finger tips from frequent lancing and injection sites for lipohypertrophy or lipoatrophy.

Regular clinic visits also provide an opportunity to review, reinforce and expand upon the diabetes self-care training begun at the time of diagnosis. The goal at each visit is to reinforce the goals of treatment while increasing the patient's and family's understanding of diabetes management, the interplay of insulin, food and exercise and their impact on BG concentrations. As cognitive development progresses, the child should become more involved in diabetes management and assume increasing age-appropriate responsibility for daily self-care. Parents are encouraged to call for advice if the pattern of BG concentrations changes between routine visits suggesting the need to adjust the insulin dose or change the regimen. Eventually, when parents and patients have sufficient knowledge and experience, they are encouraged to adjust the insulin dose(s) independently.

Goals of therapy

The microvascular complications of diabetes are caused by hyperglycemia and can be prevented or ameliorated. The aim of management is to lower glycated hemoglobin A1c (HbA1c) values to reduce the risk of development and progression of retinopathy, nephropathy and neuropathy. Treatment regimens that reduce average HbA1c to < 7% (~1% above the upper limit of normal) are associated with fewer long-term microvascular complications. Moreover, a period of improved glycemic control is associated with a sustained decreased rate of development of diabetic complications. Treatment goals are HbA1c < 7% (non-diabetic range 4–6%), pre-prandial plasma glucose 5–7.2 mmol/L (90–130 mg/dL) and peak post-prandial plasma glucose <10 mmol/L (180 mg/dL) without the occurrence of frequent or severe hypoglycemia.

The risk of microalbuminuria increases steeply with HbA1c > 8%. Less stringent treatment goals are appropriate for preschool age, children with developmental handicaps, psychosocial problems, lack of appropriate family support, children who have experienced severe hypoglycemia or those with hypoglycemia unawareness.

Insulin therapy

Most children with type 1 diabetes are severely insulin deficient. The aim is to simulate as closely as possible the normal variations in plasma insulin concentrations that occur in non-diabetic individuals but physiological replacement of insulin remains elusive. Practical considerations, including supervision of care, ability and willingness to self-administer insulin several times each day and difficulty maintaining long-term adherence, make physiological replacement of insulin challenging. There is no universal insulin regimen that can be used for all children with type 1 diabetes. The diabetes team has to design an insulin regimen that meets the needs of the individual patient and is acceptable to the patient and/or family member(s) responsible for administering insulin to the child or supervising its administration.

The initial route of insulin administration is determined by the severity of the child's condition at presentation. Insulin is given intravenously for treatment of DKA. Children who are metabolically stable without vomiting or significant ketosis may be started with SC insulin. SC insulin in the newly diagnosed child who has recently recovered from DKA is usually started with two or three injections per day of a mixture of human intermediate-acting and rapid- or short-acting insulin. Some clinicians start basal–bolus insulin therapy at the time of diagnosis, regardless of the severity of presentation or age of the child.

In addition to the severity of metabolic decompensation, the child's age, weight and pubertal status guide the initial insulin dose selection. When diabetes has been diagnosed early, before significant metabolic decompensation, 0.25–0.5 unit/kg/day is usually adequate. When metabolic decompensation is more severe (e.g. ketonuria without acidosis or dehydration), the initial dose is typically at least 0.5 unit/kg/day. After recovery from DKA, prepubertal children usually require at least 0.75 unit/kg/day, whereas adolescents require at least 1 unit/kg/day. In the first few days of insulin therapy, while the focus of care is on diabetes education and emotional support, it is reasonable to aim for premeal BG concentrations in the range 4.5–11 mmol/L (80–200 mg/dL) and to supplement, if necessary, with 0.05–0.1 unit/kg rapid- or short-acting insulin SC at 3- to 4-h intervals.

Three major categories of insulin preparations, classified according to time course of action, are available (Table 12.1). Various insulin replacement regimens, consisting of a mixture of short- or rapid-acting insulin and an intermediate- or long-acting insulin, are used in children and adolescents, typically given two to four (or more) times daily. Clear superiority of any one regimen in terms of metabolic outcome has not been demonstrated.

All regimens provide basal insulin throughout the day and night and more insulin with meals and snacks. When a two-dose regimen is used, the total daily dose is typically divided so that about two-thirds is given before breakfast and one-third is given in the evening. With a three-dose regimen, short- or rapid-acting insulin is administered before supper and the second dose of intermediate-acting insulin is given at bedtime rather than before the evening meal. The initial ratio of rapid- to intermediate-acting insulin at both times is approximately 1:2. Toddlers and young children typically require a smaller fraction of short- or rapid-acting insulin (10–20% of the total dose) and proportionately more intermediate-acting insulin. Regular insulin is given at least 30 min before eating; rapid-acting insulin (e.g. lispro insulin, insulin aspart) is given 5–15 min before eating.

The optimal ratio of rapid- or short-acting to intermediate-acting insulin for each patient is determined by the results of frequent BG measurements. At least five daily measurements are required initially to determine the effects of each component of the insulin regimen. The BG concentration is measured before each meal, before the bedtime snack and once between midnight and 04.00 h. Parents are taught to look for patterns of hyperglycemia or hypoglycemia that indicate the need for an adjustment in the dose. Adjustments are made to individual components of the insulin regimen, usually in 5–10% increments or decrements, in response to patterns of consistently elevated (above the target range for several consecutive days) or unexplained low BG concentrations, respectively. This is referred to as pattern adjustment. The insulin dose is adjusted until satisfactory BG control is achieved with most BG values in or close to the individual child's target range.

At the time of diagnosis, most children have some residual β-cells and, within a period of several days to a few weeks, may enter a period of partial remission

Table 12.1 Insulin preparations classified according to their pharmacodynamic profiles.

	Onset of action (h)	Peak action (h)	Duration of action (h)
Rapid acting			
Insulin lispro*	0.25–0.5	0.5–2.5	≤5
Insulin aspart*	<0.25	1–3	3–5
Short acting			
Regular (soluble)	0.5–1	2–4	5–8
Intermediate acting			
NPH (isophane)			
Lente (insulin zinc	1–2	2–8	14–24
suspension)	1–2	3–10	20–24
Long acting			
Ultralente	0.5–3	4–20	20–36
Insulin glargine*	2–4	Peakless	20–24
Premixed combinations			
50% NPH, 50% regular	0.5–1	Dual	14–24
70% NPH, 30% regular	0.5–1	Dual	14–24
70% NPA, 30% aspart*	<0.25	Dual	14–24
75% NPL, 25% lispro*	<0.25	Dual	14–24

*Insulin analog developed by modifying the amino acid sequence of the human insulin molecule. Data are from the manufacturers. Pharmacodynamic effects of lispro insulin and insulin aspart appear to be equivalent. NPA, neutral protamine aspart; NPL, neutral protamine lispro. Both NPA and NPL are stable premixed combinations of intermediate- and short-acting insulins.

Most of the human insulins and insulin analogs are available in insulin cartridges and/or disposable insulin pens.

These data are for human insulins and are approximations from studies in adult test subjects. Time action profiles are reasonable estimates only. The kinetics of NPH insulin may be more rapid in children. The times of onset, peak and duration of action vary within and between patients and are affected by many factors, including dose, site and depth of injection, dilution, exercise, temperature.

('honeymoon'), during which normal or nearly normal glycemic control is relatively easily achieved with a low dose of insulin. At this stage, the dose of insulin should be reduced to prevent hypoglycemia but should not be discontinued. Since destruction of the remaining β-cells occurs, the insulin dose increases ('intensification phase'), eventually reaching a full replacement dose. The average daily insulin dose in prepubertal children with long-standing diabetes is approximately 0.8 unit/kg/day and in adolescents about 1–1.5 unit/kg/day.

Technical details

Caring for young children with diabetes is challenging for many reasons, one of which is the need accurately and reproducibly to measure and inject tiny doses of insulin that is supplied in a concentration of 100 units/mL (U100 insulin). To administer a dose of 1 unit requires the ability accurately to measure 10 μL (1/100 mL) of insulin. When the dose is <2 U of U100 insulin, neither parents of children with diabetes nor skilled pediatric nurses are able to measure the dose accurately. Furthermore, a dose change of 0.25 U translates into a volume difference of 2.5 μL in a 300 μL (3/10 mL or 30 unit) syringe. When parents attempt to measure insulin doses in increments of 0.25 U of insulin (e.g. 3.0, 3.25, 3.5 U) using a standard commercial 30 unit (300 mL) syringe, they consistently measure more than the prescribed amount. Therefore, to enhance accuracy and reproducibility of small doses, insulin should be diluted to U10 (10 units/mL) with the specific diluent available from the manufacturers. Using U10 insulin, each line ('unit') on a syringe is actually 0.1 U of insulin.

To avoid intramuscular injections in infants and young children with little SC fat, syringes with 30-gauge 8 mm (short) needles or insulin pens with 31-gauge 5 mm needles should be used to administer insulin. Short needles are also desirable for use in older thin children.

Limitations of twice-daily split-and-mixed insulin regimens

Beyond the remission period, it is not generally possible to achieve near-normal glycemia with two injections per day without incurring a greater risk of hypoglycemia, especially during the overnight period. A major problem with the two-dose 'split-and-mixed' regimen (rapid- or short-acting insulin combined with intermediate-acting insulin administered before breakfast and before the evening meal) is that the peak effect of the predinner intermediate-acting insulin tends to occur at the time of lowest insulin requirement (midnight to 04.00 h), increasing the risk of nocturnal hypoglycemia (Fig. 12.4). Thereafter, insulin action declines from 04.00 to 08.00 h, when the basal insulin requirement normally increases. Consequently, the tendency for BG concentrations to rise before breakfast (dawn phenomenon) may be aggravated by waning insulin effect before breakfast and/or by counter-regulatory hormones secreted in response to a fall in BG concentrations during sleep, post-hypoglycemic hyperglycemia (Somogyi phenomenon).

A three-dose insulin regimen with mixed short- or rapid- and intermediate-acting insulins before breakfast, only short- or rapid-acting insulin before dinner and intermediate-acting insulin at bedtime may significantly reduce these problems. Intensive insulin regimens that employ intermediate-acting insulin demand consistency in the daily meal schedule, amounts of food consumed at each meal and the timing of insulin injections.

Basal–bolus regimens and continuous SC insulin infusion

Insulin therapy with at least three injections each day or with continuous SC insulin infusion (CSII) using a portable insulin pump can more closely simulate normal diurnal insulin profiles, overcome many of the limitations inherent in a two-dose regimen and permit greater flexibility with respect to timing and content of meals. A peakless long-acting insulin, insulin glargine, can be used to provide basal insulin and is used together with short- or rapid-acting insulin injected before each meal (Fig. 12.4b). Insulin glargine is an insulin analog, produced by recombinant DNA technology,

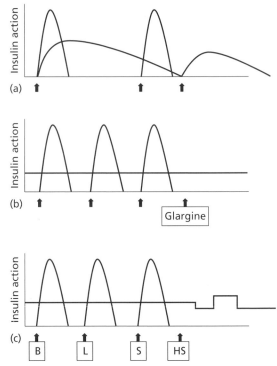

Figure 12.4 (a) Schematic representation of idealized insulin action provided by a regimen consisting of a mixture of rapid-acting insulin (lispro or aspart) and intermediate-acting insulin (NPH or Lente) before breakfast, rapid-acting insulin (lispro or aspart) before supper, and intermediate-acting insulin (NPH or Lente) at bedtime. (b) Schematic representation of idealized insulin action provided by an insulin regimen consisting of four daily injections: rapid-acting insulin (lispro or aspart) before each meal (B, L, S) and a separate injection of insulin glargine, either at bedtime (as shown here) or at dinner or breakfast. (c) Schematic representation of idealized insulin effect provided by CSII via an insulin pump with insulin aspart or lispro. In this figure, alternative basal rates are illustrated; insulin delivery is shown to decrease from midnight to 03.00 h and to increase before breakfast. B, breakfast; L, lunch; S, supper; HS, bedtime. Arrows indicate times of insulin injection or boluses before meals.

with an approximately 24-h duration of action. It has little peak activity and is typically administered once daily, usually but not invariably at bedtime. It should be injected at about the same time each day, whereas short- or rapid-acting insulin is injected separately before each meal, whenever it is eaten. Insulin glargine has been used safely in children and adolescents and, because it does not have the peak activity characteristic of NPH, lente and ultralente insulins, can reduce nocturnal hypoglycemic episodes without jeopardizing glycemic control.

An insulin pump has the ability to program changes in basal dosage to meet an anticipated increase or decrease in need (Fig. 12.4c), a unique advantage over insulin injections. This can be advantageous in combating the dawn phenomenon or preventing hypoglycemia during or after exercise. In addition to programming various basal rates, the use of dual- and square-wave bolus delivery significantly lowers 4-h post-prandial BG concentrations.

Although an insulin pump is a complex and sophisticated medical device that requires extensive training, many children can manage it. Only short- or rapid-acting insulin is used with CSII; therefore, any interruption in the delivery of insulin rapidly leads to metabolic decompensation. To reduce this risk, meticulous care must be devoted to the infusion system and BG concentrations must be measured frequently.

Increased lifestyle flexibility, reduced BG variability, improved glycemic control and reduced frequency of severe hypoglycemia are all advantages of CSII and the diabetes team should select patients who are likely to benefit. Success requires motivation, frequent BG monitoring, carbohydrate counting and frequent contact with the diabetes team. CSII therapy requires more time, effort and active involvement in diabetes care by patients and parents and considerable education and support from the diabetes team and the individual who is unable to master a multiple-dose injection regimen is not likely to be successful with CSII. Despite concerns that it might have adverse psychosocial consequences owing to the added burden of treatment, especially in adolescents, the opposite effect has been observed. Short-term studies have shown that more aggressive and successful management of their diabetes by teenagers can be accompanied by enhanced psychosocial well-being. In teenagers, CSII offers a treatment option that can lead to improved control, lower the risk of severe hypoglycemia and help prevent long-term complications.

Considerations during puberty

Owing to insulin resistance of puberty, adolescents require large doses of rapid- or short-acting insulin to control post-prandial BG excursions. However, a large increase in the dose of regular insulin markedly delays its peak effect (to 3–4 h) and prolongs its total duration of action to 6–8 h. Puberty does not cause hepatic insulin resistance; therefore, hyperinsulinemia suppresses hepatic glucose production for several hours and increases the risk of post-prandial hypoglycemia, especially at night between 22.00 and 02.00 h. This is an important reason to use rapid-acting insulin analogs (insulin lispro or insulin aspart) in preference to regular (soluble) insulin in treating adolescents, especially before the evening meal.

Technological innovations have provided patients with insulin preparations with pharmacokinetic properties that make it possible crudely to simulate physiological insulin kinetics. It is now possible for children safely to achieve unprecedented concentrations of glycemic control without excessive severe hypoglycemia. The diabetes care provider should discuss treatment options with parents and child and explain the advantages and disadvantages of each in attempting to meet the overall goals of treatment. The most suitable regimen for a given child and family should be determined by mutual consent and not by coercion.

Food

Meal planning continues to be a cornerstone of the management of all types of diabetes mellitus and education is an essential component of managing diabetes. There is no 'diabetic diet' *per se*. Nutrition should be individualized, with consideration given to the patient's usual eating habits and other lifestyle factors. Monitoring clinical and metabolic parameters, including BG, HbA1c, lipids, blood pressure and body weight, as well as quality of life, is crucial to ensure successful outcomes. Diabetes management, combining frequent SMBG with intensive insulin therapy and mastery of carbohydrate counting, enables children and adolescents to have considerable dietary flexibility while maintaining glycemic control in the target range.

There is no evidence that the nutritional needs of children with diabetes differ from those of otherwise healthy children. Total intake of energy must be sufficient to balance the daily expenditure of energy and has to be adjusted periodically to achieve an ideal body weight and to maintain a normal rate of physical growth and maturation.

Sixty to seventy percent of total energy should be from carbohydrate and monounsaturated fat. Protein requirements are not increased when diabetes is well controlled and children with diabetes should follow the recommended daily allowance guidelines, i.e. 0.9–2.2 g/kg body weight per day and 15–20% of the total daily intake of energy. The consumption of saturated fat can be reduced by eating less red meat, whole milk and high-fat dairy foods and by eating more poultry, fish and vegetable proteins and drinking more low-fat milk.

Excessive saturated fat, cholesterol and total energy lead to increased blood concentrations of cholesterol and triglycerides. Because hyperlipidemia is a major determinant of atherosclerosis and patients with type 1 diabetes eventually develop atherosclerosis and its sequelae, the meal plan should attempt to mitigate this risk factor. Children and adolescents with well-controlled type 1 diabetes are not at high risk of dyslipidemia but should be screened and monitored every 5 years. If there is a family history of hypercholesterolemia or premature atherosclerosis, screening should be more intense. If the child or adolescent is growing and developing normally and has normal plasma lipid concentrations, <10% of energy should come from saturated fat, the daily intake of cholesterol should be <300 mg/day and consumption of transunsaturated fatty acids should be minimized. Total dietary fat should be reduced in the obese child to reduce total energy consumption. Pharmacological treatment with a bile acid sequestrant or statin is recommended for a diabetic child when LDL cholesterol exceeds 4.1 mmol/L (159 mg/dL) and should be considered when LDL cholesterol is 3.3 mmol/L (129 mg/dL).

Exercise

Children with diabetes are encouraged to participate in sports and make exercise a regular part of their lives. Participation in physical exercise improves physical fitness, helps to control weight and can improve glycemic control. Regular exercise increases insulin sensitivity, cardiovascular fitness, blood lipid profiles and lowers blood pressure. For the child with type 1 diabetes, exercise is complicated by the need to prevent hypoglycemia but, with proper guidance and preparation, participation in exercise should be a safe and enjoyable experience.

Exercise acutely lowers the BG concentration by increasing utilization of glucose but increased counter-regulatory hormone secretion in response to strenuous exercise may cause hyperglycemia.

Hypoglycemia can be prevented by a combination of anticipatory reduction in pre-exercise insulin dose or temporary interruption of basal insulin infusion (with CSII) and/or supplemental snacks before, during and after physical activity. The optimal strategy depends on the intensity and duration of the activity and its timing relative to the child's meal plan and insulin schedule. A useful guide is to provide an additional 15 g of carbohydrate (one bread or fruit exchange) per 30–60 min of vigorous physical activity.

Exercising the limb into which insulin has been injected accelerates the rate of insulin absorption. If possible, the insulin injection preceding exercise should be given in a site least likely to be affected by exercise. Because physical training increases tissue sensitivity to insulin, children who participate in organized sports are advised to reduce the dose of the insulin preparation predominantly active during the period of sustained physical activity. The size of such reductions is determined by measuring BG concentrations before and after exercise and is generally in the order of 10–30% of the usual dose.

In a child with poorly controlled diabetes, vigorous exercise can aggravate hyperglycemia and ketoacid production and, accordingly, a child with ketonuria should not exercise until satisfactory biochemical control has been restored.

Adjunctive therapy

A substantial number of adolescents with type 1 diabetes are overweight or obese and have clinically significant insulin resistance. Adjunctive treatment with metformin, to improve insulin sensitivity and glycemic control without weight gain, modestly improves HbA1c concentrations but it is not yet clear whether these benefits are sustained. Metformin should not be given to individuals at high risk of ketoacidosis or to patients with impaired renal function.

Monitoring

Self-monitoring of blood glucose (SMBG)

SMBG has revolutionized management and is the cornerstone of modern diabetes care but too many patients/parents are not taught how to use the data to adjust the components of their treatment regimen. SMBG has to be performed at least 4 times in the day, before each meal and at bedtime to provide useful data. To do this every day is a considerable, and probably unattainable, burden. Nevertheless, frequency of BG monitoring is an important predictor of glycemic control in children with type 1 diabetes; the optimal frequency of SMBG should be sufficient to facilitate attainment of the individual patient's glycemic goals.

To minimize the risk of nocturnal hypoglycemia, BG should be measured between midnight and 04.00 h once each week or every other week and whenever the evening dose of insulin is adjusted. If HbA1c targets are not being met, patients should be encouraged to measure BG concentrations more frequently, including 90–120 min after meals.

Children who are able to perform SMBG independently must be properly supervised because it is not unusual for children to fabricate data with disastrous consequences.

Common reasons for deterioration of metabolic control are shown in Table 12.2.

Table 12.2 Causes of deterioration of metabolic control in children and adolescents with diabetes mellitus.

Increased insulin requirement
Progressive loss of residual β-cell function
Failure to increase dose with growth
Failure to increase dose during puberty
Increased calorie intake
Illness or significant psychological stress
Diminished physical activity (often seasonal)
Medications that cause insulin resistance (e.g. glucocorticoids)

Insulin omission (inadvertent or deliberate)

'Failure' of administered insulin
Inappropriate timing of insulin in relation to food consumption
Failure completely to suspend intermediate-acting insulin suspension
Lipohypertrophy at site of insulin injection
Loss of insulin potency (frozen, heated or expired)
Improper injection technique (intramuscular or intraepidermal injection)

Miscellaneous causes
Fabricated BG data
Glucose meter malfunction
Celiac disease
Hyperthyroidism
High-titer insulin antibodies

Continuous glucose monitoring sensors

Glucose sensors have been developed to provide frequent glucose determinations throughout the day and night in patients with diabetes. Two continuous glucose monitors, GlucoWatch® and G2™ biographer, and the continuous glucose monitoring system, CGMS™ System Gold®, are being used in children with diabetes. Both measure interstitial fluid glucose concentrations, which are normalized to approximate serum glucose values using algorithms.

Urine ketone testing

Urine should be tested for ketones during acute illness or stress, when BG concentrations are persistently elevated (e.g. two consecutive BG values >300 mg/dL) or when the patient feels unwell, especially with nausea, abdominal pain or vomiting. False-negative readings may occur when the strips have been exposed to air (e.g. improperly stored) or when urine is highly acidic (e.g. after consumption of large doses of ascorbic acid). Urine ketone tests using nitroprusside-containing reagents can give false-positive results in patients who take valproic acid or any sulfhydryl-containing drug, including captopril.

Glycated hemoglobin, HbA1c

Blood glucose and blood or urine ketone testing provide useful information for day-to-day management of diabetes, whereas HbA1c provides important information about recent overall glycemic control. It does not detect large swings so a patient with brittle control (frequent periods of high and low BG concentrations) may be falsely reassured by a relatively normal HbA1c value.

HbA1c is a minor fraction of adult hemoglobin, which is formed slowly and non-enzymatically from hemoglobin and glucose. Because erythrocytes are freely permeable to glucose, HbA1c is formed throughout the lifespan of the erythrocyte; its rate of formation is directly proportional to the ambient glucose concentration. The concentration of HbA1c, therefore, provides a 'glycemic history' of the previous 120 days, the average lifespan of erythrocytes.

In patients with hemoglobin variants (HbS, HbC, HbF), radioimmunoassay and affinity chromatography methods for measuring glycated hemoglobin must be used instead of conventional high-performance liquid or cation-exchange chromatography, which give spurious values. Several clinical conditions, including uremia and high-dose aspirin, lead to chemical modifications of hemoglobin that can spuriously increase HbA1c measurements. Average glucose concentrations are underestimated by HbA1c in conditions that shorten the average circulating red blood cell lifespan, such as hemolysis, sickle cell disease, transfusion and iron deficiency anemia. When accurate HbA1c measurement is not possible, alternative tests of chronic glycemia, such as fructosamine or glycosylated serum albumin, should be used.

HbA1c should be measured approximately every 3 months to monitor the effectiveness of glycemic therapy and as an indicator for when therapy needs to be modified.

Acute complications

Diabetic ketoacidosis

Children rarely have DKA when insulin administration is closely supervised or performed by a responsible adult and most instances of DKA in established patients are probably associated with insulin omission or treatment error, the remainder being due to inadequate insulin therapy during intercurrent illness.

DKA is the result of absolute or relative deficiency of circulating insulin and the combined effects of increased concentrations of the counter-regulatory hormones, catecholamines, glucagon, cortisol and GH. Insulin deficiency occurs in previously undiagnosed type 1 diabetes or when patients on treatment deliberately or inadvertently omit insulin. Relative insulin deficiency occurs when the concentrations of counter-regulatory hormones increase under conditions of stress such as sepsis, trauma or gastrointestinal illness with diarrhea and vomiting.

Low serum concentrations of insulin and high concentrations of the counter-regulatory hormones result in an accelerated catabolic state, the effects of which are increased glucose production by the liver and kidney (via glycogenolysis and gluconeogenesis), impaired peripheral glucose utilization resulting in hyperglycemia and hyperosmolality and increased lipolysis and ketogenesis causing ketonemia and metabolic acidosis. Hyperglycemia and hyperketonemia cause osmotic diuresis, dehydration and obligatory loss of electrolytes, which is often aggravated by

Table 12.3 Clinical manifestations of DKA.

- Dehydration
- Rapid, deep, sighing (Kussmaul) respiration
- Nausea, vomiting, abdominal pain that may mimic an acute abdomen
- Increased leukocyte count with left shift
- Non-specific elevation of serum amylase
- Fever when there is infection
- Progressive obtundation and loss of consciousness

Table 12.4 Losses of fluid and electrolytes in DKA and normal maintenance requirements.

	Average losses per kg (range)	Maintenance requirements per meter^2
Water	70 mL (30–100)	1500 mL
Sodium	6 mmol (5–13)	45 mmol
Potassium	5 mmol (3–6)	35 mmol
Chloride	4 mmol (3–9)	30 mmol
Phosphate	0.5–2.5 mmol	10 mmol

These data are from measurements in only a few children and adolescents.

vomiting (Table 12.3). DKA is characterized by severe depletion of water and electrolytes; the range of losses is shown in Table 12.4. Despite dehydration, patients continue to have considerable urine output unless they are extremely volume depleted.

Rates of hospitalization for DKA in established and new patients with type 1 diabetes have remained stable at about 10 per 100 000 children over the past 20 years. The risk of DKA in patients with established type 1 diabetes is 1–10% per patient per year. It is increased in children with poor metabolic control or previous episodes of DKA, in peripubertal and adolescent girls, in children with psychiatric disorders, including those with eating disorders, and in those with difficult family circumstances, including lower socioeconomic status. Interruption of insulin delivery by CSII, irrespective of the reason, is an important cause of DKA.

The biochemical criteria for the diagnosis of DKA include hyperglycemia (BG > 11 mmol/L (> 200 mg/dL))

Table 12.5 Goals of therapy in DKA.

- Correct dehydration
- Restore BG to near-normal levels
- Correct acidosis and reverse ketosis
- Avoid complications of treatment
- Identify and treat the precipitating event

with acidosis (venous blood pH <7.3 and/or serum bicarbonate <15 mmol/L), ketonemia with total serum ketones (β-hydroxybutyrate and acetoacetate) >3 mmol/L and ketonuria. DKA is generally categorized by the severity of the acidosis, from mild (venous pH <7.30, bicarbonate <15 mmol/L) to moderate (pH <7.2, bicarbonate <10) to severe (pH <7.1, bicarbonate <5).

Management of DKA (Table 12.5)

Initial evaluation

- Perform a clinical evaluation to establish the diagnosis and determine its cause (especially any evidence of infection). Weigh the patient and measure height or length. Determine body surface area. Assess the patient's degree of dehydration.
- Determine the BG concentration with a glucose meter and the blood or urine ketone concentration.
- Obtain a blood sample for laboratory measurement of glucose, electrolytes and TCO_2, blood urea nitrogen, creatinine, serum osmolality, venous (or arterial in critically ill patient) pH, pCO_2, pO_2, hemoglobin, hematocrit, total and differential white blood cell count, calcium, phosphorus and magnesium concentrations.
- Perform a urinalysis and obtain appropriate specimens for culture (blood, urine, throat).
- Perform an electrocardiogram for baseline evaluation of potassium status.

Supportive measures

- Secure the airway and empty the stomach by continuous nasogastric suction to prevent pulmonary aspiration in the unconscious or severely obtunded patient.
- Antibiotics should be given to febrile patients after obtaining appropriate cultures of body fluids.
- Supplementary oxygen should be given to patients with severe circulatory impairment or shock.

- Catheterization of the bladder is not usually necessary but, if the child is unconscious or unable to void on demand (e.g. infants and very ill young children), the bladder should be catheterized.
- A flow chart is essential to record the patient's clinical and laboratory data, including vital signs (heart rate, respiratory rate, blood pressure, level of consciousness (Glasgow coma scale)), details of fluid and electrolyte therapy, amount of administered insulin and urine output. A key to successful management of DKA is meticulous monitoring of the patient's clinical and biochemical response to treatment so that timely adjustments in the treatment regimen can be made when indicated by the patient's clinical or laboratory data. Frequent re-examination of laboratory parameters is required to prevent serious electrolyte imbalance and administration of either insufficient or excessive fluid.
- A heparin-locked intravenous catheter should be placed for convenient and painless repetitive blood sampling.
- A cardiac monitor should be used for continuous electrocardiographic monitoring.

Fluid and electrolyte therapy

All patients with DKA are dehydrated and suffer total body depletion of sodium, potassium, chloride, phosphate and magnesium (Table 12.4). The high osmolality of the extracellular fluid (ECF) compartment results in a shift of water from the intracellular fluid (ICF) compartment to the ECF and decreases the serum sodium concentration ~1.6 mmol/L per 5.6 mmol/L (100 mg/dL) BG above normal.

The presence of hyperlipidemia may lower the measured serum sodium concentration (depending on the methodology used to measure serum sodium concentration). Therefore, the serum sodium concentration may give a misleading estimate of the degree of sodium loss.

The osmolality (see formula below) at the time of presentation is frequently 300–350 mOsm/L. Increased serum urea nitrogen and hematocrit are useful markers of severe ECF contraction. At the time of presentation, patients are ECF contracted and clinical estimates of the deficit in patients with severe DKA are usually 7–10%. In mild to moderately severe DKA, fluid deficits are more modest, 30–50 mL/kg. Shock with hemodynamic compromise is rare in childhood.

The onset of dehydration is associated with a reduction in glomerular filtration rate (GFR), which results in decreased glucose and ketone clearance. Intravenous fluid administration expands the intravascular volume and increases glomerular filtration, which increases renal excretion of glucose and ketoanions and results in a prompt decrease in BG concentration.

Intracranial pressure rises as intravenous fluids are given. Although there is no compelling evidence showing superiority of any fluid regimen over another, there are data that suggest that rapid fluid replacement with hypotonic fluid is associated with an increased risk of cerebral edema; slower fluid deficit correction with isotonic or near-isotonic solutions results in earlier reversal of acidosis. Large amounts of 0.9% saline have also been associated with the development of hyperchloremic metabolic acidosis.

Initial intravenous fluid administration and, when necessary, volume expansion should begin immediately with an isotonic solution (0.9% saline or balanced salt solution such as Ringer's lactate). The volume and rate of administration depend on the patient's circulatory status. When volume expansion is clinically indicated, 10–20 mL/kg is given over 1–2 h and may be repeated if necessary. Subsequent fluid management should be with a solution that has a tonicity ⩾0.45% saline (0.45% saline or balanced salt solution (Ringer's lactate) or 0.45% saline with added potassium).

The rate of intravenous fluid administration should be calculated to rehydrate the patient evenly over 48 h. Since the severity of dehydration may be difficult to determine and is often overestimated, the daily volume of fluid should usually not exceed 1.5–2 times the usual daily requirement based on age, weight or body surface area (Table 12.4). Urinary losses should not be added to the calculation of replacement fluids.

The development of hyponatremia or failure to observe a progressive rise in serum sodium concentration with a concomitant decrease in BG concentration during treatment is a risk factor for cerebral edema. The composition of the hydrating fluid should be changed appropriately to increase the serum sodium concentration.

When the BG concentration reaches ~17 mmol/L (300 mg/dL), 5% dextrose is added to the infusion fluid. It may be necessary to use ⩾10% dextrose to prevent hypoglycemia. Administration of intravenous fluids should be continued until acidosis is corrected and the patient can tolerate fluids and food. Inadequate fluid administration should be evident from examination of the cumulative fluid balance and persistent tachycardia in the absence of a fever.

Insulin

Insulin is essential. Rehydration alone decreases the BG concentration but does not reverse ketoacidosis. Several routes and doses of insulin have been used but intravenous regular (soluble) insulin at a dose of 0.1 unit/kg/h achieves steady-state serum insulin concentrations of 50–200 mU/mL within 60 min, which is adequate to offset the insulin resistance characteristic of DKA, suppress glucose production, significantly increase peripheral glucose uptake and inhibit lipolysis and ketogenesis.

The dose of insulin should remain at 0.1 unit/kg/h until resolution of ketoacidosis (pH >7.30 and bicarbonate >15 mmol/L and/or closure of the anion gap). Resolution of ketoacidemia takes longer than restoration of BG concentrations so intravenous insulin must not be discontinued until ketoacidosis has resolved, even if the BG concentration is normal or near to normal. To prevent an unduly rapid fall in BG concentration and development of hypoglycemia, dextrose should be added to the intravenous fluid when the plasma glucose has fallen to <17 mmol/L (300 mg/dL).

Intravenous insulin should be administered via an infusion pump. Regular insulin is diluted in normal saline (50 units of regular insulin in 50 mL of saline) and is given at a rate of 0.1 unit/kg/h. An intravenous priming dose is not necessary but 0.1 unit/kg may be used at the start of insulin therapy if insulin treatment has been delayed.

If the BG concentration is falling but acidosis is not improving (i.e. anion gap is not decreasing) owing to severe insulin resistance, the rate of insulin infusion should be increased until a satisfactory response is achieved. Rare patients with severe insulin resistance do not respond satisfactorily to low-dose insulin infusion and require 2 or 3 times the usual dose. It is essential to monitor the BG, venous (or arterial) pH and anion gap response to insulin therapy. In addition, one should consider other possible explanations for failure to respond to insulin and especially an error in insulin preparation. When intravenous administration is not possible, the intramuscular or SC route of insulin administration may be used and rapid-acting insulin (lispro or aspart) may be preferable to regular insulin in these circumstances. Poor tissue perfusion in a severely dehydrated patient will impair SC absorption of insulin and, initially, insulin should be given intramuscularly.

The half-life of insulin in serum is 5 min so that the serum insulin concentration decreases rapidly if the insulin infusion is stopped. If the infusion were to infiltrate and this was not recognized promptly, inadequate serum insulin concentrations would ensue. Low-dose intravenous insulin therapy must be carefully supervised.

When ketoacidosis has resolved and the change to SC insulin is planned, the first SC injection should be given at an appropriate interval before stopping the infusion to allow sufficient time for the SC injected insulin to begin to be absorbed.

Potassium

Potassium is lost from the cells because of hypertonicity, insulin deficiency and buffering of hydrogen ions within the cell. During acidosis, intracellular potassium enters the extracellular compartment and is lost in urine and vomit. Serum potassium concentrations at the time of presentation vary. Hypokalemia may be related to prolonged duration of disease and persistent vomiting, whereas hyperkalemia results primarily from impaired renal function.

If the patient presents with hyperkalemia, potassium administration should be deferred until urine output has been documented and the potassium concentration has decreased to a normal level. The amount of potassium should be sufficient to maintain serum potassium concentrations in the normal range. The usual starting potassium concentration in the infusate should be 40 mmol/L and potassium administration should continue throughout the period of intravenous fluid therapy.

The plasma potassium concentration should be rechecked every hour if the plasma concentration has been outside the normal range. Potassium may be given as chloride, acetate or phosphate. Use of potassium acetate and potassium phosphate reduces the total amount of chloride administered and partially corrects the phosphate deficit.

Phosphate

Depletion of intracellular phosphate occurs in DKA because of osmotic diuresis. Deficits in adults are 0.5–2.5 mmol/kg but data in children are few.

Plasma phosphate concentrations decrease rapidly after starting therapy, because of urinary excretion and because insulin causes phosphate to re-enter cells. Low serum phosphate concentrations have been associated with a variety of metabolic disturbances but prospective studies have failed to show clinical benefit from phosphate replacement. Severe hypophosphatemia should be treated with potassium phosphate while to avoid phosphate-induced hypocalcemia.

Acidosis and bicarbonate

Severe acidosis is reversible by fluid and insulin replacement alone. Insulin stops further synthesis of ketoacids and promotes ketone utilization. The metabolism of ketoanions results in the regeneration of bicarbonate and correction of acidemia. Treatment of hypovolemia improves tissue perfusion and restores renal function, thus increasing the excretion of organic acids and reversing any lactic acidosis, which may account for 25% of the acidemia.

The indications for bicarbonate therapy in DKA are unclear. Controlled trials of sodium bicarbonate in children and adults have been unable to show clinical benefit nor a difference in the rate of rise in the plasma bicarbonate concentration.

There may be selected patients who may benefit from cautious alkali therapy, including patients with severe acidemia (arterial pH <6.9), in whom decreased cardiac contractility and peripheral vasodilatation can further impair tissue perfusion and patients with life-threatening hyperkalemia. In these circumstances, sodium bicarbonate 1–2 mmol/kg or 40–80 mmol/m^2 is infused over 2 h and the plasma bicarbonate concentration is rechecked. Bicarbonate should not be given as a bolus because this may precipitate cardiac arrhythmia.

Clinical and biochemical monitoring

Initially, plasma glucose should be measured hourly. Thereafter, plasma glucose, serum electrolytes (and calculated sodium), pH, pCO$_2$, TCO$_2$, anion gap, calcium and phosphorus should be measured every

2–4 h for the first 8 h and then every 4 h until they are normal. The data must be recorded carefully on a flow sheet.

Useful calculations for managing DKA

1 Effective osmolality 2[Na^+ + K^+] + glucose (mmol/L). Effective serum osmolality correlates with mental status abnormalities. Blood or serum urea nitrogen diffuses freely into cells and does not contribute to effective osmolality.

2 Corrected sodium = [Na^+] + {1.6 × [plasma glucose (mmol/L) – 5.6] divided by 5.6}. Corrected serum sodium assists in estimation of free water deficits.

3 Anion gap = [Na^+] – [Cl^- + HCO_3^-]. A decreasing anion gap indicates successful therapy of metabolic acidosis.

4 Evaluation for pure metabolic acidosis:

pCO_2 = last two numbers of the pH

pCO_2 + 1.5 [serum HCO_3^-] + 8±2

A lower than predicted pCO_2 indicates respiratory alkalosis and may be a clue to sepsis.

Morbidity and mortality from DKA in children (Table 12.6)

Mortality rates from DKA are 0.15–0.31%. In areas with sparse medical facilities, the risk of dying is greater and children may die before receiving treatment. Cerebral edema occurs in 0.5–1.0% of cases and the mortality rate is about 25%, accounting for the majority of deaths from DKA. Significant morbidity is evident in up to one quarter of survivors.

Other causes of DKA-related morbidity and mortality include hypokalemia, hyperkalemia, hypoglycemia, sepsis and other central nervous system (CNS) complications such as thrombosis.

Cerebral edema typically occurs 4–12 h after commencement of treatment but can occur before treatment has begun or at any time during treatment. Symptoms and signs are variable and include onset of headache, gradual decrease or deterioration in level of consciousness, inappropriate slowing of the heart rate and an increase in blood pressure. Cerebral edema is more common in children with severe DKA, new-onset type 1 diabetes, younger age and longer duration of symptoms. The cause of cerebral edema remains poorly understood (Table 12.7).

Table 12.6 Complications of DKA therapy.

- Inadequate rehydration
- Hypoglycemia
- Hypokalemia
- Hyperchloremic acidosis
- Cerebral edema

Table 12.7 Factors associated with increased risk of cerebral edema.

- An attenuated rise in measured serum sodium concentration during treatment
- More severe acidosis
- Administration of bicarbonate to correct acidosis
- More profound hypocapnia at presentation
- Increased serum urea nitrogen at presentation reflecting more severe dehydration

Treatment of cerebral edema

Treatment should be initiated as soon as the condition is suspected. The rate of fluid administration should be reduced. Intravenous mannitol (0.25–1 g/kg) should be given over 20 min and can be repeated, if necessary, in 2 h if there is no initial response. Hypertonic saline (3%), 5–10 mL/kg over 30 min may be an alternative to mannitol. Intubation may be necessary for the patient with impending respiratory failure but aggressive hyperventilation (to a pCO_2 <22 mmHg) has been associated with poor outcome and is not recommended.

Management of sick days: prevention of DKA

Even a relatively minor illness in a diabetic child can cause rapid deterioration of metabolic control. The stress of infection, surgery, injury or severe emotional distress increases counter-regulatory hormone concentrations, which cause hyperglycemia and stimulate lipolysis and ketogenesis. Even when carbohydrate consumption is reduced by illness, BG concentrations usually increase and these metabolic disturbances can rapidly progress to DKA. The aim of sick day management is to minimize deterioration of metabolic control and prevent DKA.

Failure to administer insulin can have disastrous consequences and supplemental injections of rapid- or short-acting insulin are often required to prevent or correct hyperglycemia and/or ketosis. The child who has a gastrointestinal illness with nausea, vomiting or diarrhea and low, normal or near-normal BG concentrations is a special case because there is an increased risk of hypoglycemia. The dose of rapid- or short- and intermediate-acting insulins may have to be reduced. Ketonuria with BG concentrations that are normal or near to normal usually signifies starvation ketosis but must be distinguished from 'euglycemic ketoacidosis.'

Fluid requirements increase as a result of osmotic diuresis and increased insensible fluid losses due to fever; dehydration can develop rapidly if insufficient fluid is consumed. The child should be encouraged to drink at least 1 mL per kg of body weight per hour (or a minimum of 1500 mL/m^2/24 h, the usual maintenance fluid requirement). The child should receive fluids that provide sodium, glucose and potassium to replace urinary losses of these electrolytes that occur with metabolic decompensation. Fluids suitable for sick days are broth or bouillon (high salt content), water, carbonated beverages (Coca Cola, ginger ale) and fruit juices. Sugar-free fluids are recommended if the child is able to continue to follow his/her meal plan and/or BG is >11 mmol/L (200 mg/dL). However, when the child is unable to eat solid foods and the BG is <11 mmol/L (200 mg/dL), the liquids should contain a source of glucose. Weight loss is a reliable sign of dehydration and, if a bathroom scale is available, the child should be weighed carefully several times each day.

BG should be measured every 2–4 h throughout the day and night and ketone concentrations checked each time the child urinates. If the BG concentration is <4.5 mmol/L (80 mg/dL), measurements should be repeated hourly until it is >4.5 mmol/L (80 mg/dL). Cotton balls placed in the diaper can be used to obtain urine for ketone testing in infants and toddlers.

BG concentrations and severity of ketonuria or ketonemia are used to guide the administration of supplemental insulin. Rapid-acting insulin (lispro or insulin aspart) may be given every 2.5–3 h or short-acting (regular) insulin every 3–4 h until BG is <11 mmol/L (200 mg/dL) and ketonuria has been reduced to negative or trace or blood β OHB <0.5 mmol/L.

Table 12.8 Signs and symptoms in an ill child with diabetes mellitus requiring urgent medical attention.

- Signs of dehydration: dry mouth or tongue, cracked lips, sunken eyes, dry flushed skin, decreased urine output, weight loss
- Inability to consume the recommended amount of fluid or carbohydrate
- Persistent or recurrent vomiting for more than 4 h
- Symptoms suggestive of DKA: nausea, abdominal pain, vomiting, hyperventilation, drowsiness
- BG >14 mmol/L (250 mg/dL) and ketonuria for more than 12 h; for a child using an insulin pump after 6–8 h
- Inability to maintain BG >4.5 mmol/L (80 mg/dL)

Evidence that continued management of the child at home may no longer be safe and the child requires urgent medical attention is listed in Table 12.8. Assiduous attention to these guidelines enables most intercurrent childhood illnesses to be managed successfully at home.

Illness in the child managed with an insulin pump

The child using an insulin pump requires additional specific attention during sick day management. Because nausea and vomiting may be the earliest manifestations of interrupted insulin delivery and impending ketoacidosis, the patient may incorrectly assume that the symptoms are caused by a viral illness and not recognize the insulin-deficient state. Therefore, the patient who experiences nausea or vomiting must immediately check blood or urine for ketones.

Ketosis is evidence of a potential impending medical emergency because, when insulin delivery is interrupted, DKA can develop within 4–6 h. Rapid-acting insulin must immediately be given SC with a syringe. The dose may be based on the child's usual 'correction factor' to reduce the BG concentration to 6 mmol/L (110 mg/dL).

The infusion set should be replaced and the pump examined carefully to look for possible causes of failure to deliver insulin. These include battery failure, mechanical failure, an empty insulin reservoir, leakage at the site where the catheter connects to the syringe, occlusion of the catheter and withdrawal of the catheter from its SC insertion site on the skin. A temporary increase in the basal rate of insulin infusion may be required during illness. If BG concentrations exceed the target range, a 4-h trial of a 25% increase in the basal rate may be sufficient to restore the BG to an acceptable level. If the BG level has not decreased after 4 h, the basal rate should be increased by 50%.

Side-effects of treatment

Weight gain

Subjects treated intensively have a considerably increased risk of becoming overweight, due to reduced glycosuria and a reduction in daily energy expenditure. Furthermore, frequent symptomatic hypoglycemia necessitating consumption of carbohydrate to restore normoglycemia also contributes to weight gain in some individuals. It has also been suggested that intermittent hyperinsulinemia and lack of amylin to regulate appetite may underlie the propensity to weight gain in type 1 diabetes.

There is a J-shaped curve relating body mass index (BMI) to mortality in type 1 diabetes, with the highest relative all-cause mortality in those with the lowest BMI. It is generally accepted, therefore, that the long-term benefits of intensive glycemic control greatly outweigh the adverse effects of weight gain.

Children and adolescents who adopt basal–bolus insulin therapy may be tempted to eat more liberally and increase their calorie consumption because they are no longer obliged to follow a regimented meal plan. The highly motivated patient should be advised to take advantage of the flexibility of a basal–bolus regimen to balance insulin replacement with calorie intake to avoid obesity or even to lose weight.

Local effects of insulin

Lipohypertrophy, the accumulation of excess adipose tissue at the sites of SC insulin injection, is the most common cutaneous side-effect, occurring in 25–50% of individuals. Lipoatrophy is much less common but rotation of injection sites, thereby avoiding repeated insulin injections in a single area, prevents both lipo-hypertrophy and -atrophy. In addition to undesirable cosmetic appearances, it is important to avoid these complications because both cause erratic absorption of insulin.

Lipoatrophy may be treated by injecting insulin into the perimeter of the affected area and topical glucocorticoid injection into and around the site may be helpful in severe cases. If the patient is using animal-source insulin, switching to human insulin may prevent further atrophy and lead to gradual filling in of the atrophic area.

Insulin allergy may result in local or systemic effects. Severe reactions, including generalized urticaria and anaphylaxis, are extremely rare. Switching to synthetic human insulin may prevent further allergic reactions. This should be done after preliminary skin testing in a supervised setting. Insulin delivery by pump has been reported to stop local reactions in some cases. In rare instances, insulin desensitization may be necessary.

Cellulitis or abscess may occur at the injection site but is rare when patients use a sterile technique. Injection through clothing is strongly discouraged. Insulin pump therapy is associated with increased rates of cellulitis, abscess and local scarring at the sites of SC catheter insertion. It is essential to replace the catheter every 2–3 days and remove a catheter immediately if the site becomes red or painful.

Hypoglycemia

Hypoglycemia is the most common acute complication of treatment in children and adolescents and concern about hypoglycemia is a central issue. It is the principal factor limiting attempts to achieve near-normal glycemic control and patients, parents and the diabetes team have continuously to balance the risks of hypoglycemia against those of long-term hyperglycemia.

After an episode of severe hypoglycemia, the confidence of the patient and parents is often shaken and fear of a recurrence may induce the patient or parents to change their diabetes management. Altered patient behaviors may include overeating and/or deliberate selection of inadequate doses of insulin to maintain higher BG concentrations perceived as being safe, resulting in deterioration of glycemic control. Concern about nocturnal hypoglycemia causes more anxiety for some parents than any other aspects of diabetes, including the fear of long-term complications. Some parents believe that an episode of severe hypoglycemia during the nighttime may go undetected or not be treated in a timely fashion and lead to permanent brain damage or death.

The glucagon response to hypoglycemia is lost early in the course of the disease and patients with type 1 diabetes depend on sympathoadrenal responses to prevent or correct hypoglycemia. Mild hypoglycemia itself reduces epinephrine responses and symptomatic awareness of subsequent episodes of hypoglycemia. Little is known about counter-regulatory responses in preschool-aged children.

Symptoms and signs of hypoglycemia

Symptoms of hypoglycemia are caused by neuronal deprivation of glucose and have been categorized into autonomic (sweating, palpitations, shaking, hunger), neuroglycopenic (confusion, drowsiness, odd behavior, speech difficulty, inco-ordination) and non-specific malaise (hunger and headache). The most common signs and symptoms of hypoglycemia are pallor, weakness, tremor, hunger, fatigue, drowsiness, sweating and headache.

Autonomic symptoms are less common in children <6 years of age whose symptoms are more often neuroglycopenic or non-specific in nature. Behavioral changes are often the first manifestation of hypoglycemia in young children and this has implications for parent education. Also, in contrast to adult patients who are usually able to distinguish between autonomic and neuroglycopenic symptoms, children and their parents report that symptoms tend to cluster. The coalescence of autonomic and neuroglycopenic symptoms in children may indicate that both types of symptoms are generated at similar glycemic thresholds.

Hypoglycemia is classified as mild, moderate or severe. Most episodes are mild and cognitive impairment does not usually accompany them. Older children are able to treat themselves. Mild symptoms abate within about 15 min of treatment with rapidly absorbed carbohydrate.

Moderate hypoglycemia has neuroglycopenic and adrenergic symptoms, such as headache, mood changes, irritability, decreased attentiveness, drowsiness and behavior change. Young children typically require assistance with treatment because they are often confused and have impaired judgment. Weakness and poor co-ordination may make self-treatment difficult. Moderate hypoglycemia causes more protracted symptoms and may require a second treatment with oral carbohydrate.

Severe hypoglycemia is characterized by unresponsiveness, unconsciousness or convulsions and requires emergency treatment with parenteral glucagon or intravenous glucose.

Children who have had diabetes for several years may describe a change in symptomatology over time: autonomic symptoms occur less frequently and are more muted and neuroglycopenic symptoms (drowsiness, difficulty concentrating, lack of co-ordination) are more common. Patients must learn to recognize the change in symptoms to prevent severe episodes.

The BG concentration at which symptoms occur varies among patients and the threshold may vary in the same individual in parallel with antecedent glycemic control. Children with poorly controlled diabetes experience symptoms of hypoglycemia at higher BG concentrations than those with good glycemic control.

Impact of hypoglycemia on the child's brain

Numerous studies have documented cognitive impairment in diabetic children and adolescents. Global intellectual deficits have been described as well as specific neurocognitive impairments in memory, visuospatial skills and attention. Neuropsychological complications have been detected within 2 years of onset of diabetes. Children with long-term diabetes, especially those who developed the disease before the age of 6 years, appear to be at greatest risk but it is difficult to dissect the contributions of metabolic disturbances (hyperglycemia and hypoglycemia) and the psychosocial effects of the chronic disease in a young child.

Impaired intellectual development without a clear relationship to experienced hypoglycemia has been reported and cognitive impairments in children with early-onset diabetes mellitus may result from a number of factors, including severe hypoglycemia, recurrent asymptomatic hypoglycemia, psychosocial effects of chronic illness and chronic hyperglycemia, the relative importance of which is unclear. The cognitive sequelae of intensive diabetes management in children whose brains are still developing are still largely unknown but preliminary findings suggest poorer memory skills, presumably the consequence of recurrent and severe hypoglycemia.

Even in the absence of typical symptoms, cognitive function deteriorates at low BG concentrations. Moderate and severe hypoglycemia is disabling, affects school performance and makes driving a car or operating dangerous machinery hazardous, which should be avoided. Repeated or prolonged severe hyperinsulinemic hypoglycemia can cause permanent CNS damage especially in very young children but, fortunately, hypoglycemia is a rare cause of death in diabetic children.

Nocturnal hypoglycemia

Hypoglycemia, often asymptomatic, frequently occurs during sleep. Moderate and severe hypoglycemia is more common during the night and early morning (before breakfast) than during the daytime. Episodes of hypoglycemia during sleep often exceed 4 h in duration and up to half these episodes may be undetected because the subject does not wake. The incidence of hypoglycemia on any given night may be affected by numerous factors, including the insulin regimen, the timing and content of meals and snacks, and antecedent physical activity. The highest frequency of asymptomatic nocturnal hypoglycemia occurs in children less than 10 years old. Low BG concentrations in the early morning (before breakfast) are associated with a higher frequency of preceding nocturnal hypoglycemia and knowledge of this fact is useful in counseling patients to modify the evening insulin regimen and bedtime snack.

Sleep impairs counter-regulatory hormone responses to hypoglycemia in normal subjects and in patients with diabetes. Because a rise in plasma epinephrine is normally the main hormonal defense against hypoglycemia in patients with diabetes, impaired counter-regulatory hormone responses to hypoglycemia explain the increased susceptibility to hypoglycemia during sleep. Asymptomatic nocturnal hypoglycemia may impair counter-regulatory hormone responses and so may contribute to the vicious cycle of hypoglycemia, impaired counter-regulatory responses and unawareness of hypoglycemia either awake or asleep. Recurrent asymptomatic nocturnal hypoglycemia is an important cause of hypoglycemia unawareness, which, in turn, leads to more frequent and severe hypoglycemia because of failure to experience autonomic warning symptoms before the onset of neuroglycopenia.

Treatment

Except in preschool-aged children, most episodes of symptomatic hypoglycemia are self-treated with rapidly absorbed carbohydrate such as glucose tablets, juices, soft drinks, candy, crackers or milk. Glucose tablets, which raise BG concentrations more rapidly than orange juice or milk, are the treatment of choice for children old enough to chew and safely swallow large tablets.

The recommended dose is 0.3 g of glucose per kg of body weight. BG should be remeasured 15 min after treatment and, if the BG level does not exceed 3.9–4.4 mmol/L (70–80 mg/dL), treatment should be repeated. The glycemic response to oral glucose usually lasts <2 h so, unless a scheduled meal or snack is due within 1 h, the patient should be given either a snack or a meal containing carbohydrate and protein.

Hypoglycemia frequently occurs when a child with diabetes is unable to consume or absorb oral carbohydrate because of nausea and vomiting associated with an intercurrent illness (e.g. gastroenteritis) or oppositional behavior. To maintain BG concentrations in a safe range, parents either seek emergency medical attention or attempt to force feed oral carbohydrate to an ill child, which often leads to more vomiting.

Mini-dose glucagon raises BG by 3.3–5 mmol/L (60–90 mg/dL) within 30 min and its effect lasts approximately 1 h. This method is effective in managing most situations of impending hypoglycemia at home. Using a U100 insulin syringe and after dissolving 1 mg of glucagon in 1 mL of diluent, children <2 years receive 2 'units' (20 μg) of glucagon SC and children older than 2 year, receive 1 unit (10 μg) per year of age up to 15 units (150 μg). If the BG concentration does not increase within 30 min, double the initial dosage should be administered.

Severe reactions (unresponsiveness, unconsciousness or convulsions) require emergency treatment with parenteral glucagon (IM or SC). Glucagon raises BG concentrations within 5–15 min and usually relieves symptoms of hypoglycemia. Symptoms of experimentally induced hypoglycemia in children with diabetes are relieved within 10 min of giving glucagon by either SC or IM injection. Mean BG and plasma glucagon concentrations are slightly but not significantly higher after IM than after SC injection. Both 10 and 20 μg/kg glucagon relieve clinical signs and symptoms but the increment in BG concentration after 10 min is less after a dose of 10 μg/kg. However, after 20 and 30 min, the differences in BG concentrations are not significant. Nausea and/or vomiting occur after the injection in a minority of children who receive a dose of 20 µg/kg but does not often occur after 10 µg/kg. Excessively high plasma glucagon concentrations are more likely to cause nausea and/or vomiting and the recommended dose is 15 µg/kg to a maximum of 1.0 mg.

In children with diabetes and in healthy adults, there appears to be no important difference between the effects of glucagon injected either SC or IM. Plasma glucagon concentrations are higher than those in peripheral venous or portal blood of healthy adults during insulin-induced hypoglycemia and are probably higher than is necessary for maximal effect. The increase in BG concentration after glucagon administration is sustained for at least 30 min. Therefore, it is unnecessary to repeat the dose or force the child to eat or drink for at least 30 min. Intranasal glucagon has a similar effect.

In an emergency department or hospital, the preferred treatment is intravenous glucose (0.3 g/kg). Because the glycemic response is transient after bolus administration of glucose, intravenous glucose infusion should be continued until the patient is able to swallow safely.

If severe hypoglycemia was prolonged and the patient had a seizure, complete recovery of mental and neurological function may take many hours, despite restoration of normal BG concentrations. Permanent hemiparesis or other neurological sequelae are rare but the post-ictal period may be complicated by headache, lethargy, nausea, vomiting and muscle ache.

Driving a motor vehicle

Hypoglycemia increases the rate of driving mishaps among adults with diabetes due to failure to measure the BG level before driving and a lower BG level at which subjects choose not to drive. Driving is impaired at plasma glucose concentrations of <3.3 mmol/L (60 mg/dL).

The adolescent with diabetes who is learning to drive should be counseled always to measure BG before driving and not to drive unless BG is greater than 4 mmol/L (70 mg/dL). Furthermore, patients should be advised to stock the glove compartment with a source of rapidly absorbed carbohydrate and non-perishable snacks and to and stop the car when symptoms of hypoglycemia are detected.

Dead in bed

Sudden unexplained deaths during sleep have been described in adolescents with type 1 diabetes but are rare. Young adult males are at highest risk. Lethal cardiac arrhythmias triggered by hypoglycemia may be responsible for some cases and severe hypoglycemia related to recreational drug abuse may account for others.

Chronic complications of diabetes

Non-vascular complications

Cataracts

Cataracts rarely occur in children with diabetes and, when present at the time of diagnosis, may regress after treatment of diabetes has been instituted.

Limited joint mobility

Limited joint mobility (LMJ), also referred to as cheiroarthropathy, is caused by glycosylation of collagen in the connective tissue of skin and tendons. It manifests as inability to extend the fingers and/or wrists normally because of loss of skin elasticity and contraction of tendons. LMJ is a sign of chronic poor glycemic control and is associated with increased risk of microvascular complications.

Growth

Growth failure in children with diabetes is uncommon even with only 'average' glycemic control. Nonetheless, abnormality of the GH–IGF-I axis is common. With average BG control, GH secretion is increased and serum concentrations of IGF-I and IGF binding protein (BP)-III tend to be reduced. Delayed puberty and growth failure occur typically only when a child or adolescent experiences chronic very poor glycemic control.

Mauriac syndrome (growth failure, delayed puberty, a cushingoid pattern of fat distribution and hepatosteatosis) is thought to be due to recurrent cycles of adequate alternating with inadequate insulinemia.

Skin

Necrobiosis lipoidica diabeticorum is an uncommon poorly understood complication that causes unsightly lesions in the pretibial area. Treatment is generally unsatisfactory but intralesional injection of corticosteroids often results in some improvement.

Disordered eating and eating disorders

Adolescent females with type 1 diabetes have a twofold increased risk of developing an eating disorder compared with their peers without diabetes. Eating disorders are associated with poor metabolic control and earlier onset and progression of microvascular complications. This problem should be suspected in adolescent females who are unable to achieve and maintain BG targets or who have unexplained weight loss or deterioration of metabolic control. Screening should be conducted by asking non-judgmental questions about weight and shape concerns, dieting, episodes of binge eating and insulin omission for the purpose of controlling weight. Patients with eating disorders or deliberate misuse of insulin should receive intensive multidisciplinary care that includes a mental health professional with relevant expertise. Use of a basal–bolus insulin regimen allows increased meal flexibility.

Vascular complications

The vascular complications of diabetes are classified as microvascular (retinopathy, nephropathy and neuropathy) or macrovascular, which include coronary artery, peripheral and cerebral vascular disease. The microvascular complications can develop within 5 years of the onset of type 1 diabetes mellitus but rarely before the onset of puberty. Clinically significant macrovascular complications are virtually never seen until adulthood.

Intensive glycemic control decreases the risk of microvascular disease (retinopathy, nephropathy and neuropathy) but several other modifiable risk factors contribute to the risk of vascular complications. Tobacco considerably increases the risk of onset and progression of retinopathy, nephropathy and macrovascular disease. Hypertension increases risk and rate of progression of retinopathy, nephropathy and macrovascular disease. Dyslipidemia (increased ratio of LDL to HDL cholesterol) greatly contributes to the risk of macrovascular disease and may increase retinopathy. A family history of hypertension or nephropathy increases the risk of nephropathy.

Microvascular

Retinopathy

Damage to the microvasculature of the retina is the most common cause of acquired blindness in economically developed countries. Although improvement in glycemic control delays the onset of retinopathy and retards its progression, nearly all individuals with diabetes eventually develop mild non-proliferative retinopathy which may progress to moderate or severe non-proliferative retinopathy, characterized by abnormal blood flow in the retinal microvasculature.

Proliferative retinopathy, characterized by growth of new vessels, carries a high risk of visual loss due to hemorrhage or retinal detachment. Macular edema may occur at any stage of retinopathy and threaten visual acuity. Screening detects early disease and leads to effective treatment with laser retinal photocoagulation before vision is impaired.

Nephropathy

Diabetes is the most common cause of endstage renal disease in western countries and eventually occurs in 30–40% of persons with type 1 diabetes. Improving glycemic control and treating hypertension delays the onset of nephropathy and slows its progression.

Microalbuminuria, defined as $\geq 30\,mg/day$ or $\geq 20\,\mu g/min$ albumin in the urine, is the earliest stage of clinical nephropathy. Sustained microalbuminuria is highly predictive of progression to overt nephropathy (clinical albuminuria), defined as $\geq 300\,mg/24\,h$ or $\geq 200\,\mu g/min$ albumin in the urine but microalbuminuria may be less predictive in adolescents during the first decade of diabetes.

Overt albuminuria is accompanied by systemic hypertension and progressive impairment of glomerular filtration and typically precedes the development of endstage renal disease by 10 years. Progression of nephropathy can be delayed by improving glycemic control, controlling hypertension and by treatment with an angiotensin-converting enzyme (ACE) inhibitor. If an ACE inhibitor is used, it is important to monitor plasma potassium concentrations.

Neuropathy

Neuropathy resulting from diabetes is rare in children. Early signs include loss of ankle reflexes and decreased vibration sense or touch sensation to monofilament in the great toe. Although sensitive cardiovascular testing may detect subtle autonomic abnormalities in some adolescents with diabetes, they tend to be transient and are of unknown clinical importance. As with other microvascular complications, improvements in HbA1c decrease the risk of onset of neuropathy.

Macrovascular

Both men and women whose diabetes commences in childhood are at high risk of macrovascular disease. Women with type 1 diabetes lose the protective effect of their gender. Although the absolute risk is low until 30 years of age, macrovascular events are the most common cause of mortality in persons with type 1 diabetes and individuals with renal complications have an especially high risk. Other predictors of macrovascular risk and/or progression include dyslipidemia, hypertension and smoking.

It is not yet clear to what extent intensive glycemic control reduces the risk of macrovascular events. Long-term progression of carotid artery intimal thickening is slower in intensively treated patients. Strategies to reduce lifetime risk of macrovascular disease in children with diabetes include avoiding use of tobacco, early and vigorous treatment of hypertension, treatment of dyslipidemia, intensive glycemic control and, of course, a life style of healthy eating and exercise.

Screening for long-term complications

Development of diabetic complications is insidious but can usually be detected years before the patient has symptoms or organ function is impaired. Systematic screening can detect abnormality at an early stage when intervention to arrest, reverse or retard the disease process will have the greatest impact. Diabetic retinopathy is rare before the onset of puberty or in patients who have had type 1 diabetes for <5 years.

An annual dilated retinal examination by an ophthalmologist should begin 3–5 years after diagnosis once the child is age 10 years or older. Temporary rapid progression of retinopathy may occur when metabolic control improves drastically and, in these circumstances, retinal examinations should be performed more frequently.

After the child has had diabetes for 5 years, annual screening for urine albumin and creatinine concentrations should be performed to detect microalbuminuria. Several methods can be used, the most convenient of which is to measure the albumin-to-creatinine ratio in a random spot urine specimen. First-void collections upon arising in the morning avoid the confounding effect of increased albumin excretion induced by upright posture.

Timed collections, either 24h or timed overnight, are more accurate but less convenient than spot samples. Standard hospital laboratory assays for urinary protein are not sufficiently sensitive and measurement should be performed by an assay that specifically detects microalbuminuria. Albumin excretion is transiently elevated by hyperglycemia, exercise and febrile illness. Because of marked day-to-day variability in albumin excretion, microalbuminuria should be confirmed in at least two of three collections over a 3- to 6-month period to establish the diagnosis of diabetic nephropathy and before instituting treatment. Circulatory and neurological complications of diabetes are seldom clinically significant during childhood and adolescence.

In contrast to the above recommendations for type 1 diabetes in children, monitoring lipids, urinary albumin excretion and screening eye examinations should begin at diagnosis in type 2 diabetes.

The first consideration before an endocrine test is arranged is its indication and how its result will inform diagnosis and treatment. A blanket approach is not only often unhelpful but it constitutes an unwarranted assault on a child. The efficacy of endocrine tests depends on the choice of tests, the preparation of the patients, the integrity of the specimens, the quality of the measurements and the validity of the reference data. The measurement of basal hormone concentrations is often of limited use and the investigation of endocrine disorders frequently involves the use of dynamic tests to check the ability of individual axes to respond to suppressive or stimulatory effects of a variety of provocative agents. The performance of such tests is complicated and invariably involves some discomfort and, in certain cases, risk to the patient.

General principles for all endocrine tests

Safety considerations

For all tests, there should be:

- Performance or supervision by a pediatric endocrinologist.
- Detailed knowledge of the particular test protocol and provocative agents.
- Specialized nursing staff familiar with the tests.
  - An environment where full pediatric emergency resuscitation facilities are available.
  - Adjustment of protocols for particular individuals or circumstances.

Handbook of Clinical Pediatric Endocrinology, 1st edition. By Charles G. D. Brook and Rosalind S. Brown. Published 2008 by Blackwell Publishing, ISBN: 978-1-4501-6109-1.

- Appropriate laboratory back-up, particularly for tests involving fasting, induction of hypoglycemia or water deprivation.
- Glucose meters with acceptable accuracy/precision in the hypoglycemic range for immediate glucose monitoring in the testing area.
- A physician readily available and, for certain tests (e.g. insulin hypoglycemia), immediately available.
- Experienced personnel to site intravenous (IV) cannulae.

Patient preparation

1 Confirm (by discussion with a pediatric endocrinologist) that the test to be undertaken is appropriate. Ensure that all relevant baseline tests (endocrine and non-endocrine) have been performed (e.g. renal function tests to exclude renal failure, electrolytes and glucose in suspected adrenal or pituitary disease).

2 Ensure that up-to-date protocols are available in the clinical area, that medical and nursing staff are competent in the performance of the test(s) and briefed on sample collection and transportation to the laboratory.

3 Ensure that liaison has occurred with the laboratory, which is thereby prepared for urgent processing/analysis of samples.

4 Confirm that the patient and parent understand the reasons for the test, the test protocol and that the patient has been suitably prepared (e.g. fasted where this is a requirement of the procedure).

5 Measure the height and weight of the child (essential that this is done on the day of the test) and calculate the correct doses of provocative agents. Surface area can be calculated using the formula:

$$\text{Surface area (m}^2) = \sqrt{\frac{\text{height (cm)} \times \text{weight (kg)}}{3600}}$$

6 Confirm that the dose of the provocative agent has been calculated correctly and checked by another member of staff. Also confirm that the agent has been prepared correctly and that this too has been checked by another member of staff.

Sample collection

Blood

1 Most tests require the insertion of an IV cannula for serial blood sampling. Apply local anesthetic cream (EMLA cream or patch or equivalent) for a minimum of 1 h, clean the site with sterile water and insert the cannula. Maintain patient with a heparin/saline solution (1 U/mL).
2 Collect basal samples, including a sample taken at the time of cannulation (e.g. $t = -60$ min). This is essential as the stress generated by the procedure may be sufficient to stimulate hormone production, which may be followed by a period of quiescence. This has the potential to generate false-positive results if sampling only commences at $t = 0$.
3 Ensure that the correct sample tubes are available and labeled appropriately. The local laboratory will provide a policy indicating minimum requirements for sample labeling, which will include patient ID, ward/clinic, date of test and sample test time (e.g. 0, 30, 60 min).
4 Check the blood volumes required at each time. Additional samples are frequently required at $t = 0$ and volumes may vary at different times throughout the test (e.g. combined pituitary function tests).
5 Complete the request form supplied by your local laboratory legibly and fully, providing information on patient ID, gender, ward/clinic, times of samples, tests requested at each time and clinical details stating indication for tests. Give contact details of the doctor to be contacted in the event of any problem with the samples collected.

Urine

1 Provide written instructions for the patient and parents on how to collect a timed (usually 24 h or overnight) urine sample and ensure that these written instructions are explained verbally and understood.

2 Ensure that the appropriate container (plain or with the correct preservative) is obtained from the local laboratory and supplied to the patient.
3 Ensure that the container is correctly labeled and the accompanying request form is completed in full.

Pituitary

The anterior pituitary gland secretes six known hormones: growth hormone (GH), adrenocorticotrophic hormone (ACTH), luteinizing hormone (LH), follicle-stimulating hormone (FSH), thyroid-stimulating hormone (TSH) and prolactin. Each of these is regulated by releasing or inhibitory hormones from the hypothalamus. A summary of the anterior pituitary hormones and their control is provided in Table 13.1.

The posterior pituitary is responsible for the release of oxytocin and arginine vasopressin (AVP). The principal stimulus for AVP secretion is an increase in plasma osmolality.

Indications for testing pituitary function

There are three broad groups of pediatric patients for whom pituitary function tests are required:
1 Patients with short stature and/or abnormal growth velocity in whom other causes of growth failure (e.g. hypothyroidism, chronic systemic disease, Turner syndrome, skeletal disorders) have been excluded.
2 New patients with suspected hypopituitarism. This includes patients with target organ failure not associated with appropriate elevation of the relevant pituitary trophic hormone, patients with suspected

Table 13.1 Hormones of the anterior pituitary gland and their control.

Cell type	Hormone	Hypothalamic hormone
Thyrotroph	TSH	TRH (if available) (+)
		Somatostatin (−)
Corticotroph	ACTH	CRH (+)
Gonadotroph	LH/FSH	GnRH (if available) (+)
Somatotroph	GH	GHRH (+)
		Somatostatin (−)
Lactotroph	Prolactin	Dopamine (−)
		TRH (if available) (+)

(+) stimulatory, (−) inhibitory.

diabetes insipidus (DI), patients presenting with clinical features of hypothalamo-pituitary tumors (e.g. headaches, visual failure), patients with optic nerve hypoplasia or septo-optic dysplasia and patients in whom a hypothalamic–pituitary mass is found incidentally during the course of radiological investigations.

3 Patients with known hypothalamo-pituitary disease in whom an evolving endocrine deficit is anticipated. This group mainly comprises patients who have received radiotherapy for a pituitary tumor.

Anterior pituitary

Growth hormone deficiency

The diagnosis of GH deficiency (GHD) in childhood requires clinical and auxological assessment, combined with biochemical tests of the GH insulin-like growth factor (IGF) axis and radiological evaluation. The components of the GH–IGF axis are depicted in Fig. 13.1. GHD may present as an isolated problem or in combination with multiple pituitary hormone deficiency (MPHD). Criteria to initiate immediate investigation for GHD have been defined and include:

1 Severe short stature, defined as a height more than 3 SD below the mean.

2 Height more than 1.5 SD below mid-parental height.

3 Height more than 2 SD below the mean and a height velocity over 1 year more than 1 SD below the mean for chronological age or a decrease in height SD of more than 0.5 over 1 year in children over 2 years of age.

4 In the absence of short stature, a height velocity more than 2 SD below the mean over 1 year or more than 1.5 SD sustained over 2 years.

5 Signs of an intracranial lesion.

6 Signs of MPHD.

7 Neonatal symptoms and signs of GHD (e.g. hypoglycemia, prolonged jaundice).

Single GH estimations are rarely helpful in diagnosing or excluding GHD. Hence, a variety of provocation tests have been used. There is no "gold standard" test against which biochemical tests can be evaluated. GH secretion is a continuum from normality to complete deficiency so defining the point at which mild GH insufficiency becomes normality is not possible. Arbitrary cutoffs have been used, which define inadequate GH secretion

as a peak GH concentration during a stimulation test of <15 or 20 mU/L (10 ng/mL in the USA).

All provocation tests have poor specificity (50–80%) with a high incidence of false positives. In an attempt to overcome this problem, it has been common practice to carry out two tests either separately or sequentially but the outcome of this is merely to compound the errors. Alternative approaches to assessing GH secretion have proved either too demanding (e.g. 12- or 24-h GH profiles) or to offer no advantage in terms of predictive value (e.g. urinary GH). It has been argued that provocative tests are reliable only in patients in whom the clinical signs and symptoms are clear and that they should be abandoned. However, guidelines on the use of human GH in children with growth failure recommend the performance of provocation tests to support the clinical diagnosis of GHD.

Stimulation tests may be combined with one or more other measures of the GH axis, namely IGF-I and/or IGF binding protein-III (IGFBP-III) to improve diagnostic efficiency.

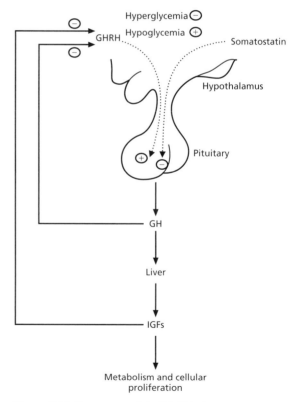

Figure 13.1 Components of the GH–IGF axis.

Sex steroid priming

In peripubertal children who have a subnormal response to provocative testing, sex steroid priming may increase the response to that seen in late puberty and should be considered because of the estrogen-induced rise in GH during puberty.

Oral ethinylestradiol should be given (20 mg in the evening) to girls daily for 3 days and the test carried out on day 4. Be aware that ethinylestradiol will almost certainly cause nausea. In boys, give testosterone (as enanthate, cypionate or mixed esters (e.g. Sustanon)) 100 mg intramuscularly (IM) as a single injection 5–7 days before the test.

Insulin tolerance test

Background

Insulin-induced hypoglycemia suppresses the somatostatin tone and stimulates the α-adrenergic receptors. It induces not only GH but also ACTH release and a rise in serum cortisol concentrations. The advantage of the insulin tolerance test (ITT) is that, in addition to stimulating GH secretion, it also tests the integrity of the entire hypothalamo-pituitary–adrenal axis. This test has been associated with morbidity and mortality, mainly because of the use of inappropriate amounts of hyperosmolar fluid to correct hypoglycemia. The decision to undertake an ITT should be considered carefully.

Precautions

1 The test is contraindicated in children with diagnosed epilepsy or a history of unexplained blackouts and in children <2 years of age, for whom a glucagon provocation test may be more appropriate.
2 Hypothyroidism impairs the GH and cortisol response. Patients with adrenal and thyroid insufficiency should have corticosteroid replacement commenced before thyroxine, as thyroxine may precipitate an adrenal crisis. The insulin provocation test may need to be repeated after 3 months of thyroxine therapy in patients with confirmed thyroid or dual insufficiency.
3 Special precautions are required in children suspected of having panhypopituitarism.
4 IV 10% dextrose (never 50%) must be immediately available.

5 A glucose meter with acceptable performance in the hypoglycemic range must be available and staff performing the test must be certified competent to use it.

Preparation

1 Check that thyroid function tests are normal.
2 Prime with sex steroids if indicated.
3 The child should be fasted for 8 h before the test, only water is allowed.
4 The child should be weighed prior to the test, in order to calculate accurately the dose of insulin to be administered.
5 Insert IV cannula (see section on blood collection) and maintain patent with heparinized normal saline. The stress of cannulation can cause an increase in GH, making interpretation of the test difficult. After cannulation, wait for 30–60 min before commencing the test and take a blood sample at −30 min to aid interpretation if the basal sample is found to be elevated.

Protocol

1 $t = -30$ min; take blood (plain tube) for GH and cortisol estimation.
2 $t = 0$ min; give soluble insulin 0.10–0.15 U/kg IV, using the lower dose if there is a strong suspicion of panhypopituitarism or if the child has had previous cranial surgery or radiotherapy. The dose may need to be increased in patients with diabetes mellitus, insulin resistance or obesity.
3 Take samples as shown in Table 13.2. Measure glucose concentrations on the glucose meter but also send a sample to the laboratory for urgent analysis.
4 Observe child closely for clinical signs and symptoms of hypoglycemia (e.g. sweating and drowsiness).
5 The results can be interpreted only if adequate hypoglycemia has been achieved. This is defined as a laboratory glucose half the fasting value or <2.2 mmol/L (40 mg/dL). If there have been no clinical signs of hypoglycemia by 45 min, the dose of insulin should be repeated and the test continued with blood samples timed again from 0 min.
6 Once hypoglycemia has occurred, the child should be given glucose drinks. If the child remains persistently hypoglycemic or loses consciousness or fits, he/she should be treated with an IV bolus of 200 mg/kg glucose (2 mL/kg 10% dextrose) over

Table 13.2 Sampling for ITT.

Time (min)	Meter glucose	Laboratory glucose (fluoride oxalate tube)	GH (plain tube)	Cortisol (plain tube)
−30 (before insulin)	+	+	+	+
0 (before insulin)	+	+	+	+
30	+	+	+	+
45	+	+	+	+
60	+	+	+	+
90	+	+	+	+
120	+	+	+	+

3 min followed by an IV infusion using 10% dextrose at 2.4–4.8 mL/kg/h (4–8 mg/kg/min glucose). Check glucose concentrations on the glucose meter after 4–5 min and adjust dextrose infusion to maintain blood glucose at 5–8 mmol/L (90–144 mg/dL). If there is no improvement in conscious concentration after normal glucose concentration is restored, an alternative explanation should be sought. Do not stop sampling.

7 If panhypopituitarism is suspected, give 100 mg of hydrocortisone IV at the end of the test or earlier if recovery from hypoglycemia is slow.

8 The child must not be sent home until an adequate high-carbohydrate meal has been eaten without vomiting and the blood glucose has been maintained at 4 mmol/L (145 mg/dL) for a minimum of 2 h.

9 This test may be conducted as part of a combined ITT/thyrotrophin-releasing hormone (TRH) (if available)/gonadotropin-releasing hormone (GnRH (if available)) pituitary function test, in which case the sampling protocol is shown in Table 13.3.

Interpretation

Interpretation is not possible unless adequate hypoglycemia has been achieved.

A GH concentration of >20 mU/L (10 ng/mL in the USA) excludes GHD but there is no precise cutoff. Biochemical data must be interpreted in conjunction with clinical and auxological data in order to make decisions about GH treatment in an individual patient. Combining the test with measurement of IGF-I and its binding proteins is one approach that has been recommended to aid the decision in patients

Table 13.3 Sampling for combined ITT/TRH (if available)/ GnRH (if available) test.

	Glucose	Cortisol	GH	LH	FSH	TSH
−30	+	+	+			
0	+	+	+	+	+	+
Give soluble insulin 0.10–0.35 U/kg, GnRH (if available) 2.5 mg/kg, TRH (if available) 5 mg/kg IV						
30	+	+	+	+	+	+
45	+	+	+			
60	+	+	+	+	+	+
90	+	+	+			
120	+	+	+			

Additional samples at 0 min: prolactin, free thyroxine, testosterone or estradiol.

with peak GH concentrations in the partially deficient range (>7.5 but <15 mU/L, >3 but <10 ng/mL).

Interpretation of the cortisol response is possible only if hypothyroidism has been excluded. An adequate cortisol response is defined as a peak concentration of >550 nmol/L (20 µg/dL). Patients with peak concentrations <550 (20) but >400 nmol/L (15 µg/dL) may need steroid cover only for major illnesses and stress.

Glucagon stimulation test

Background

Glucagon stimulates the release of GH and ACTH by a hypothalamic mechanism and therefore indirectly stimulates cortisol secretion. The test is useful for the assessment of GH and cortisol reserve in children <2 years and others in whom the ITT is contraindicated. The timing of the peak GH response depends on whether the glucagon is injected IV or IM. Subcutaneous administration is not recommended because absorption is unreliable.

Precautions

1 The test is contraindicated in patients suspected of having pheochromocytoma or hyperinsulinism and is unreliable in patients with diabetes mellitus.
2 As for the ITT, hypothyroidism impairs the GH and cortisol response.
3 Glucagon may cause nausea, vomiting and abdominal pain.

Preparation

As for the ITT.

Protocol

1 $t = -30$ min; take blood (plain tube) for GH and cortisol estimation.
2 $t = 0$ min; give glucagon IV or IM 20 mg/kg up to a maximum of 1 mg.
3 Take samples as shown in Table 13.4.
4 In children with suspected hypopituitarism, prolonged fasting may induce hypoglycemia. Blood glucose should be checked using a glucose meter in these patients whenever a sample is taken for GH/cortisol. If the patient shows signs/symptoms of hypoglycemia, send an urgent sample to the laboratory for glucose analysis.

Table 13.4 Sampling for glucagon stimulation test.

Time (min)	Meter glucose	GH (plain tube)	Cortisol (plain tube)
−30 (before glucagon)	+	+	+
0 (before glucagon)	+	+	+
60	+	+	+
90	+	+	+
120	+	+	+
150	+	+	+
180	+	+	+

5 If hypoglycemia is confirmed, treatment should be instigated as described for the ITT.
6 This test may be performed as a combined glucagon/TRH (if available)/GnRH (if available) pituitary function test.

Interpretation

For interpretation of GH and cortisol concentrations, see ITT.

Arginine stimulation test

Background

The injection of various amino acids (e.g. ornithine, arginine) is followed by an increase in GH concentrations in blood. Arginine stimulates GH secretion by reducing somatostatin tone and possibly by stimulation of α-adrenergic receptors with GHRH release.

Precautions

1 Hypothyroidism impairs the GH response.
2 Arginine may cause nausea and some irritation at the infusion site.
3 Vomiting has been described in a few patients.

Preparation

As for the ITT.

Protocol

1 $t = -30$ min: take blood (plain tube) for GH estimation.
2 $t = 0$ min; give arginine 0.5 g/kg up to a maximum of 30 g. This is given by infusion IV of a 10% solution of arginine monochloride in 0.9% NaCl at a constant rate over 30 min.
3 Take samples at 15 min intervals to 60 min and then at 90 and 120 min.
4 In children with suspected hypopituitarism, blood glucose should be checked as described in the glucagon stimulation test protocol.
5 This test may be performed as a combined arginine/TRH (if available)/GnRH (if available)/synacthen (Cosyntropin) dynamic function test.

Interpretation

For interpretation of peak GH concentrations, see ITT. Usually, the peak GH concentration is reached about 60 min after staring the arginine infusion.

Measurement of IGF-I and IGF binding proteins

GH action is mediated via the production of IGF-I and -II. Hepatic synthesis of these growth factors is mainly regulated by GH and severe GHD is associated with a reduction in their concentrations. IGF-I circulates bound to IGFBP-III.

IGF-I and IGFBP-III concentrations in the circulation are valuable markers of GH insufficiency and are frequently used as an adjunct to provocative testing. Their concentrations are more stable and their circulating half-lives are much longer than GH itself, although concentrations are affected by nutritional status, liver and renal disease, hypothyroidism, diabetes mellitus and sex steroids. Studies have shown the markers to have high specificity but low sensitivity so low concentrations are highly indicative of GHD but normal concentrations do not necessarily exclude the diagnosis. In cases of congenital (Laron syndrome) and acquired GH insensitivity, GH concentrations are elevated and IGF-I and IGFBP-III concentrations very low. IGF-I and IGFBP-III concentrations are highly method dependent and are affected by age, sex and pubertal status. Comprehensive reference ranges must be developed locally to enable data to be interpreted.

IGF-I generation test

Indication

Diagnosis of congenital or acquired GH insensitivity. The former is usually due to a defect in the GH receptor but may also be the result of defective intracellular GH signaling. Conditions that may result in acquired GH insensitivity include malnutrition and liver disease.

Patient preparation

Ensure that nutritional intake is adequate prior to and during the performance of this test.

Protocol

1 Day 1: take blood for IGF-I and IGFBP-III estimation.
2 Days 1–4: give SC GH (0.1 IU/kg/day=33 μg/kg/day).
3 Day 5: take blood for IGF-I and IGFBP-III estimation.

Interpretation

An incremental increase in IGF-I of >20 mg/L and IGFBP-III of >0.4 mg/L above the baseline excludes GH insensitivity.

Radiological investigations in growth failure

Radiological investigations are indicated when GHD has been identified and also if clinical symptoms suggestive of a pituitary lesion are present, e.g. persistent early morning headaches, visual disturbance and/or field defect or overt hypopituitarism without explanation. High-resolution computed tomography (CT) or magnetic resonance (MR) scanning can be used. Midline calcification on CT scan is highly suggestive of craniopharyngioma. Structural abnormalities within the midline, as demonstrated by MR scan, are most commonly due to septo-optic dysplasia, a condition frequently associated with pituitary dysfunction. Reduced anterior pituitary height, an attenuated or interrupted pituitary stalk and/or an ectopically positioned posterior pituitary are all associated with pituitary dysfunction. Germinomas may occur in the hypothalamic region – tumor marker concentrations (α-fetoprotein and β-hCG) are key to the diagnosis of these tumors.

A radiological skeletal survey may diagnose a skeletal dysplasia if body proportions suggest this as a possibility for short stature.

Growth hormone excess

Growth hormone excess presenting as pituitary gigantism or juvenile acromegaly is rare and is caused by a GH-secreting pituitary adenoma in most instances. Most tall children are not suffering from a pathological condition but all children with an unexplained height velocity >97th centile over 1 year or >75th centile over 2 years require investigation. It is important to assess whether growth is disproportionate, since this is more commonly associated with an underlying genetic syndrome.

Single random GH measurements are not a reliable diagnostic indicator of GH excess because of the sporadic nature of GH secretion and its increase in response to stress may result in an abnormally high random GH concentration in a normal patient. IGF-I and IGFBP-III concentrations are elevated in GH excess. IGF-I concentrations are less variable than GH concentrations and it has been proposed that they should be used as a screening test for GH hypersecretion. Confirmation of the diagnosis must be made on the basis of failure of GH to suppress during an oral glucose tolerance test (OGTT).

Hyperprolactinemia

Any process that interferes with dopamine synthesis, disrupts the hypothalamo-pituitary connection or prevents dopamine binding to its receptors can cause hyperprolactinemia. The etiology of hyperprolactinemia is diverse and includes drugs, stress, pituitary tumors, polycystic ovary syndrome (PCOS) and primary hypothyroidism. Drugs include tricyclic antidepressants, phenothiazines, metaclopramide, methyldopa and reserpine. Pituitary tumors are an important cause of hyperprolactinemia – they may be prolactin-secreting tumors or non-functioning pituitary tumors that secondarily increase prolactin concentrations by interfering with the transport of dopamine.

Radiological evaluation is necessary in all cases of hyperprolactinemia. Skull radiographs may be abnormal because of an expanded fossa associated with the empty sella syndrome and high-resolution CT should be performed in all patients with abnormal plain skull radiographs and elevated serum prolactin concentrations.

Secretion of prolactin is pulsatile and at least three measurements are required to make the diagnosis. Serum thyroxine and TSH concentrations should be measured to exclude hypothyroidism. Interpretation of raised concentrations of prolactin is difficult but some guidelines are defined in Table 13.5. In the case of prolactinomas, the serum prolactin concentration generally correlates with the size of tumor. If the CT scan shows a large pituitary tumor but the serum prolactin concentration is only mildly elevated, this suggests that the tumor is non-secretory.

Other releasing hormone tests

TRH test (Note: TRH not available in US)

Indications
1 Investigation of secondary hypothyroidism.
2 Differentiation of TSH-secreting pituitary tumors and the pituitary variant of resistance to thyroid hormones (TSH and thyroxine are elevated in both these conditions).

Precautions
1 TRH may cause minor side-effects including flushing, a desire to micturate, headache, abdominal and chest discomfort, nausea and a metallic taste in the mouth.

Table 13.5 Guidelines for interpretation of serum prolactin concentrations.

Prolactin concentration (mU/L) (×0.05 for ng/mL)	Interpretation
<425	Normal
425–1000	Suggest repeat sample Does not normally indicate serious pathology
1000–2000	Suggest repeat sample The raised prolactin concentration may be secondary to stress, drugs, PCO, hypothalamic disorders, GH hypersecretion, primary hypothyroidism or chronic renal failure Patients with 'non-functioning' pituitary tumors often have a serum prolactin in this range
2000–4000	Suggestive of microprolactinoma or a hypothalamic disorder Drug treatment is less likely to give this degree of prolactin elevation but is possible
4000–6000	Likely to be a prolactinoma or possibly a hypothalamic disorder
>6000	Almost always indicates the presence of a macroprolactinoma

2 TRH can also cause smooth muscle spasms, so caution must be exercised in patients with asthma or ischemic heart disease.

Preparation
Thyroxine and triiodothyronine therapy must be stopped for 3 weeks prior to the test. The patient does not need to be fasted (unless TRH combined with a test of GH secretion).

Protocol
1 $t = 0$ min: insert a reliable cannula and take blood samples for TSH and free thyroxine (plain bottle).
2 Give a bolus dose of TRH, 5 mg/kg IV (up to a maximum of 200 mg).
3 $t = 20, 60$ min: take blood samples for TSH and free thyroxine.

4 This test may be performed as combined ITT/TRH/ GnRH, glucagon/TRH/GnRH and arginine/TRH/ GnRH/synacthen (Cosyntropin) dynamic function tests. The sampling protocols are shown in Table 13.3.

Interpretation

1 In normal individuals, a rise in TSH concentration at 20 min with a fall at 60 min is observed.

2 Basal TSH: 0.5–5.0 mU/L.

3 Increment: 5–25 mU/L.

4 A blunted response is seen in hypopituitary disease.

5 A slightly increased basal concentration with a delayed and exaggerated response (60 min value higher than 30 min) is suggestive but not conclusive of hypothalamic hypothyroidism.

6 In TSH-secreting pituitary tumors, the response is flat whereas a brisk response is obtained in thyroid hormone resistance.

GnRH test (Note: GnRH not available in the USA; use leuprolide as below)

Indications

1 Investigation of hypogonadotrophic hypogonadism suspected prepubertally.

2 Investigation of precocious puberty.

3 Monitoring of children with precocious puberty treated with GnRH analogs.

Precautions

GnRH may rarely cause nausea, headache and abdominal pain.

Preparation

No specific patient preparation is required. Patient does not need to be fasted (unless GnRH is combined with a test of GH secretion).

Protocol

1 $t = 0$ min: insert a reliable cannula and take blood samples for LH, FSH, testosterone or estradiol and sex hormone binding globulin (plain bottles).

2 Give a bolus dose of GnRH, 2.5 mg/kg IV (up to a maximum of 100 mg).

3 $t = 20, 60$ min: take blood samples for LH/FSH.

4 This test may be performed as combined ITT/TRH/ GnRH, glucagon/TRH/GnRH and arginine/TRH/

GnRH/synacthen (Cosyntropin) dynamic function tests. The sampling protocols are shown in Table 13.3.

Note: In the USA, where GnRH is not available, leuprolide can be used (20 μg/kg, maximum 500 μg) and blood samples drawn at 0, 60, 120 and 180 min.

Interpretation

1 In normal prepubertal children, there is an incremental rise in LH of 3–4 U/L and in FSH of 2–3 U/L above the basal concentration.

2 In peripubertal children, higher increments, especially if LH dominant, provide evidence of a pubertal pattern of gonadotropin response.

Pubertal delay and pubertal failure In children with suspected hypogonadotrophic hypogonadism, lack of response supports the diagnosis. A low response has limited predictive value. In gonadal failure, the basal LH/FSH is elevated and the response to GnRH (if available) exaggerated.

Precocious puberty In gonadotropin-independent precocious puberty (and in the presence of excess endogenous or exogenous sex steroids), spontaneous gonadotropin secretion is suppressed by the autonomous sex steroid secretion, basal LH/FSH concentrations are low and response to GnRH flat.

In gonadotropin-dependent precocious puberty, basal LH/FSH concentrations are elevated and response to GnRH exaggerated.

Precocious puberty (treated) Suppressed basal LH/FSH and a flat response to GnRH indicate adequate treatment with GnRH analogs.

Corticotrophin-releasing hormone test

Indications

1 Differentiation of hypothalamic and pituitary causes of secondary adrenal insufficiency.

2 Differentiation of Cushing syndrome (pituitary vs. ectopic).

3 In conjunction with petrosal sinus sampling, to confirm pituitary ACTH-dependent Cushing disease.

Precautions

Corticotrophin-releasing hormone (CRH) may cause mild facial flushing, marked transient hypotension and occasional allergy.

Preparation

The patient should not be on steroid therapy. Prednisolone must be discontinued for 3 days and hydrocortisone for 24 h prior to the test. If steroid cover is essential, switch to dexamethasone, which does not interfere with the test.

The patient should be fasted from midnight.

If both CRH and high-dose dexamethasone test are to be performed, the CRH test should be completed first.

Protocol

1 An indwelling cannula should be inserted 30 min before the test.
2 $t = -15$ min (before administration of CRH): take blood samples for cortisol (plain tube) and ACTH. ACTH samples must be collected into a plastic lithium heparin tube and sent to the laboratory immediately on ice.
3 $t = 0$ min (before administration of CRH): take blood samples for cortisol and ACTH. Give CRH IV 1 mg/kg (up to a maximum of 100 mg) over 30 s.
4 Take further blood samples for cortisol and ACTH at $+15$, $+30$, $+45$, $+60$, $+90$, $+120$ min after CRH.
5 This test may be performed as combined GHRH/ TRH/GnRH/CRH stimulation test. The sampling protocols are shown in Table 13.8.

Interpretation

ACTH peaks at about 30 min and cortisol at 45–60 min after CRH administration. Reported normal responses vary and should therefore be established locally.

Secondary adrenal insufficiency A flat ACTH and cortisol response to CRH is consistent with a pituitary cause whereas, in hypothalamic disease, the ACTH response is delayed and exaggerated.

Cushing syndrome Patients with pituitary Cushing disease typically show an exaggerated response with an increase in ACTH >50% above the basal concentration and an increase in cortisol concentration >20% above the basal concentration. In ectopic causes of Cushing syndrome, the basal ACTH is high but there is no response to CRH. The false-negative rate of the test (i.e. patients with pituitary Cushing disease who do not show the typical response) is 10–15%. It should be noted that, because of the overlap between the response in control subjects and patients with

Cushing disease, the CRH test must not be used for initial diagnosis of Cushing syndrome.

Petrosal sinus sampling combined with CRH A central-peripheral ACTH ratio of >2 basally and >3 after CRH stimulation is necessary to diagnose Cushing disease with confidence.

Posterior pituitary
(See Chapter 8, page 146).

Diabetes insipidus

A patient with a differential diagnosis that includes DI will by definition complain of polyuria and polydipsia. The first step should be to confirm polyuria. An early morning paired blood and urine osmolality should be checked. If the plasma osmolality is high and the urine osmolality low, the diagnosis of DI is made without further tests.

Polyuria may have other causes (e.g. diabetes mellitus or renal failure). Plasma urea and electrolytes, glucose and calcium should be measured, which may reveal hypokalemia, hypercalcemia, hyperglycemia or renal impairment.

Water deprivation/desamino-D-arginine vasopressin test

Background/indication

1 To determine the urine-concentrating ability in patients with polydipsia and polyuria.
2 To investigate suspected DI and differentiate from compulsive water drinking (CWD) (psychogenic polydipsia).
3 The water deprivation test measures urine-concentrating ability, which is lost in patients with DI but maintained in CWD. Pituitary and nephrogenic DI may be differentiated by giving a test dose of desamino-D-arginine vasopressin (DDAVP).

Precautions

1 This test must be arranged in advance with the local laboratory as it requires their close collaboration. Osmolality values are required urgently on all specimens collected.
2 Care must be taken in patients in whom the likelihood of DI is very high. Tests on these patients must be started later.
3 Thyroid and adrenal reserve must be normal or adequately replaced.

4 The patient must be kept under close surveillance throughout the test to avoid surreptitious water drinking and monitored for any signs of dehydration. If 5% weight loss or extreme distress occurs, the test must be terminated and DDAVP (5 mg intranasally or 0.3 mg IM) and free fluids given immediately.

Preparation The night before the test, take blood for urea, electrolytes and osmolality. If the osmolality is >300 mosmol/kg, the water deprivation test must not be undertaken because the diagnosis has already been made.

If the test is to proceed, weigh the patient undressed, record the weight and insert a reliable IV cannula.

Protocol

1 Stop all fluid intake at 24.00 h (or later in infants or in patients who are polyuric or borderline hyperosmolar).

2 If there is a high index of suspicion of DI in a child <2 years, fluid restriction should commence in the morning.

3 At 09.00 h, weigh the child again undressed and record the weight. Collect blood and urine for osmolality. Send specimens to the laboratory immediately.

4 Continue to weigh the child hourly. Ensure that the child is undressed on each occasion.

5 Collect blood and urine samples for osmolality if possible each time the child is weighed. Liaise with the laboratory throughout.

6 The test is normally continued until midday or until:
- The urine osmolality exceeds 600 mosmol/kg (or 500 mosmol/kg in infants).
- 5% of initial weight is lost.
- Plasma osmolality exceeds 300 mosmol/kg.

7 It may be necessary to prolong the test in CWD, especially if the child has been drinking excessively prior to the start.

8 At 12.00 h or when the test is terminated, take blood samples for urea, electrolytes and osmolality.

9 If urine osmolality remains below 600 mosmol/kg, proceed with the DDAVP test.

Protocol DDAVP test

1 Allow the patient to drink but not excessively or a dilutional hyponatremia may ensue. Fluid intake should be no more than twice the volume of urine passed during fluid restriction.

2 Give DDAVP 5 mg intranasally or 0.3 mg IM.

3 Collect blood and urine samples for osmolality hourly (if possible) for the next 4 h.

Interpretation In normal subjects, the plasma osmolality does not exceed 295 mosmol/kg and the urine osmolality rises to above 600 mosmol/kg (urine: plasma osmolality >2:1).

Central (cranial) DI: Plasma osmolality >295 mosmol/kg with inappropriately dilute urine (<300 mosmol/kg). DDAVP produces a normally concentrated urine.

Nephrogenic DI: As for central DI but DDAVP fails to increase urine osmolality more than 100 mosmol/kg.

Partial DI: Patients have moderate elevation of plasma osmolality and urine osmolality typically between 300 and 600 mosmol/kg.

It is important to exercise caution in interpretation of the test. Any patient with a prolonged polyuria from any cause will have some impairment of urine-concentrating ability because of medullary washout. The majority of patients under investigation will have either central DI or CWD. Patients with CWD often have low serum osmolality at the start of the test but otherwise may behave similarly to patients with partial cranial DI. In difficult cases, the plasma and urine AVP measurements on samples taken at the end of the water deprivation may aid diagnosis. However, a hypertonic saline infusion test with serial plasma AVP measurement may be necessary to differentiate the two conditions.

Adrenal axis (see Chapter 6, page 99)

Adrenocortical insufficiency

There are a number of abnormalities of routine laboratory tests that provide clues to the diagnosis of adrenal insufficiency. In primary adrenal insufficiency, hyponatremia, hyperkalemia and acidosis are common consequences of aldosterone deficiency. Hyponatremia also occurs in secondary adrenal insufficiency but is due, in this case, to cortisol deficiency, increased AVP secretion and water retention.

Other laboratory abnormalities associated with adrenal insufficiency include hypoglycemia, hypercalcemia (rare), mild normocytic anemia, lymphocytosis and mild eosinophilia. Basal early morning cortisol concentrations (between 08.00 and 09.00 h) may be useful in establishing a diagnosis. Morning plasma cortisol concentrations of <138 nmol/L (5 μg/dL) are highly suggestive of adrenal insufficiency, whereas concentrations >525 nmol/L (20 μg/dL) rule out the disorder. Random cortisol concentrations are of no value except in a patient suffering from acute illness requiring intensive care when a concentration of >700 nmol/L (25 μg/dL) probably rules out adrenal insufficiency.

Simultaneous measurement of cortisol and ACTH identifies most patients with primary adrenal insufficiency – ACTH concentrations are high while cortisol concentrations are low. Normal plasma ACTH rules out primary but not mild secondary, adrenal insufficiency.

Adrenal cortex antibodies should be measured in all cases of biochemically confirmed primary adrenal insufficiency. In boys who are antibody negative, serum concentrations of very long-chain fatty acids should be measured to exclude adrenoleukodystrophy.

Short synacthen (Cosyntropin) test

Indications
1 Screening test for suspected adrenal insufficiency.
2 Investigation of non-classical congenital adrenal hyperplasia (CAH).

Precautions
1 Severe allergic reactions to synacthen have been described, particularly in children with a history of allergic disorders but are very rare.
2 The dose of synacthen used is excessive and only of value in assessing severe adrenal insufficiency. The standard short synacthen test is insensitive to minor degrees of adrenal suppression (e.g. in children with asthma on inhaled steroid).
3 The test is unreliable if performed within 4 weeks of pituitary surgery as ACTH deficiency may not have been sufficiently prolonged to result in adrenal atrophy.

Preparation
The patient does not need to be fasted.

All steroid therapy (other than dexamethasone or betamethasone) interferes with the assay of cortisol. If the patient is on prednisolone therapy, this must be discontinued for 3 days prior to the test; hydrocortisone must be discontinued for 24 h. If steroid cover is essential, switch to a maintenance dose of dexamethasone.

Insert a reliable cannula and rest patient for 30 min.

Protocol
1 $t = 0$ min: take basal blood samples for cortisol and 17-hydroxyprogesterone (17-OHP) (if test is for investigation of non-classical CAH).
2 Give synacthen (ACTH 1–24) IV 250 μg (or 36 μg/kg for children <1 year old).
3 Take further blood samples for cortisol and 17-OH progesterone (if indicated) at +30, +60 min after administration of synacthen.

Interpretation
1 Plasma cortisol concentration at 30 min should be >550 nmol/L (20 μg/dL). It is extremely important that the 30-min concentration is used for interpretation. There is a significant difference between cortisol responses at 30 min compared with 60 min. Only the 30 min value has been validated against the ITT and use of the 60-min value can give misleading interpretation. It should also be noted that the use of a cutoff of 550 nmol/L (20 μg/dL) is somewhat arbitrary and was established using earlier studies in which cortisol was measured by a fluorimetric method. Cortisol values are highly method dependent and bias differences between methods do not show consistency at different time points. There are greater method-related differences in specimens taken after synacthen, probably due to release of steroids (other than cortisol), which cross-react to different degrees in different assays. Where possible, locally derived decision concentrations should be defined, which should be reassessed with any change in methodology.
2 An impaired response does not distinguish between adrenal and pituitary failure, as the adrenal glands may be atrophied secondary to ACTH deficiency. Traditionally, the long synacthen test has been used to distinguish between primary and secondary adrenal failure but, with the improved availability and reliability of ACTH assays, this test has become redundant.
3 Patients with pituitary-dependent cortisol insufficiency require dynamic testing of the pituitary

gland. Use of the CRH test may allow differentiation of hypothalamic and pituitary causes of secondary adrenal insufficiency.

4 A normal 17-OHP response to synacthen is an incremental increase of <10 nmol/L (3 μg/L) above the basal concentration at 60 min. Patients with late-onset or non-classical CAH show an incremental increase of >20 nmol/L (6 μg/L), while heterozygotes have an intermediate response with considerable overlap into the normal range.

Low-dose (1 μg) synacthen (Cosyntropin) test

Background/indications

This is a modified version of the short synacthen test, which uses a physiological rather than a pharmacological dose of synacthen. It may be indicated in children who have a normal response to the standard short synacthen test but a clinical history (e.g. chronic steroid therapy) or symptoms (e.g. hypoglycemia) suggesting adrenocortical insufficiency.

Preparation

The patient does not need to be fasted.

All steroid therapy (other than dexamethasone or betamethasone) interferes with the assay of cortisol. If the patient is on prednisolone therapy, this must be discontinued for 3 days prior to the test; hydrocortisone must be discontinued for 24 h. If steroid cover is essential, switch to a maintenance dose of dexamethasone.

Insert a reliable cannula and rest patient for 30 min.

Protocol

1 Prepare 1 μg solution of synacthen from 250 μg vial as follows:
   – Dilute 1–50 mL with normal saline giving 250 μg in 50 mL.
   – Take 1 mL of above solution and dilute with 9 mL of saline giving 5 μg in 10 mL.
2 $t = 0$ min: take basal blood samples for cortisol.
3 Administer 2 mL of above solution (1 μg of synacthen) to patient IV.
4 Flush the line with 5 mL of saline to ensure that the whole dose has been administered.
5 Take further blood samples for cortisol at +20, +30 and +40 min after administration of synacthen.

Interpretation

1 Normal response is a peak cortisol concentration of >550 nmol/L (20 μg/dL), which may occur at 20, 30 or 40 min. The definition of this cutoff may vary locally and is influenced by the particular cortisol assay as for the standard short synacthen test.

2 Peak concentrations below the defined cutoff indicate a degree of adrenal insufficiency.

Assessment of glucocorticoid replacement therapy

Adequate assessment of patients on glucocorticoid replacement therapy is important to avoid the consequences of undertreatment (e.g. poor response to stress, electrolyte disturbances) or overtreatment (e.g. glucose intolerance, hypertension, osteoporosis). Twenty-four-hour urine free cortisol (UFC) concentrations can be used as an initial screen to detect overreplacement but a full detailed assessment of therapy requires a day curve. Day curves are often performed in children with CAH when 17-OHP concentrations are also measured.

Hydrocortisone day curve

Preparation

1 Omit the morning dose of hydrocortisone until the first sample has been taken.
2 There is no requirement for the patient to be fasted.
3 Insert an IV cannula at 08.00–08.30 h.

Protocol

1 At 09.00 h, collect blood sample for cortisol estimation.
2 Administer morning dose of hydrocortisone.
3 Collect blood sample at 10.00 h and then at 2-hourly intervals until 24.00 h for cortisol estimation. Administer hydrocortisone therapy according to the patient's normal regime.

Interpretation

The aim is to achieve adequate concentrations throughout the day, avoiding excessive peaks after each dose. The trough concentrations before each dose should not be below 100 nmol/L (3.6 μg/dL).

Laboratory tests for detection and monitoring of CAH

Diagnosis of CAH relies mainly on the measurement of plasma concentrations of 17-OHP. Most pediatric cases of 21-hydroxylase deficiency have grossly elevated concentrations (typically 300–800 nmol/L, 100–250 μg/L): unaffected neonatal concentrations are <15 nmol/L. In late-onset or non-classical CAH, concentrations may be only marginally elevated and it may be necessary to measure the response of 17-OHP to synacthen stimulation in order to make a diagnosis. Modest increases in 17-OHP can also occur in deficiencies of 11μ-hydroxylase and 3μ-hydroxysteroid dehydrogenase. Stressed normal newborn babies may have 17-OHP concentrations as high as 100 nmol/L (30 μg/L) and this, together with interference in the assay by fetal adrenal zone steroid sulfates, can lead to diagnostic confusion if 17-OHP is measured in the first few days after birth.

Assays for plasma/serum 17-OHP exhibit large and consistent differences in bias; it is essential therefore that laboratories employ reference ranges appropriate to their assay. Elevated plasma 11-deoxycortisol concentrations (>60 nmol/L, 2 μg/L) are found in 11β-hydroxyslase deficiency and androstenedione is raised in both 21-hydroxylase and 11β-hydroxylase deficiencies. CAH may be confirmed by urinary steroid metabolite profile, which will also identify the site of the block from the pattern of metabolites.

Biochemical monitoring of CAH patients on treatment should include blood spot 17-OHP to assess glucocorticoid replacement and plasma renin or plasma renin activity (PRA) to assess mineralocorticoid replacement.

Urinary steroid profile

Background/indication

A urine steroid profile examines many steroid metabolites simultaneously and provides specific diagnostic information. It is useful for investigating adrenal and gonadal tumors and as an aid in the diagnosis of children with ambiguous genitalia, precocious puberty, premature adrenarche, abnormal virilization and salt-losing states. It can also assist in the differential diagnosis of Cushing syndrome, hypertension and adrenal suppression.

Protocol

For quantification of urinary steroid excretion rates, a 24-h collection is required. Where this is difficult, a spot or random urine collection will in most cases still be helpful as the finding of abnormal proportions of specific metabolites may allow biosynthetic defects to be identified. A sample of 20 mL of urine should be collected into a plain tube for analysis.

If the child is on hydrocortisone replacement, switch to dexamethasone and inject a depot preparation of synacthen (Cosyntropin) before urine collection. In this way, the patient can be controlled while stimulating the adrenal to secrete large amounts of steroids, which are excreted in urine.

In children with suspected 5α-reductase deficiency, the ratio of 5α to 5β metabolites can be measured in urine after stimulation of androgen by human chorionic gonadotropin (hCG).

Interpretation

1 CAH
 – *21-Hydroxylase deficiency* – in newborn urine, many unusual derivatives of 17-OHP are found, several products being hydroxylated at C-15. In patients >6 months of age, there are three major peaks (17-hydroxypregnenolone, pregnanetriol and 11-oxo-pregnanetriol).
 – *11β-hydroxylase deficiency* – elevated tetrahydro-11-deoxycortisol (THS) and 6-hydroxy-THS.
 – *3β-hydroxysteroid dehydrogenase deficiency* – excess dehydroepiandrosterone (DHEA) and pregnenolone; cortisol metabolites very low or absent.
 – *17α-hydroxylase deficiency (rarely presents in childhood)* – corticosterone metabolites elevated; adrenal androgen and cortisol metabolites absent.
 – *Lipoid adrenal hyperplasia* – no steroids in urinary steroid profile.

2 Tumors of the adrenal gland
 – Excess of adrenal androgen and/or cortisol metabolites.

3 Defects in testosterone biosynthesis or action
 – *5α-reductase deficiency* – low 5α:5β ratio.
 – 17-Ketosteroid reductase deficiency – high ratio androsterone:etiocholanolone.

4 Hypertension
 – *CAH* – 11β-hydroxylase deficiency, 17α-hydroxylase deficiency.
 – *11β-hydroxysteroid dehydrogenase deficiency (converts cortisol to inactive cortisone)* – excess of tetrahydrocortisol:tetrahydrocortisone.
 – *Dexamethasone-suppressible hyperaldosteronism* – high excretion of 18-hydroxycortisol and 18-oxo-cortisol.

5 Defects of aldosterone synthesis or action
  – Aldosterone biosynthetic defects.
  – 18-Hydroxylase deficiency – high concentrations of corticosterone.
  – 18-Oxidation defects – high concentration of 18-hydroxycorticosterone with low plasma aldosterone concentrations.
  – Defects of aldosterone action.
  – High aldosterone and 18-hydroxycorticosterone concentrations.
6 Adrenal suppression
  – From a 24-h urine collection the sum of individual cortisol metabolites in the urine can be calculated. This can give a better indication of adrenal suppression in patients on inhaled steroids in whom plasma cortisol concentrations are equivocal.
7 Cushing syndrome
  – Due to adrenal tumors – excess adrenal androgen metabolites will be detected. Steroid pattern can be used to detect recurrence following resection.
  – Due to ectopic ACTH-secreting tumor – total steroid output much higher than in Cushing disease or adrenal tumor. Increased cortisol:cortisone metabolites.

Adrenal hyperfunction

Cushing syndrome (Fig. 13.2)

Examination of the circadian rhythm of cortisol secretion (24.00 and 08.00 h) and 24-h UFC estimations are useful preliminary investigations prior to provocative tests. A single sleeping midnight cortisol, 48 h after admission to hospital and asleep prior to venipuncture, of <50 nmol/L (2 μg/dL) excludes a diagnosis of Cushing syndrome. UFC measurements have the advantage of providing an integrated measure of cortisol secretion. The test has a sensitivity of 95% but, in order to attain this, requires multiple collections (ideally four but a minimum of two) from each patient. Many assays lack specificity, with a large number of urinary metabolites exhibiting significant cross-reactivity; it is essential to ascertain that the local laboratory employs an extraction step prior to measurement of urinary cortisol.

Dexamethasone suppression tests

Dexamethasone is a synthetic glucocorticoid many times more potent than cortisol. It suppresses ACTH by negative feedback; consequently, cortisol production falls to very low concentrations. Patients with Cushing syndrome lose the normal negative feedback control and cortisol fails to suppress.

Overnight dexamethasone suppression test

Background/indications
The test can be performed as an outpatient investigation and, as a result, is widely used as a screening test. It has good diagnostic sensitivity but poor specificity; hence, all patients who fail to suppress will require a formal low-dose dexamethasone suppression test (LDDST).

Precautions
1 The patient should not be on steroid therapy or suffering from major infection or psychological stress.
2 Patients on enzyme-inducing drugs, e.g. anticonvulsants and rifampicin, may rapidly metabolize dexamethasone and give a false-positive result, i.e. no suppression. Ideally, these drugs should be stopped for several weeks prior to investigation.

Preparation
None required.

Protocol
1 Patient takes dexamethasone (15 mg/kg) orally at 23.00 h.
2 At 09.00 h the following morning, a sample is collected for plasma/serum cortisol. Plasma cortisol normally falls after 09.00 h and false-positive tests may occur if blood sampling is delayed.

Interpretation
1 A normal response is suppression of 09.00 h cortisol to <50 nmol/L (2 μg/dL), which excludes Cushing syndrome.
2 All patients who fail to suppress should undergo a formal LDDST.

Low-dose dexamethasone suppression test

Indications
Diagnosis of Cushing syndrome.

Precautions/preparation
As for overnight dexamethasone suppression test.

Protocol
1 Day 1: take blood samples for cortisol and ACTH at 09.00 and 24.00 h. Note that ACTH is unstable, should be collected in plastic tubes (it adheres to glass) and normally requires immediate transportation to the

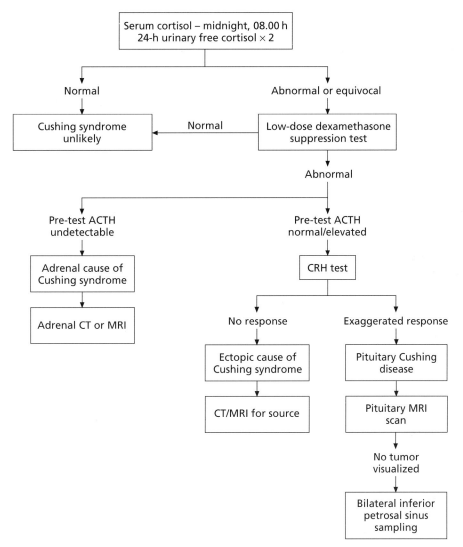

Figure 13.2 Flow chart for the investigation of Cushing's syndrome.

laboratory on ice. Contact the local laboratory for precise details regarding specimen collection and transportation.

2 Days 2 and 3: give oral dexamethasone 0.5 mg (or 10 μg/kg/dose in children <10 years) strictly 6 hourly.

3 Day 4: collect blood at 09.00 h for cortisol estimation.

Interpretation

In normal individuals, cortisol concentrations suppress to <50 nmol/L (2 μg/dL).

Patients with Cushing syndrome, from whatever cause, exhibit detectable plasma cortisol concentrations

after dexamethasone administration. Very rarely, patients with Cushing syndrome show normal suppression and, if there is a high index of suspicion in such cases, the patient should be investigated further.

In patients who fail to suppress, a pretest ACTH of <5 ng/L is highly suggestive of an adrenal cause of Cushing syndrome.

Differential diagnosis of Cushing syndrome

Plasma ACTH concentrations

ACTH measurement is the first step in the differential diagnosis of Cushing syndrome. Patients with adrenal tumors or non-ACTH bilateral adrenal hyperplasia (very rare) will have undetectable plasma ACTH. In these patients, proceed directly to CT or MRI scanning of the abdomen to localize the lesion.

High-dose dexamethasone suppression test

Indications To differentiate pituitary-dependent and ectopic causes of Cushing syndrome.

Precautions/preparation As for overnight and LDDST.

Protocol

1 Day 1: take blood samples for cortisol and ACTH/ACTH precursors at 09.00 and 24.00 h.
2 Days 2 and 3: give oral dexamethasone 2 mg (or 40 μg/kg/dose in children <10 years) 6 hourly.
3 Day 4: take blood at 09.00 h for cortisol measurement.
4 LDDST and HDDST may be performed sequentially if desired.

Interpretation Plasma cortisol suppresses to 50% or less of the basal value in pituitary-dependent Cushing syndrome (Cushing disease) but not in adrenal tumors. However, approximately 10% of patients with Cushing disease fail to suppress, whereas 10% of those with ectopic ACTH secretion will suppress.

ACTH precursor concentrations may be helpful in the diagnosis: elevated concentrations in patients previously diagnosed with Cushing syndrome suggest ectopic secretion.

Corticotrophin-releasing hormone (CRH) test See anterior pituitary.

Mineralocorticoid deficiency and excess

Background The adrenal cortex is also concerned with the maintenance of normal sodium homeostasis via the renin–angiotensin–aldosterone axis. The major disorders that are associated with abnormalities of this axis are summarized in Table 13.6.

Investigation of the axis is indicated:

• When a patient presents with hypertension and hypernatremia.
• When a patient presents with salt loss.
• To assess the control of a disease associated with salt loss, e.g. congenital adrenal hypo- or hyperplasia, isolated mineralocorticoid deficiency, Addison disease.

Table 13.6 Disorders associated with the renin–angiotensin–aldosterone axis.

Disorder	Renin	Aldosterone
Conn syndrome	Lowered	Raised
Renal artery stenosis	Raised	Raised
Bartter syndrome	Raised	Raised
Renin-secreting tumors	Raised	Raised
Pseudohypoaldosteronism	Raised	Raised
Primary aldosterone deficiency	Raised	Lowered
Secondary aldosterone deficiency	Lowered	Lowered
CAH	Raised	Lowered

Protocol Baseline tests include plasma sodium, potassium, creatinine, bicarbonate and pH, together with the measurement of sodium, potassium and creatinine concentrations in a 24-h urine. Ambulant and recumbent PRA and aldosterone should be measured. The tests should ideally be performed before and after a 3–5 day low-sodium diet (10–20 mmol/day).

Interpretation In mineralocorticoid deficiency due to Addison disease, CAH or congenital adrenal hypoplasia, the plasma aldosterone concentration is low with an elevated PRA. Pseudohypoaldosteronism is associated with high PRA and high plasma aldosterone concentration. If a low-sodium diet fails to reduce urinary sodium excretion to less than 20 mmol/day, a trial of fludrocortisone should be given and sodium excretion reassessed. Fludrocortisone will have no effect in the case of pseudohypoaldosteronism but will reduce sodium excretion in all cases of true mineralocorticoid deficiency.

In primary hyperaldosteronism (Conn syndrome), hypernatremia, hypokalemia, hyperkaluria and alkalosis are associated with an elevated plasma aldosterone and a suppressed PRA.

Gonadal axis

Testis

In inborn errors of testosterone biosynthesis, demonstration of precursor hormones immediately prior to the block is key to making a diagnosis. In 5α-reductase deficiency, the ratio of testosterone to dihydrotestosterone (DHT) is elevated, in 17β-hydroxysteroid dehydrogenase, there is an increase in androstenedione:testosterone and in 3β-hydroxysteroid dehydrogenase deficiency, the concentration of DHEA is elevated. The measurement of basal testosterone is also of value in the investigation of hypogonadism in late adolescence when subnormal concentrations indicate a need for further investigation. In other situations in the pediatric patient, basal gonadal steroids may be undetectable and further investigation requires hCG stimulation.

hCG stimulation test

Indications

1 To detect functioning testicular tissue (e.g. in undescended testes or cryptorchidism).
2 To define enzyme blocks in testosterone biosynthesis.

Precautions/preparation
None.

Protocol

1 Between 08.00 and 09.00 h (day 1), collect baseline samples for testosterone. Collect samples for androstenedione and DHT if a biosynthetic defect is suspected.
2 Immediately following collection of baseline blood samples, give hCG IM as follows: 500 IU if weight <5 kg; 1000 IU if weight between 5 and 10 kg; 1500 IU if weight between 10 and 15 kg; 3000 IU if weight above 15 kg.
3 Repeat blood samples 72 h after hCG injection (day 4) for testosterone (plus androstenedione and DHT if indicated).
4 Collection of 24-h urine samples before and after hCG stimulation for measurement of steroid metabolites may be useful in investigation of defects in testosterone biosynthesis.

Interpretation
The normal testosterone response depends on the age of the patient. In infancy, a normal testosterone increment may vary from 2- to 10- or even 20-fold. During childhood, the increment is between 5- and 10-fold. During puberty, as the basal concentration is higher, the increment is less, i.e. 2- to 3-fold.

Testosterone will respond normally to hCG in cases of complete or partial androgen insensitivity or in 5α-reductase deficiency. In 5α-reductase deficiency, the ratio of testosterone (T) to DHT is elevated following hCG stimulation and this may be helpful in cases in which basal T/DHT ratios are not diagnostic.

A T/DHT ratio >27 after hCG stimulation suggests 5α-reductase deficiency.

An absent response with an exaggerated LH/FSH response to LHRH stimulation indicates primary gonadal failure or anorchia. If there is a defect in testosterone biosynthesis, there will be an increase in precursor steroid secretion following hCG stimulation.

Prolonged hCG stimulation test

If there is no response to the short hCG test, a more prolonged test may be performed. hCG (2000 IU) is administered twice-weekly for 3 weeks. A 5- to 10-fold increment from the basal testosterone constitutes a normal response. The size of the phallus should be recorded at the start and on completion of the test to assess whether there has been an increase.

Ovary

Unfortunately, current estradiol assays are insufficiently sensitive to enable the use of basal estradiol to detect failure of the ovary to produce the hormone in childhood. There is also no good or reliable dynamic test comparable to the hCG stimulation test for testicular endocrine function in boys. Laboratory tests are of value in polycystic ovarian disease in which ovarian insufficiency occurs together with hyperandrogenism.

Polycystic ovarian disease

The PCOS phenotype may include three major components: anovulation, hyperandrogenism and hyperinsulinemia. However, the clinical presentation is variable and not all components are necessarily present. Insulin resistance is a common finding in PCOS independent of obesity. Hormonal tests are an essential component of the workup for a patient suspected of having the syndrome. Table 13.7 summarizes the key endocrine investigations and changes that are consistent with PCOS.

Table 13.7 Key endocrine investigations and changes in PCOS.

Endocrine test (serum/plasma)	Nature of abnormality in PCOS
LH/FSH	Increased LH concentrations, LH/FSH ratio >2
Androgens	Increased testosterone and androstenedione
SHBG	Decreased
Free androgen index	Increased
Estradiol and estrone	Increased
Prolactin	Often moderately increased
Fasting insulin	Increased
Insulin response to OGTT	Increased

Disorders of puberty

(see Chapter 4, page 59)

Thyroid axis (see Chapter 5, page 84)

Hypothyroidism

Investigation of infants and older children with suspected hypothyroidism requires measurement of plasma fT_4 or total T_4 and TSH. A reduction in T_4 with a rise in TSH indicates primary hypothyroidism. Elevated TSH with a normal T_4 is defined as 'subclinical' hypothyroidism. Measurement of T_3 is not generally helpful as T_3 may be only slightly reduced in patients with hypothyroidism because of increased peripheral conversion of T_4 to T_3. 'Non-thyroidal illness' also commonly causes a reduction in the concentration of T_3.

Secondary hypothyroidism (caused by hypothalamo/pituitary disease) is indicated by a low T_4 and a normal or low TSH, although this picture is also frequently seen in patients with 'non-thyroidal illness" or in those on corticosteroid or anticonvulsant drug therapy. In patients with suspected secondary hypothyroidism, a TRH (if available) test will confirm the diagnosis and is helpful in distinguishing hypothalamic and hypopituitary causes (see anterior pituitary section).

Some laboratories have a strategy of measuring only TSH as a first-line test in all samples from patients under investigation for thyroid disorders. It is important to be aware that this strategy will fail to recognize secondary hypothyroidism and, if this is to be excluded, a T_4 concentration should be specifically requested. TSH measurements should be used for monitoring patients with hypothyroidism on T_4 replacement therapy – a TSH at the lower end of the reference range usually coincides with an optimal symptomatic response. Suppressed concentrations are consistent with overreplacement with associated potential deleterious effects on bone. Measurement of antithyroid antibodies is helpful in establishing the etiology of hypothyroidism. Antibodies to thyroglobulin or thyroid peroxidase (microsomal antibodies) are typically strongly positive in Hashimoto's thyroiditis.

Hyperthyroidism

TSH is the single most useful test in confirming the diagnosis of hyperthyroidism. Plasma TSH concentrations are suppressed (0.1 mU/L) except in cases of a TSH-secreting pituitary tumor or thyroid hormone resistance. Low but detectable concentrations of TSH may be found in 'subclinical hyperthyroidism,' and suppressed (and sometimes undetectable) TSH concentrations can also be found in 'non-thyroidal illness.' In most cases of suspected hyperthyroidism, a suppressed TSH in combination with a raised tT_4 or fT_4 confirms the diagnosis and T_3 measurement is superfluous. T_3 measurement is however indicated when TSH is suppressed in the presence of a normal T_4, in order to diagnose T_3 toxicosis. T_3 measurements are valuable in monitoring treatment of hyperthyroidism, as elevated concentrations indicate persistent thyroid hormone excess, despite normal or even subnormal T_4 concentrations.

Detection of TSH receptor antibodies (TRAb) in the serum of patients with hyperthyroidism is useful for establishing a diagnosis of Graves' disease in those patients in whom the clinical picture is unclear. Unfortunately, most assays are unable to distinguish antibodies with stimulating activity (found in Graves' disease) from those with blocking activity. Radioiodine uptake used to be a first-line procedure in the investigation of hyperthyroidism. It is no longer performed universally in all patients but may still be of value for the identification of 'hot' nodules.

Thyroid cancer

Serum concentrations of thyroglobulin are useful for long-term follow-up of patients treated for differentiated thyroid cancer. Thyroglobulin concentrations should be undetectable in patients who have had total thyroid ablation and detectable concentrations indicate persistent or recurrent disease. It is important that samples analyzed for thyroglobulin are also screened for the presence of antithyroglobulin antibodies because, if present, these will interfere with thyroglobulin quantitation, most commonly leading to falsely low results.

Calcitonin measurement is increased in medullary thyroid cancer and, thus, serum calcitonin should be measured in patients with a family history of this condition (see multiple endocrine neoplasia (MEN)).

Calcium, parathyroid and vitamin D

(See Chapter 7, page 123).

Endocrine pancreas

Hypoglycemia
(See Chapter 10, page 172).

Hyperglycemia
(See Chapter 12, page 189).

Obesity

(See Chapter 11, page 179).

Oral glucose tolerance test

Indications

1 *Tall stature*
The OGTT may be used to assess whether a tall, rapidly growing child has pituitary gigantism. In pituitary gigantism, as in acromegaly, GH secretion is persistently elevated and is not suppressed by the ingestion of an oral glucose load. A paradoxical GH response to the administration of TRH is often seen and for this reason a TRH test may be used in the assessment of children with tall stature, although the response is variable in normal children in puberty and so lacks specificity.

2 *Hypoglycemia*
Glucose leads to secretion of insulin from the pancreas. If there is abnormal regulation of insulin release, e.g. PHHI, there is an exaggerated release of insulin in response to the glucose load, and insulin secretion fails to switch off in spite of the blood glucose concentrations returning to normal values, leading to rebound hypoglycemia.

3 *Insulin insensitivity*
The diagnosis of diabetes mellitus is not often in doubt in childhood, and GTT are rarely needed. An OGTT may be used to assess insulin insensitivity, which is rarely symptomatic in children, in a number of situations:
- obesity,
- acanthosis nigricans,
- PCOS,
- insulin receptor defects,
- children with a strong family history of insulin resistance.

Contraindications
None.

Special precautions
The test is hazardous in children with hyperinsulinism, in whom excessive insulin secretion may lead to rebound hypoglycemia.

Patient preparation
1 The child should have had a normal balanced diet for at least 5 days prior to the test. The child should be fasted from midnight. Drinks of water are allowed. Small children should be encouraged to have a late snack during the evening before the test.
2 On admission to the ward, the child should be assessed clinically, and local anesthetic cream should be applied over the proposed IV access site.
3 The weight of the child should be recorded at admission.
4 30 min after the application of the local anesthetic cream, an IV cannula should be inserted using as large a gauge device as possible. It is important to

Table 13.8 Sampling for a GTT.

Time (min)	−30	0	30	60	90	120	150	180
BM stix	☐	☐	☐	☐	☐	☐	☐	☐
Glucose	☐	☐	☐	☐	☐	☐	☐	☐
GH[a]	☐	☐	☐	☐	☐	☐	☐	☐
Insulin[b]	☐	☐	☐	☐	☐	☐	☐	☐

[a]When assessing children for tall stature.
[b]Liaise with laboratory in advance.

realize that the stress of cannulation can cause an increase of GH that may make interpretation of the results difficult. Therefore, after insertion of the cannula, a period of 1 h should elapse before the commencement of the study.

Test procedure

An oral glucose load is administered at a dose of 1.75 g/kg (maximum 75 g). This calculation may result in a relatively low dose of glucose in the very obese and this must be taken into consideration.

Sampling

See Table 13.8.

In certain situations, C-peptide measurements can be helpful in suspected hyperinsulinism because the half-life of C-peptide is much longer than that of insulin. Proinsulin and insulin split products may also be of use in some circumstances.

IGF-I and IGFBP-III should be measured in children being investigated for tall stature.

Interpretation

1 Tall stature (GH response).
During the OGTT, the serum GH concentration should become undetectable after 30 or 60 min of the test. As the studies are often carried up to 180 min, a slight increase in serum GH concentrations can often be observed toward the end of the test (i.e. at the 150- and 180-min samples) as glucose concentrations decline secondary to the excessive secretion of insulin.
2 Hypoglycemia
Usually in children with hyperinsulinism. Continue sampling at 30-min intervals until 300 min, or even longer if required.

3 Insulin insensitivity
Diagnosis of diabetes
Fasting plasma glucose >7.0 mmol/L (130 mg/dL) and/or 2-h sample >11.1 mmol/L (200 mg/dL).
Diagnosis of impaired glucose tolerance
Fasting plasma glucose <7.0 mmol/L (130 mg/dL) and 2-h sample >7.8 (140 mg/dL) and <11.1 mmol/L (200 mg/dL).
Diagnosis of impaired fasting glycemia
Fasting blood glucose >6.1 (110 mg/dL) and <7.0 mmol/L (130 mg/dL).

The homeostatic model assessment (HOMA) provides a measure of basal insulin resistance

$$\text{HOMA-IR} = \frac{\text{fasting insulin (mU/L)} \times \text{fasting glucose (mmol/L)}}{22.5}$$

Lower HOMA-IR values indicate greater insulin sensitivity, whereas higher HOMA-IR values indicate lower insulin sensitivity (insulin resistance). Although the HOMA-IR is simple and practical, it suffers from the major disadvantage that it is based on measurements of basal glucose and insulin, whereas in a significant proportion of individuals with insulin resistance, the fasting insulin concentrations are normal but stimulated insulin concentrations are raised.

A simple approach to assessing stimulated insulin secretion is to undertake insulin measurements at 0 and 30 min in a standard 75 g OGTT and to calculate the ratio of the 30-min increment in insulin concentration to the 30-min increment in glucose concentration. This has been shown to correlate with the first-phase insulin response in an IV GTT.

Procedure at the end of test

1 Lunch should be provided for the child, who should not be sent home until an adequate meal has been taken and the BM is stable, because of the risk of rebound hypoglycemia.
2 The IV cannula should be left *in situ* until lunch has been completed.
3 Ascertain that the child has an outpatient appointment for review of the results.

Multiple endocrine neoplasia

MEN syndromes are characterized by the presence of tumors involving two or more endocrine glands. They

Table 13.9 Characteristic tumors in MEN syndromes.

Type	Characteristic tumors
MEN1	**Parathyroid glands**
	Pituitary
	Gland prolactinomas (most common)
	GH secreting (much less common)
	Pancreatic islets
	Insulinoma
	Glucagonoma
	Gastrinoma
	VIPoma
	PPoma
	Other associated tumors
	Adrenal cortical
	Carcinoid
	Lipomas
	Thyroid adenomas
MEN2A	MTC
	Pheochromocytoma
	Parathyroid
MEN2B	MTC
	Pheochromocytoma
	Associated abnormalities
	Ganglioneuromatosis
	Marfanoid habitus
Familial MTC	MTC

may be inherited in an autosomal-dominant fashion or may occur sporadically as a result of somatic mutations. There are two major forms of MEN – types 1 and 2 (which is further subdivided into types 2A and 2B). Each type is characterized by the occurrence of tumors in specific endocrine glands (Table 13.9), although 'overlap' syndromes may occur, which feature a combination of tumors from both types. Familial medullary thyroid carcinoma (MTC) may also occur without any additional endocrinopathy. The MEN syndromes commonly present clinically in early adulthood or later but may cause significant disease in childhood. Genetic and biochemical testing has a key role in these conditions – it identifies those children in affected families who are at risk of developing the disorder and allows close monitoring and, where appropriate, early surgical intervention in those at-risk individuals.

Pentagastrin stimulation test
(*Note*: pentagastrin not available in the USA)

Background
Medullary carcinoma of the thyroid secretes excess calcitonin, the hormone normally secreted by thyroid parafollicular (C) cells to lower plasma calcium. Sometimes, patients with C-cell disease may have a normal basal plasma calcitonin and basal calcitonin concentration may be increased in patients other than those with MTC. Therefore, calcitonin secretion following pentagastrin stimulation has been used as a diagnostic test of calcitonin hypersecretion.

Indication
1 For screening families with clinical symptoms of MEN2 in whom no RET mutation has been identified.
2 Post-operative follow-up of patients with C-cell hyperplasia or MTC.
3 To monitor patients with lowest risk mutations in whom thyroidectomy has been postponed.

Precautions
Pentagastrin may cause chest tightness, abdominal cramping and nausea.

Preparation
The fasting plasma calcium should be measured to exclude hypocalcemia. The patient should be fasted and an IV cannula inserted.

Protocol
1 0 min: collect plasma sample for baseline calcitonin estimation.
2 Inject pentagastrin 0.5 mg/kg in 2 mL of saline IV over 10–20 s.
3 Take a further sample for pentagastrin at 3, 5, 10, 15 and 20 min after administration of pentagastrin.

Interpretation
Assay characteristics and reference ranges of laboratories measuring calcitonin are different and should not be compared. It is important to liaise with the laboratory regarding appropriate local values and test interpretation. An exaggerated response suggests a diagnosis of medullary carcinoma of the thyroid,

Table 13.10 Molecular genetics of endocrine disorders (this list is far from exhaustive and is growing rapidly).

Disorder	Defective gene
Transcription factors in endocrine development	
Septo-optic dysplasia/pituitary hypoplasia	HESX1
Pituitary hypoplasia with GH, prolactin, TSH and gonadotropin deficiency	PROP-1
Pituitary hypoplasia ± GH, prolactin and TSH deficiency	POU1F1 (PIT1)
Congenital adrenal hypoplasia	DAX1
XY sex reversal	øSRY, WT1, SF-1, SOX9
X-linked Kallmann syndrome	KALIG-1
Congenital hypothyroidism	TTF1, TTF2, PAX8
Defects in hormone biosynthesis	
Isolated GHD	GH-1
IUGR with poor postnatal growth	IGF-I
Cranial DI	Prepro-AVP-NPII
CAH	CYP21A2, CYP11A1, CYP11B1, CYP11B2, StAR, 3b-HSD2, CYP17
Ambiguous genitalia	17,20-lyase, 17β-hydroxysteroid dehydrogenase, 5α-reductase, LH receptor
Defects associated with abnormalities of hormone secretion	
Tall stature	Aromatase, estrogen receptor
Persistent hyperinsulinemic hypoglycemia of infancy	SUR-1, Kir 6.2, glucokinase, glutamate dehydrogenase hepatic nuclear factor-4α, glucokinase
MODY	Hepatic nuclear factor-1α, insulin promoter factor-1, hepatocyte nuclear factor-1β
Hypoparathyroidism	PTH
Familial hypocalciuric hypercalcemia	Calcium-sensing receptor
Beckwith–Wiedemann	Loss or imprinting of 11p15 region (H19, p57KIP2 and IGF-II genes)
Li–Fraumeni	p53
MEN1	MENIN
MEN2	RET proto-oncogene
Obesity	POMC, PC1, LEPTIN
Prader–Willi syndrome	70% paternal 15q11–q13 deletion, 25% maternal uniparental disomy, 5% imprinting defect
Vitamin D-resistant rickets type 1	25-Hydroxylase, 1α-hydroxylase
Polyglandular autoimmune syndrome	APECED
Defects in hormone receptor	
GH resistance (Laron-type dwarfism)	GH receptor
GHD with pituitary hypoplasia	GHRH receptor
Hypogonadotrophic hypogonadism	GnRH (if available) receptor
Delayed puberty	FSH-β, LH-β
Thyroid hormone resistance	TR-β receptor
Nephrogenic DI	V_2 receptor, aquaporin 2 gene
Androgen insensitivity	Androgen receptor
McCune–Albright syndrome	Gsa
Familial male precocious puberty	LH receptor
Insulin resistance	Insulin receptor
Familial glucocorticoid deficiency	ACTH receptor
Obesity	Leptin receptor, MC4R
Pseudohypoparathyroidism type 1α	Gsa

although both false positives and false negatives may occur. Following total thyroidectomy, basal and stimulated calcitonin concentrations should be maintained within the reference range. A high basal concentration or an exaggerated response to stimulation suggests recurrence of the disease.

Molecular genetic analysis

Table 13.10 lists some disorders in which DNA analysis can be useful. The list is not exhaustive and is growing rapidly.

Appendix 1: Syndrome-Specific Growth Charts

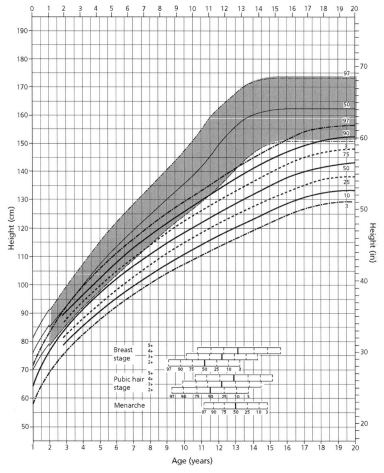

Figure A1.1 Height centiles for girls with untreated Turner syndrome aged 1–20 years. The gray-shaded area represents the 3rd to 97th centiles for normal girls. Pubertal staging is for normal girls. Adapted from Lyon A, Preece M, Grant D. Growth curves for girls with Turner syndrome. *Arch Dis Child* 1985; 60: 932–5.

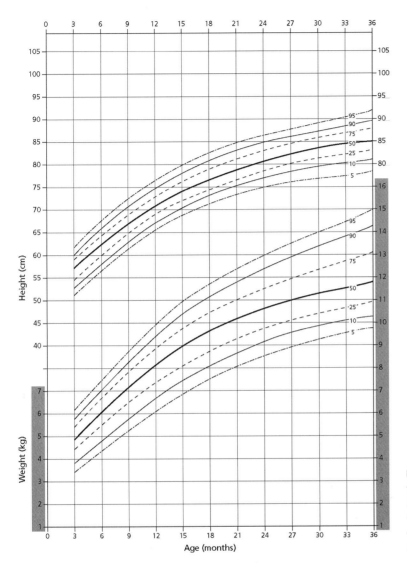

Figure A1.2 Height and weight centiles for boys with trisomy 21 syndrome aged 3–36 months. Adapted from Cronk C, Crocker A, Peushel S *et al*. Growth charts for children with Down syndrome. *Pediatrics* 1988; 81: 102–10.

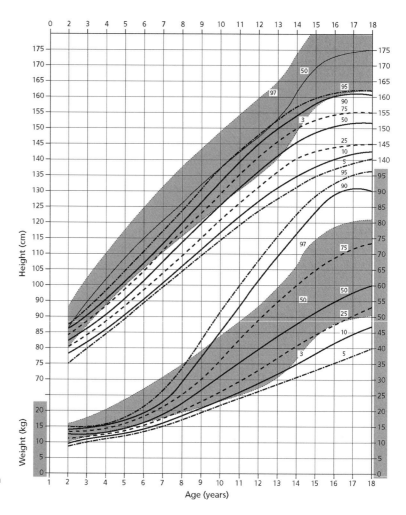

Figure A1.3 Height and weight centiles for boys with trisomy 21 syndrome aged 2–18 years. The gray-shaded areas represent the comparable values for the 3rd to 97th centiles for normal children. Adapted from Cronk C, Crocker A, Peuschel S *et al*. Growth charts for children with Down syndrome. **Pediatrics** 1988; 81: 102–10.

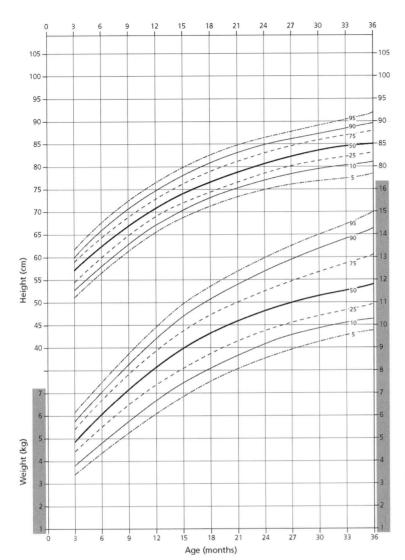

Figure A1.4 Height and weight centiles for girls with trisomy 21 syndrome aged 3–36 months. Adapted from Cronk C, Crocker A, Peuschel S *et al*. Growth charts for children with Down syndrome. *Pediatrics* 1988; 81: 102–10.

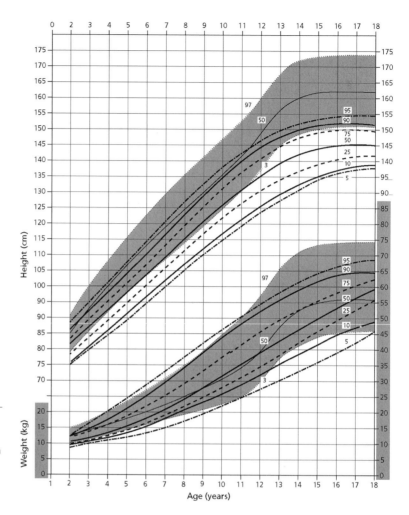

Figure A1.5 Height and weight centiles for girls with trisomy 21 syndrome aged 2–18 years. The gray-shaded areas represent the comparable values for the 3rd to 97th centiles for normal children. Adapted from Cronk C, Crocker A, Peuschel S *et al.* Growth charts for children with Down syndrome. *Pediatrics* 1988; 81: 102–10.

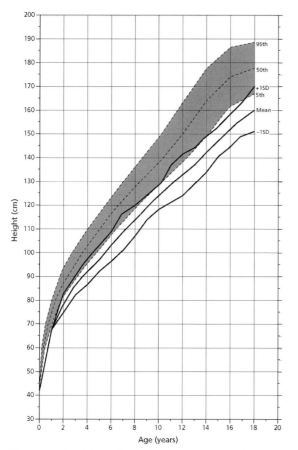

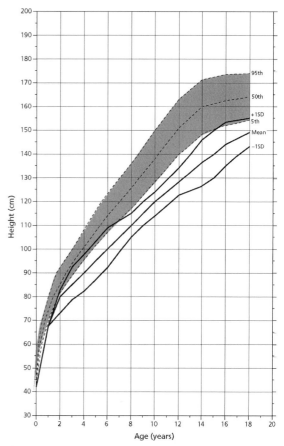

Figure A1.6 Height centiles for boys with Noonan syndrome aged 0–18 years compared with normal values (dashed lines). The data were obtained from 64 Noonan syndrome males in a collaborative retrospective review. Adapted from Witt D, Keena B, Hall J *et al*. Growth curves for height in Noonan syndrome. *Clin Genet* 1986; 30: 150–3.

Figure A1.7 Height centiles for girls with Noonan syndrome aged 0–18 years compared with normal values (dashed lines). The data were obtained from 48 Noonan syndrome females in a collaborative retrospective review. Adapted from Witt D, Keena B, Hall J *et al*. Growth curves for height in Noonan syndrome. *Clin Genet* 1986; 30: 150–3.

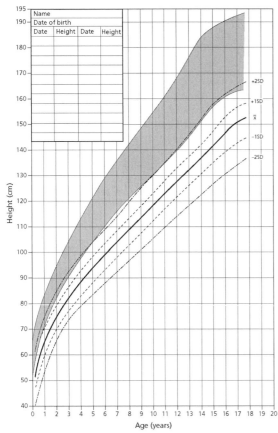

Figure A1.8 Height centiles for boys with Silver–Russell syndrome. The gray-shaded area indicates normal boys ±2 standard deviations (SD). Adapted from Wollman H, Kirchner T, Enders H *et al*. Growth and symptoms in Silver–Russell syndrome: review on the basis of 386 patients. *Eur J pediatr* 1995; 154: 958–68.

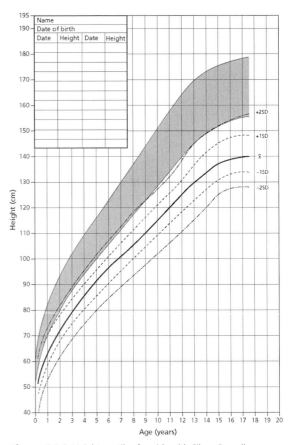

Figure A1.9 Height centiles for girls with Silver–Russell syndrome. The gray-shaded area indicates normal girls ±2 standard deviations (SD). Adapted from Wollman H, Kirchner T, Enders H *et al*. Growth and symptoms in Silver–Russell syndrome: review on the basis of 386 patients. *Eur J pediatr* 1995; 154: 958–68.

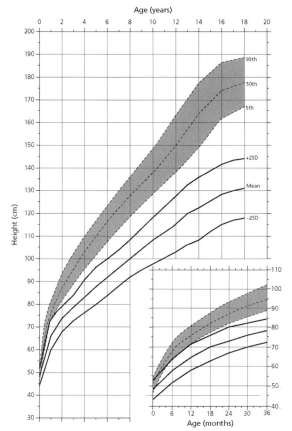

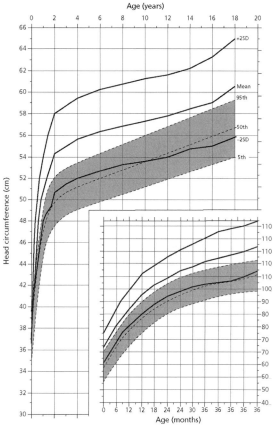

Figure A1.10 Height centiles for boys with achondroplasia (mean ±2 SD) compared with normal standard curves (dashed lines). Data derived from 189 males. Adapted from Horton W, Rotter J, Rimoin D *et al*. Standard growth curves for achondroplasia. *J Pediatr* 1978; 93: 435–8.

Figure A1.11 Head circumference centiles for boys with achondroplasia compared with normal curves (dashed lines). Data derived from 114 males. Adapted from Horton W, Rotter J, Rimoin D *et al*. Standard gowth curves for achondroplasia. *J Pediatr* 1978; 93: 435–8.

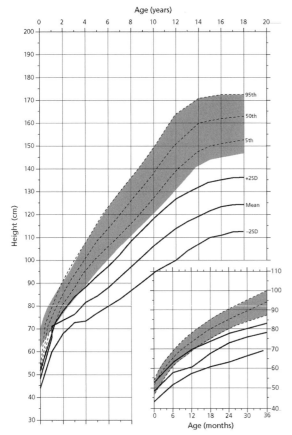

Figure A1.12 Height centiles for girls with achondroplasia (mean ±2 SD) compared with normal standard curves (dashed lines). Data derived from 214 females. Adapted from Horton W, Rotter J, Rimoin D *et al.* Standard growth curves for achondroplasia. *J Pediatr* 1978; 93: 435–8.

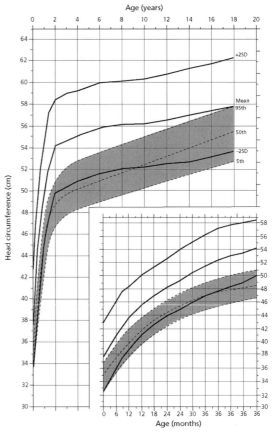

Figure A1.13 Head circumference centiles for girls with achondroplasia compared with normal curves (dashed lines). Data derived from 145 females. Adapted from Horton W, Rotter J, Rimoin D *et al.* Standard growth curves for achondroplasia. *J Pediatr* 1978; 93: 435–8.

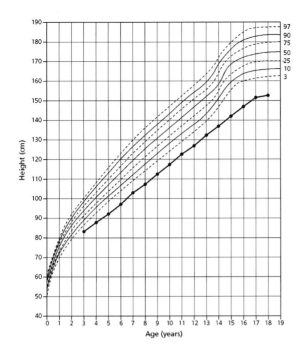

Figure A1.14 Linear growth in hypocondroplasic boys (solid line). Adapted from Appan S, Laurent S, Champan M *et al.* Growth and growth hormone therapy in hypochondroplasia. *Acta paediatr Scand* 1990; 79: 796–803.

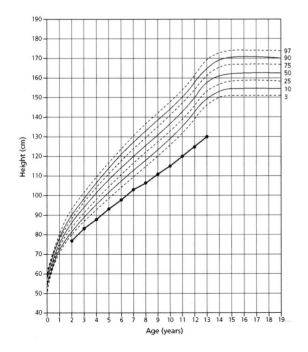

Figure A1.15 Linear growth in hypocondroplasic girls (solid line). Adapted from Appan S, Laurent S, Champan M *et al.* Growth and growth hormone therapy in hypochondroplasia. *Acta paediatr Scand* 1990; 79: 796–803.

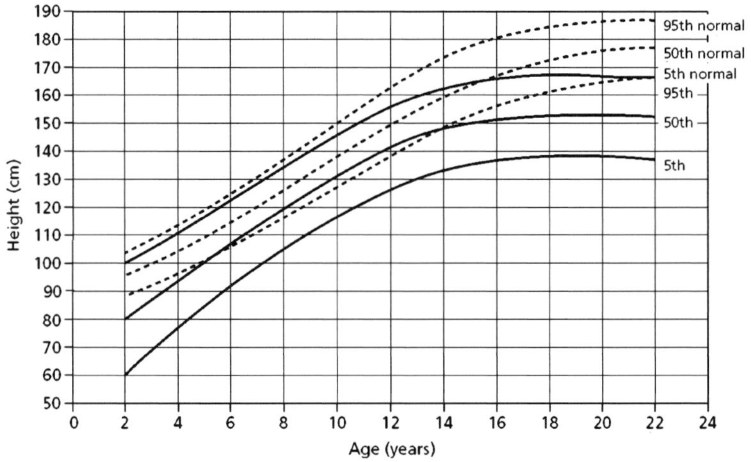

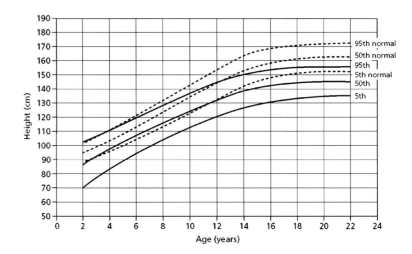

Figure A1.16 Standardized curves for height in Prader–Willi syndrome (PWS) in male patients (solid line) and healthy individuals (broken line). Adapted from Butler MG, Brunschwig A, Miller LK *et al*. Standards for selected anthropometric measurements in Prader–Willi syndrome. *Pediatrics* 1991; 88: 853–60.

Figure A1.17 Standardized curves for height in Prader–Willi syndrome (PWS) in female patients (solid line) and healthy individuals (broken line). Adapted from Butler MG, Brunschwig A, Miller LK *et al*. Standards for selected anthropometric measurements in Prader–Willi syndrome. *Pediatrics* 1991; 88: 853–60.

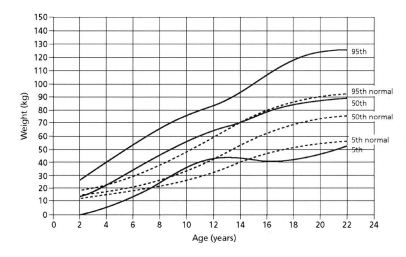

Figure A1.18 Standardized curves for weight in Prader–Willi syndrome (PWS) in male patients (solid line) and healthy individuals (broken line). Adapted from Butler MG, Brunschwig A, Miller LK *et al.* Standards for selected anthropometric measurements in Prader–Willi syndrome. *Pediatrics* 1991; 88: 853–60.

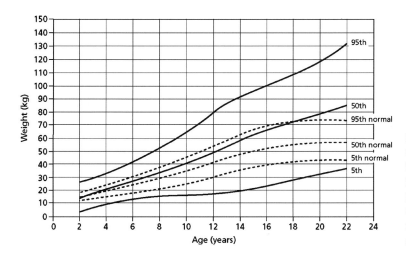

Figure A1.19 Standardized curves for weight in Prader–Willi syndrome (PWS) in female patients (solid line) and healthy individuals (broken line). Adapted from Butler MG, Brunschwig A, Miller LK *et al.* Standards for selected anthropometric measurements in Prader–Willi syndrome. *Pediatrics* 1991; 88: 853–60.

Appendix 2: Normal Values

Hormones	Traditional units	Conversion factor	SI units
Pituitary			
GH			
Basal	Low, often undetectable		
Peak (after appropriate stimulation)	>6 ng/mL	Dependent on standard used – approximately 2.6 for IS 80/505	>15 mU/L (assay dependent)
Prolactin (PRL)	<20 ng/mL	Approximately 21 for IS 84/500	<425 mU/L
TSH			
Basal			
<1 month	Up to 10 μU/mL	1	Up to 10 mU/L
Child and adult	0.5–5.0 μU/mL		0.5–5.0 mU/L
Stimulated	5.5–30 μU/mL		5.5–35 mU/L
FSH			
(highly method dependent)			
Basal			
Female			
Prepubertal	0.4–3.0 mIU/mL	1	0.4–3.0 IU/L
Tanner stage II	1.6–7.0 mIU/mL		1.6–7.0 IU/L
Tanner stage III	4.0–7.0 mIU/mL		4.0–7.0 IU/L
Tanner stage IV	3.0–8.0 mIU/mL		3.0–8.0 IU/L
Adult (follicular phase)	2.0–6.6 mIU/mL		2.0–6.6 IU/L
Adult (luteal phase)	1.6–5.7 mIU/mL		1.6–5.7 IU/L
Male			
Prepubertal	0.4–1.6 mIU/mL		0.4–1.6 IU/L
Tanner stage II	0.5–4.0 mIU/mL		0.5–4.0 IU/L
Tanner stage III	2.5–4.5 mIU/mL		2.5–4.5 IU/L
Tanner stage IV	3.0–5.5 mIU/mL		3.0–5.5 IU/L
Adult	1–7 mIU/mL		1–7 IU/L
Incremental rise following			
GnRH (if available) stimulation			
Prepubertal	2–3 mIU/mL		2–3 IU/L
Post-pubertal	>3 mIU/mL		>3 IU/L

Hormones	Traditional units	Conversion factor	SI units
LH			
(highly method dependent)			
Basal			
Female			
Prepubertal	<0.5 mIU/mL	1	<0.5 IU/L
Tanner stage II	1–7 mIU/mL		1–7 IU/L
Tanner stage IV	2–8 mIU/mL		2–8 IU/L
Adult (follicular phase)	2.0–6.6 mIU/mL		2.0–6.6 IU/L
Adult (mid-cycle)			
Adult (luteal phase)	14–72 mIU/mL	14–72 IU/L	
Male	1.6–5.7 mIU/mL	1.6–5.7 IU/L	
Prepubertal	<0.5 mIU/mL	<0.5 IU/L	
Tanner stage II	1–4 mIU/mL	1–4 IU/L	
Tanner stage IV	2–8 mIU/mL	2–8 IU/L	
Adult	1–10 mIU/mL	1–10 IU/L	
Incremental rise following			
GnRH (if available) stimulation			
Prepubertal	3–4 mIU/mL	3–4 IU/L	
Post-pubertal	>4 mIU/mL	>4 IU/L	
ACTH	*(LH dominant)*	*(LH dominant)*	
At 09.00 h			
RIA	<80 pg/mL	0.22	<18 pmol/L
IRMA	<50 pg/mL		<11 pmol/L
ADH (not routinely available)			
Basal	1–6 pg/mL	0.92	1–5 pmol/L
Plasma osmolality	275–295 mosmol/kg	1	275–295 mmol/kg

Growth factors

IGF-I	Normal ranges are dependent on age, sex and stage of puberty. Information must be provided with the request.		Consult reference laboratory for details

Adrenal cortex

Cortisol			
Basal			
09.00 h	7–25 µg/dL	27.6	200–700 nmol/L
24.00 h (sleeping)	1.8 µg/dL		<50 nmol/L
Following ACTH stimulation	Peak concentration (at 30 min) >20 µg/dL or increment of at least 7.2 µg/dL		Peak concentration (at 30 min) <550 nmol/L or increment of at least 200 nmol/L
Urinary free cortisol	<87 µg/24 h	2.76	<240 nmol/24 h
17-OHP (highly assay dependent)			
Basal	<5 µg/L	3.03	<15 nmol/L

(Continued)

Hormones	Traditional units	Conversion factor	SI units
Stressed newborn	Up to 33 µg/L		Up to 100 nmol/L
Following ACTH stimulation	Incremental increase		Incremental increase
	<3.3 µg/L at 60 min		<10 nmol/L at 60 min
11-Deoxycortisol	<1 µg/dL	29	<30 nmol/L
DHEAS			
Female			
<8 years	<222 µg/L	0.0027	<0.6 µmol/L
<8–10 years	111–593 µg/L		0.3–1.6 µmol/L
10–12 years	296–1185 µg/L		0.8–3.2 µmol/L
12–14 years	370–1852 µg/L		1–5 µmol/L
Adult	1100–4400 µg/L		3–12 µmol/L
Male			
<8 years	<222 µg/L		<0.6 µmol/L
8–10 years	74–1037 µg/L		0.2–2.8 µmol/L
10–12 years	333–1407 µg/L		0.9–3.8 µmol/L
Adult	750–3700 µg/L		2–10 µmol/L
Androstenedione			
Prepubertal	8.6–52 ng/dL	0.0349	0.3–1.8 nmol/L
Adult	57–230 ng/dL		2–8 nmol/L
Aldosterone			
(should be interpreted in conjunction with PRA)			
Up to 1 week	Up to 181 ng/dL	27.7	Up to 5000 pmol/L
1 week–1 year	11–54 ng/dL		300–1500 pmol/L
1–2 years	7–54 ng/dL		200–1500 pmol/L
2–10 years	4–29 ng/dL		100–800 pmol/L
10–15 years	2–22 ng/dL		60–600 pmol/L
Adult			
Normal sodium diet			
Upright (4 h)	7–30 ng/dL		190–830 pmol/L
Supine (30 min)	3–16 ng/dL		80–444 pmol/L
Low-sodium diet	Levels increase two- to fivefold		
PRA			
Up to 1 week	Up to 26 ng/h/mL	0.77	Up to 20 pmol/h/mL
1 week–1 year	2.6–9.1 ng/h/mL		2–7 pmol/h/mL
1–2 years	2.6–7.8 ng/h/mL		2–6 pmol/h/mL
2–10 years	1.9–5.2 ng/h/mL		1.5–4 pmol/h/mL
10–15 years	1.0–2.6 ng/h/mL		0.8–2 pmol/h/mL
Adult			
Normal sodium diet			
Upright (4 h)	1.6–7.4 ng/h/mL		1.2–5.7 pmol/h/mL
Supine (30 min)	0.1–3.1 ng/h/mL		0.1–2.4 pmol/h/mL
Low-sodium diet			
Upright (4 h)	5.6–14.2 ng/h/mL		4.3–10.9 pmol/h/mL
Supine (30 min)	2.1–5.4 ng/h/mL		1.6–4.2 pmol/h/mL

Hormones	Traditional units	Conversion factor	SI units
Gonads			
Estradiol			
Female			
<12 months	<80 pg/mL	3.67	<300 pmol/L
Prepubertal	<16 pg/mL		<60 pmol/L
Adult			
Follicular	20–70 pg/mL		70–260 pmol/L
Mid-cycle	95–410 pg/mL		350–1500 pmol/L
Luteal	50–300 pg/mL		180–1100 pmol/L
Adult male	<40 pg/mL		<150 pmol/L
Progesterone			
Female			
Prepubertal	<60 ng/dL	0.0318	<2 nmol/L
Follicular	<315 ng/dL		<10 nmol/L
Mid-luteal	940–2515 ng/dL		30–80 nmol/L
Male (all ages)	<60 ng/dL		<2 nmol/L
Testosterone			
Male			
Birth	115–400 ng/dL	0.03467	4–14 nmol/L
First week	Falls to 10–35 ng/dL		Falls to 0.5–1.5 nmol/L
15–60 days	115–230 ng/dL		4–10 nmol/L
Prepubertal (from 7 months)	<10 ng/dL		<0.5 nmol/L
Adult	230–865 ng/dL		10–30 nmol/L
Adult female	10–75 ng/dL		0.5–2.5 nmol/L
Dihydrotestosterone			
Male			
Birth	5–60 ng/dL	34.4	172–2064 pmol/L
First week	Falls rapidly		Falls rapidly
15–60 days	12–85 ng/dL		413–2924 pmol/L
Prepubertal (from 7 months)	<3 ng/dL		<103 pmol/L
Adult	30–85 ng/dL		1032–2924 pmol/L
Adult female	4–22 ng/dL		138–757 pmol/L
Thyroid			
FT_4			
<1 month	1.17–2.64 ng/dL	12.87	15–34 pmol/L
<1 year	0.76–2 ng/dL		10–26 pmol/L
Adult	0.7–1.55 ng/dL		9–20 pmol/L
FT_3			
<1 month	1.4–5.5 pg/mL	1.54	2.2–8.5 pmol/L
<1 year	2.0–6.9 pg/ml		3.1–10.6 pmol/L
Adult	2.3–5.5 pg/ml		3.5–8.5 pmol/L
Total T_4			
<1 month	5.9–21.5 µg/dL	12.87	76–276 nmol/L
<1 year	4.9–13.9 µg/dL		63–179 nmol/L
Adult	4.7–12.4 µg/dL		60–160 nmol/L

(Continued)

Hormone/analyte	Traditional units	Conversion factor	SI units
Total T$_3$			
<1 month	15–210 ng/dL	0.0154	0.2–3.2 nmol/L
<1 year	50–275 ng/dL		0.8–4.2 nmol/L
Adult	70–180 ng/dL		1.1–2.8 nmol/L
TBG	14–30 µg/mL	1	14–30 mg/L
Perchlorate discharge	<10% at 1 h		
Calcitonin			
Basal			
Hammersmith	<30 pg/mL	1	<30 ng/L
Newcastle	<100 pg/mL		<100 ng/L
After pentagastrin stimulation			
Hammersmith	<80 pg/mL		<80 ng/L
Newcastle	<200 pg/mL		<200 ng/L

Electrolytes, parathyroid and vitamin D

Sodium			
Up to 1 month			130–145 mmol/L
>1 month			135–145 mmol/L
Potassium			
Up to 1 month			3.5–6.0 mmol/L
>1 month			3.4–5.0 mmol/L
Chloride			98–110 mmol/L
bicarbonate			
1–4 years			17–25 mmol/L
4–8 years			19–27 mmol/L
>8 years			21–29 mmol/L
Urea			2.5–7.5 mmol/L
creatinine			
1 week			40–125 µmol/L
2 weeks			35–105 µmol/L
3 weeks			25–90 µmol/L
4 weeks			20–80 µmol/L
6 months			20–50 µmol/L
2 years			25–60 µmol/L
6 years			30–70 µmol/L
10 years			30–80 µmol/L
Adult male			65–120 µmol/L
Adult female			50–110 µmol/L
Total protein			63–83 g/L
Albumin			30–51 g/L
Total calcium			
Premature			1.50–2.50 µmol/L
Up to 2 weeks			1.90–2.80 µmol/L
Child			2.20–2.70 µmol/L

Hormone/analyte	Traditional units	Conversion factor	SI units
Ionized calcium			1.13–1.18 μmol/L
phosphate			
1 month			1.4–2.8 mmol/L
1 year			1.2–2.2 mmol/L
3 years			1.1–2.0 mmol/L
12 years			1.0–1.8 mmol/L
15 years			0.95–1.50 mmol/L
Adult			0.8–1.4 mmol/L
Magnesium			0.7–1.2 mmol/L
ALP			
(highly method dependent)			
IFCC method			
Up to 1 month			48–406 U/L
1 month–2 years			82–383 U/L
2–8 years			69–325 U/L
Puberty			74–390 U/L
Adult			28–94 U/L
PTH	9–54 pg/mL	0.1053	<5 pmol/L
(should be interpreted in conjunction with calcium concentration)			
25-OH vitamin D	2–50 ng/mL	2.599	50–130 nmol/L (seasonal)
Urine calcium/creatinine			<0.56 mol/mmol

Endocrine, pancreas hormones

Hormone/analyte	Traditional units	Conversion factor	SI units
Glucose (fasting)			
Up to 1 month	45–100 mg/dL	0.055	2.5–5.5 mmol/L
Child	55–110 mg/dL	0.055	3.0–6.1 mmol/L
Insulin			
Fasting	2.3–26 mU/L	Dependent on standard used – approximately 6.0 for IS 83/500	14–156 pmol/L
In presence of hypoglycemia (blood glucose <2.6 mmol/L, 45 mg/dL)	<2 μU/L		<12 pmol/L
C-peptide			
Fasting	0.36–3.6 ng/ml	333	119–1189 pmol/L
In presence of hypoglycemia	<0.6 ng/ml		<200 pmol/L
Glucagon	<175 pg/mL	0.28	<50 pmol/L

IS, International Standard; DHEAS, dehydroepiandrosterone sulfate; PRA, plasma renin activity; ALP, alkaline phosphatase.

Index